D0837648

NEVER GOOD ENOUGH

A VOLUME IN THE SERIES

The Culture and Politics of Health Care Work

Edited by Suzanne Gordon and Sioban Nelson

NEVER GOOD ENOUGH

*Health Care Workers and the False
Promise of Job Training*

ARIEL DUCEY

ILR PRESS

AN IMPRINT OF
CORNELL UNIVERSITY PRESS
ITHACA AND LONDON

Copyright © 2009 by Cornell University

All rights reserved. Except for brief quotations in a review, this book, or parts thereof, must not be reproduced in any form without permission in writing from the publisher. For information, address Cornell University Press, Sage House, 512 East State Street, Ithaca, New York 14850.

First published 2009 by Cornell University Press
First printing, Cornell Paperbacks, 2009

Printed in the United States of America

Library of Congress Cataloging-in-Publication Data

Ducey, Ariel, 1972–
    Never good enough : health care workers and the false promise of job training / Ariel Ducey.
        p.   cm.—(The culture and politics of health care work)
    Includes bibliographical references and index.
    ISBN 978-0-8014-4459-3 (cloth : alk. paper)—
    ISBN 978-0-8014-7504-7 (pbk. : alk. paper)
    1. Hospitals—Employees—Training of—New York (State)—
New York. 2. Health facilities—Employees—Training of—
New York (State)—New York. 3. Hospitals—Employees—Labor
unions—New York (State)—New York. 4. Health facilities—
Employees—Labor unions—New York (State)—New York.
I. Title. II. Series.

    RA971.35.D83 2009
    362.11068'3097471—dc22   2008023736

Cornell University Press strives to use environmentally responsible suppliers and materials to the fullest extent possible in the publishing of its books. Such materials include vegetable-based, low-VOC inks and acid-free papers that are recycled, totally chlorine-free, or partly composed of nonwood fibers. For further information, visit our website at www.cornellpress.cornell.edu.

Cloth printing   10   9   8   7   6   5   4   3   2   1
Paperback printing   10   9   8   7   6   5   4   3   2   1

For Ty

Contents

ACKNOWLEDGMENTS

In the years spent writing this book, I have acquired many debts. In the first phase of this project, there are the colleagues, mentors, and friends from the City University of New York Graduate Center. Patricia Clough, Stanley Aronowitz, and Barbara Katz Rothman made a lasting impact on me, intellectually, personally, and politically. Patricia encouraged me to think faster and provided a rare space for experimentation and creativity. Stanley made it possible for me to pay for food and shelter while doing research—indeed, he gave me the gift of time. From Barbara I learned how to be a compassionate and critical academic—which is not always encouraged—as well as how to teach and breathe medical sociology.

Most important to me was the extraordinary group with whom I marked all significant personal and academic events for about six years: Jeffrey Bussolini, Penny Lewis, Lorna Mason, Ananya Mukherjea, Gina Neff, Michelle Ronda, and Elizabeth Wissinger. Among the many others (mostly at the Graduate Center) to whom I am indebted are the late Robert Alford, Chun-Mei Chuang, Melissa Ditmore, Deborah Gambs, Heather Gautney,

Karen Gilbert, Jean Halley, Hosu Kim, Micki McGee, Michael Menser, Grace Mitchell, Nicole Rudolph, Jennifer Smith Maguire, Joel Vandevusse, Jami Weinstein, Dominic Wetzel, Craig Willse, Jonathan Wynn, and Margaret Yard. Thanks are due as well to Michelle Fine, Colette Daiute, and the Spencer Foundation Social Justice and Social Development in Education Studies Training Grant, of which I was a recipient. And from my student days at the University of Minnesota I'd like to acknowledge John Archer and my friends Carrie Rentschler and Jonathan Sterne.

I am also grateful to my colleagues at the University of Calgary, who have been so welcoming and provided invaluable support. In particular, Tom Langford, Daniel Béland, and Arthur Frank each read portions of this manuscript as it was under preparation and provided substantive comments, in addition to much practical advice. The graduate students at the University of Calgary have also been a joy to teach and get to know. I have learned much from Dominika Boczula, Mike Corman, Jessica Gish, Becky Godderis, Roland Simon, and Stephanie Talbot and their stimulating projects. Sophie Bonneau and Mike Corman provided research assistance for this book.

I would also like to thank several people who have been involved (as participants or observers) with the health workforce training and education industry and helped me carry out my research or pointed me to questions that were important and interesting: Nick Bedell, Helen Chappell, Judy Cicurel, Niev Duffy, Bill Ebenstein, John Garvey, Fran Boren Gilkenson, Dr. Samuel Heller, Betty Jaiswal, Ruth Leon, Kate Quinn-Miller, and most especially, Natalie Hannon and Judy Wessler. In addition, I am thankful to everyone who allowed me to interview or observe them for this study—for their thoughtful and open attitudes toward me and my questions.

Several other people read portions of this manuscript. Particularly crucial was the encouragement and editorial direction of Grey Osterud, who steered the project through a difficult passage. I also learned much from the comments of Robb Burlage, Jonathan Cutler, and Steve Early. Three reviewers from Cornell University Press—Eileen Boris, Gordon Lafer, and Steven Lopez—also made invaluable suggestions, providing both criticism and encouragement at each stage of the publishing process. Then, of course, there are the editors at Cornell—Fran Benson, whose support for this project gave me the will to go on, and the series editors, Sioban Nelson and Suzanne Gordon. Suzanne is an inspiration and her guidance made this project, finally, into a book. Naturally, none of the people who have shared their advice and comments are to blame for any faults in what follows, but they can share in its strengths.

I was exposed to the ethnographic eye early in my life, from my father, Michael Ducey, sociologist and incessant observer of the world. My sisters Aimee Ducey and Jeni Houser, mother Emily Osborn, and second father, David Houser, have always given me sound advice, even when I was too stubborn to listen. Finally, I am fortunate to have had the support and love of my husband, Ty Eggenberger. He is my connection to honesty and absurdity, and a second pair of eyes. He is also the reason I enjoy the company of such a wonderful (and expanding) pack—Rita and Rayen, of course, but now too our son, Terrence, who will always be perfect to me.

Introduction

Health Care and Getting By in America

Hospitals are the economic and social centers of many urban neighborhoods in the United States, but in New York their number and size is unusual. The campuses of major academic medical centers occupy entire city blocks and their buildings loom over the apartment buildings, brownstones, tenements, and public housing projects that surround them. Seen from above, hospital campuses are as easy to pick out as famous city landmarks; approaching them on the street, they are like magnets, drawing in thousands of workers and patients each day.

Inside these metropolises, medical students shuffle between lecture halls, the medical library, and patient units, and physicians conduct procedures, check patient charts, and write orders. Doctors, however, are only a minority of people working in such hospitals. Many spend only a few hours of the day there before returning by car service to their private offices in more serene settings. They are even less numerous in the smaller community hospitals that dot the city. Nurses and nursing assistants, overwhelmingly women, make up the bulk of the hospital workforce, and they arrive to work by subway and bus in their scrubs and thick-soled shoes, an ID card hanging around their necks—many on a colored cord that identifies their union. There are other workers too, overwhelmingly people of color and immigrants: maintenance workers, food service workers, housekeepers, laundry workers, technicians of many types, social workers, paramedics, therapists, and therapy assistants—workers whose experiences claim less scholarly and journalistic attention, perhaps because their work seems less crucial to patient care. Patients and their loved ones are tourists in these places (though some unfortunately become like members of the community), who disrupt the movement of hospital staff when they stop short in busy corridors to look at the signs hanging from the ceilings or the colored lines on the floors intended to guide them through the labyrinth of buildings.

New Yorkers work hard in a variety of service industries, old and new: as retail salespeople, waitresses, cab drivers, street vendors, garment workers, teachers. But health care is unusual because it offers the possibility of economic security for entire communities. The proliferation of health care jobs available to women, immigrants, and people of color constitutes the possibility of reversing, or at least slowing, the growing inequality that characterizes contemporary America. Already, over one in ten employed Americans work in health care settings or occupations, while in New York City, where health care is the largest employer, that number is closer to one in eight.[1] At the peak of the dot-com bubble, in 2000, business services briefly surpassed health care as the city's number one private employer, but the bubble's collapse shortly thereafter returned health care to its traditional leading position.[2]

In hospitals and the neighborhoods they dominate you can still feel the buzz of working-class New York, the city that was for a long time defined as much by the tradespeople, craftsman, and semiskilled laborers in its sprawling and diverse manufacturing sector as it was by Wall Street traders and real estate brokers.[3] Health care has produced the working-class jobs that make up for the evisceration of the manufacturing sector in the traditional industrial strongholds of the northeast—at least partially. In New York City, health care added 21,400 jobs between 2000 and 2003, while manufacturing lost 50,000 jobs in approximately the same period.[4] The northeast corridor stretching from Baltimore to Boston, the "nation's health epicenter," added 50,000 jobs between 2000 and 2002 while all other industries combined shed 220,0000.[5] Even in Manhattan, hub of the nation's financial and commercial networks, health care is the social and economic anchor.

Not only is health care today the largest employer in New York City, but it is of central importance for workers in the "sub-baccalaureate labor market," those who have at least a high school diploma but not a baccalaureate degree, who may or may not have some college education.[6] Despite the hype about the "knowledge economy" and postindustrial, flexible, creative workplaces of advanced capitalist nations, three-quarters of workers in the United States do not have a baccalaureate degree.[7] Most of these workers are employed in the growing service sector, and the rate of growth of health care jobs nationally has even surpassed job growth in the service sector as a whole in all but a few years.[8] In 2004, six of the ten occupations projected to grow most quickly between 2002 and 2012 were in health care: medical assistants, physician assistants, home health aides, medical records and health information technicians, physical therapist aides, and physical therapy assistants.[9] Only one of those occupations, physician assistant (PA), typically requires a credential beyond the associate's degree. In New York City, estimates are that over one-third of the 375,000 jobs in health care are open to people with an associate's degree or less.[10]

There is no satisfactory term to denote this segment of the health care workforce, but I generally refer to those in it as "allied" health care workers.[11] Some of the health care workers included in my research started working in health care before they had a high school diploma, others have gone on to achieve credentials higher than an associate's degree; but they hold the kind of jobs that are the core of the sub-baccalaureate labor market. Sometimes I refer to them as "frontline" health care workers, which captures the fact that they are responsible for the day-to-day tasks that keep hospitals and health facilities running, from mopping the floors to bathing patients. Much of the social science literature on health care still gives the impression that physicians and registered nurses are the only care providers at the bedside, but the workers I profile in this book make fundamental contributions to patient care, sometimes at the bedside but also when they are not directly interacting with patients.

The quality of frontline health care jobs—their working conditions, status, wages—not only affects patient care, but determines the well-being of a growing number of Americans and their families. The quality of life among those who do health care jobs in the sub-baccalaureate labor market is a litmus test of the U.S. economy and whether the recent transition from an economy based on manufacturing to one based on services warrants the optimistic outlook that corporate leaders and managerial theorists urge us to adopt. Health care work is a life-support system for the contemporary working class, and health care workers' experiences tell us just how much of the American dream can still be realized.

Labor unions' struggles are the reason the health care sector in New York City offers some of the most stable and secure work possible in the sub-baccalaureate labor market. In particular, New York City–based Local 1199—the union examined mostly closely in this book—has become one of the most influential labor organizations in the country. Merged with the Service Employees International Union (SEIU) in 1998 and known officially as "1199SEIU United Healthcare Workers East," its membership throughout the northeast totals nearly 300,000. In New York City, where its core membership remains allied health care workers in private hospitals, 1199's contracts and wages establish the standard to which all other city health care workers aspire, including more than 10,000 health care workers in the public hospital system, the Health and Hospitals Corporation (HHC), represented by District Council 37—an affiliate of the American Federation of State, County and Municipal Employees (AFSCME). Many smaller unions representing workers in nursing homes and home care agencies have merged with 1199 in recent years, and while DC37 was unable to prevent the gutting of the public hospital system in the 1990s, 1199 managed to protect most of its jobs.

1199's strategies toward the health care sector and how health care is financed and delivered, particularly under past president Dennis Rivera, have also become a template for other health care unions nationally. Indeed Rivera, who lead the union from 1989 to 2007, resigned only to head a new one million–member health care workers division within SEIU— called SEIU Health Care. That "union within a union" will unite 1199 with nearly forty other SEIU branches, representing hospital and nursing home workers around the country, and try to unionize more of America's nine million unorganized health care workers.

In the 1990s, resurgent neoliberal pundits and politicians in New York initiated a number of policy reforms intended to increase the role of markets and competition in the health care sector. As a result, consultants, policy specialists, and regulators encouraged hospitals to undergo the same sort of "restructuring" and "reengineering" by then ubiquitous in the corporate sector. Unsurprisingly, this was really an attempt to cut costs and shift more work onto the least-paid health care workers. Hospital leaders also used this political context to argue that layoffs were inevitable and substantial wage increases inconceivable. In the face of this hostile environment, 1199's key strategy was to form a common cause with hospital leaders to lobby against pro-market reforms and shore up state funding for the hospital sector. 1199's pivotal 1992 contracts with New York City hospitals formalized a labor–management partnership and "endorsed the notion of labor and management working together to confront the challenges facing the healthcare industry."[12] Foremost among the support the union leveraged from the state beginning in the mid-1990s was hundreds of millions of dollars for training and education programs directed at frontline workers, reaching $1.3 billion by 2005[13] and creating a veritable health care workforce training industry. The union's decision to embrace job training programs as the solution to hospitals' threats of layoffs, as well as workers' demands for higher pay, better working conditions, and more meaningful employment, has since become pivotal to 1199's identity. The health care workforce training industry in New York City is the subject of this book, an assessment of who gains—and who does not—from it. Remarkably, the union emerged from the tumultuous 1990s as one of the most powerful labor unions in the country. Its expanding influence, however, was not accompanied by improvements in the working conditions faced by its members or the organization of the city's health care services.

These elements of the 1199 model under Rivera—forming partnerships with employers, lobbying for greater health care financing, and offering prospective management partners the opportunity for their employees to participate in training programs, many of them publicly funded—now form the strategic basis for SEIU's projected expansion around the country. Job training and upgrading is not only a signature piece of the negotiated benefit package advertised to prospective members, it is one of the major ways the union tries to demonstrate that it can "add value" to the health care industry and convince the latter to drop its opposition to organizing efforts. As Rivera explained to the *Boston Globe* in 2005, when the union was wooing top executives of Boston's major teaching hospitals, SEIU's pitch to nonunion managers is: "We've got to get to know each other. We want to convince you that we are the best thing that could ever happen to you and your institution."[14] Boston Mayor Thomas Menino indicated he supported the union's organizing efforts, surely because the union endorsed his 2004 reelection campaign, but also because 1199 promised to provide workers with valuable training. "It's about workers' rights and workers' ability to move up in the economy," he said.[15]

1199's efforts to develop programs to train and retrain its members are, in some respects, confirmation of the union's foresight and concern for the rank and file. Nonetheless, the elaborate and extensive training and education system established for health care workers in New York in the 1990s, and the envy of labor unions around the country, largely failed to address, and in some instances reinforced, key problems in health care work and the health care system more broadly. The most heavily funded training programs could not fulfill their promise to provide more meaningful and better-paid work, better-skilled workers, and better jobs, especially since meeting these goals became the responsibility of training alone—training directed almost exclusively at frontline health care workers. Indeed these programs seemed to substitute for efforts to address other aspects of health care that required change, and upon which the working conditions and quality of life of 1199ers hinged: a fractured system of delivering patient care; organizational dysfunction; the disproportional and, from the perspective of medical needs, irrational emphasis on acute care rather than community-based services. Training programs deflected attention from these systemic problems and instead blamed them on the skills and attitudes of allied health care workers. Some training programs even cajoled workers to accommodate the market-driven health care reforms that had produced and aggravated the aspects of their working conditions they found most frustrating.

Frontline health care workers are always most vulnerable to the perpetual tides of health care "reform," but the particular conjuncture of policy and politics in mid-1990s New York meant that they bore the brunt of change in a new way. They were obliged to tweak their skills by "multi-skilling," to recalibrate their attitudes through "soft skills" training, and, if those failed to fix the problems with their work, to take advantage of training and upgrading programs for an ostensibly better job. Through training and education, allied health care workers became not only targets of pro-market policy and restructuring mantras, but were blamed for many of the problems in health care, from the organization of work and patient care to the financial viability of entire institutions. Both the content of many training and education programs and the sheer commitment of time they require reveal how individual health care workers are pressured to compensate for the irrationalities of America's health care "system," for the fact that their work is devalued, and for the inequities of an economy driven by the relentless creation of low-wage service jobs. For some individuals, the health care workforce training and education industry established in the 1990s created unprecedented opportunities for advancement. When viewed from the perspective of the consequences for health care workers as a whole, however, who in New York are also predominantly those who have been historically disadvantaged—workers of color, immigrants, women—the opportunities created by training and education also seem to be an unequal obligation to continually work more.

At the same time training programs expanded, workers' wages stagnated. Although the wages of 1199 members are better than those in many other service occupations and above the national average for health care workers, for most entry-level jobs they still hover near subsistence levels. Marie, an 1199 member and nursing assistant in a Bronx hospital, was making $14 an hour, or roughly $29,000 a year (before taxes) when we spoke in 2002—and wages in hospitals are significantly better than in home care or nursing homes. In the same year, the minimum hourly wage necessary for someone in Marie's position—a single adult with a school-age child living in the Bronx—to attain self-sufficiency was estimated at $14.44 an hour. Marie was in some ways better off than this measure suggests because she paid nothing for health care through 1199's benefit plan; she did not often have to pay for child care since her mother, who worked the night shift, cared for her eleven-year-old son after school; and her apartment was publicly subsidized (though her rent was about to be doubled). Her one-bedroom apartment was small, although she had made it comfortable. It was crammed with children's books and toys and the day I visited filled with the smell of baking banana bread. Nonetheless, Marie was able to get by in part because she lived in a cheap—and unsafe—neighborhood. She was afraid to let her son go outside alone. Marie was certainly not destitute, but she struggled to stay on top of her bills and earn enough to support her son's education. The self-sufficiency measure, while more realistic than other measures of wages and costs of living such as the federal poverty level, assumes only minimum spending on the bare necessities each month—housing, child care, food, transportation to and from work (by bus or subway), health care, and taxes. For a family of Marie's size in the Bronx, the measure assumes they need to spend only $192 a month on everything else—the "miscellaneous" category. The measure makes no allowances for vacations, owning a car, any travel other than getting to and from work, entertainment, or even savings.[16]

Marie's experience exemplifies the insecurities of the sub-baccalaureate labor market, the pivotal role of health care jobs in that labor market, and the limitations of training and upgrading as an ostensible remedy to those insecurities. A thirty-year-old single mother born in Brooklyn (to parents from Puerto Rico), Marie had been laid off from the two jobs she obtained after dropping out of high school, first by a company where she performed clerical duties for over two years. The company reviewed hospital patient records for coding and billing accuracy but closed down after losing several major contracts. While working there from 1986 to 1988, Marie took home $365 in pay every two weeks. "I thought I was rich!" she laughed as she told me the story. In the meantime, she had obtained her general equivalency diploma (GED), so after being laid off she started college part-time while making due on her severance pay and eventually took another clerical job with a firm on Wall Street. When the firm learned she was pregnant, they "said that they couldn't keep on training me because I was due to give birth. They said that they needed somebody who was going to be in the position permanently...so they let me go." Marie said she became depressed, and after the birth of her son enrolled in public assistance, which she found to be a demeaning experience. She paid about $1,000 out of pocket for a certified nursing assistant (CNA) course in the early 1990s, but did not take the final exam because she was afraid she would not pass. A few years later, however, she completed and passed a different CNA training course, to which New York State sent her as part of its efforts to reduce its welfare rolls. She was then hired for her first nursing assistant job by a hospital just north of the city, in Westchester County, where her starting wage was $8.50 an hour.

For women like Marie, the stakes for success or failure in health care are high. Health care is one of the only avenues, perhaps the only one, for women in the sub-baccalaureate labor market to increase their earnings. According to an analysis of several surveys of income and educational achievement, economic returns for most sub-baccalaureate certificates and associate degrees (wage gains above what workers would obtain with only a high school degree) vary widely, and "some kinds of postsecondary education provide no economic advantage at all." However, some health-related sub-baccalaureate credentials are consistent exceptions. Health-related occupations are the only field in which sub-baccalaureate certificates showed statistically significant positive economic returns for women over time; at the associate degree level, only health and business-related fields showed such returns for women.[17] Workers in health care who are able to advance beyond entry-level positions may achieve meaningful improvements in their quality of life. In 2001, the median hourly wage for a respiratory therapist in the New York City metropolitan area was $22.91 and for a registered nurse, $28.20,[18] and both occupations require only an associate's degree for employment. Health care occupations are furthermore one of the only exceptions to the finding that work involving caring labor is subject to a wage penalty of 5 to 6 percent for both men and women.[19] In sum, some jobs in health care are crucial sources of stable wages and benefits for women without a bachelor's degree. This is particularly true in wake of welfare reform, which placed strict limits on the number of years people can receive benefits and abruptly transferred many women into the ranks of the working poor. For many immigrant women, health care jobs are also by far the best alternative to domestic work.

Marie, not surprisingly, had regularly sought more education and training to improve the quality of her life, and she was aware of the union-driven opportunities seemingly sprouting up around her. In particular, all of the college and university officials I interviewed for this study had begun to offer contract courses for specific employers in the wake of federal and state support for the training of the health care workforce. (One study has found that over 90 percent of community colleges in the United States now offer contract training.[20]) Administrators and planners in postsecondary education in New York City now think strategically about the health care sector and its workforce as a stable source of students and revenue.

Most important is the City University of New York (CUNY), the largest urban institution of higher education in the country with seventeen undergraduate colleges and over 400,000 students. As the city's public institution of higher education, the extent of CUNY's involvement in the training industry has major implications for poor, minority, and working-class New

York City residents. In 1997, almost half of CUNY's first-time freshmen were foreign-born and over three-quarters were non-white, with blacks and Hispanics each approaching one-third of enrollment.[21] The doors that CUNY chooses to open and close to its students and the city's residents are therefore central in determining the quality of life for students who have been historically denied equal access to education and the labor market.[22] What does it mean, then, that by 2003, nearly half of CUNY's total enrollment, or 238,379 students, were in continuing education and workforce programs?[23]

Marie had enrolled at CUNY on a number of occasions, but faced some obstacles. Though she had passed several English and sociology classes at a four-year college, she could not continue toward a bachelor's degree without passing all sections of the CUNY entrance exam, a controversial admissions requirement implemented in 2000 for all four-year CUNY colleges. Largely because of a math phobia that had followed her since high school and seemed to get worse as years passed, she failed the math portion of the exam. When we spoke, Marie had quit college in frustration and was hoping to qualify for a nine-month, noncredit, licensed practical nurse (LPN) program offered at 1199 and CUNY's new training facility in the Bronx.

Plans for the new training facility were announced early in 2002 when, shortly before Dennis Rivera rewarded the Republican Governor George Pataki for his largesse toward the health care system by endorsing his bid for a third term in office, Pataki provided a $3 million grant to 1199 and CUNY to turn an abandoned department store on the once-illustrious Grand Concourse in the Bronx into a health care workforce training center. Financially, $3 million was a drop in the bucket, but symbolically, the training center was a means for these political actors to demonstrate their commitment to the well-being of health care providers, who in effect stood for hard-working New Yorkers as a whole.

Yet Marie's situation, and what she needs and desires, cannot be solved through more training and education alone. Looking at her credentials, Marie might seem to lack skills, yet in important ways her talents and abilities had never been adequately used. Marie, whom I observed several times at work, is a highly competent caregiver. She took great satisfaction in caring for people and wanted to become a nurse, both for the higher wages and to be a better role model for her son, to whom she was devoted.

She was capable of completing college-level academic work, but her fear of math exams would make it difficult to pass even the entrance test for LPN programs used in New York, widely judged to be more difficult than the standard entrance exam for more advanced RN programs. Marie's ability was not the problem. In junior high she had been accepted to one of the city's elite public high schools, which admit students on the basis of a competitive, citywide exam, but she did not recognize the import of that opportunity, nor apparently did those around her. She chose instead to attend another high school with a cousin, where she was bullied and eventually dropped out.

Even if Marie became an LPN, her daily responsibilities would be similar to those of an RN but her wages closer to those of a nursing assistant. In 2001, the median hourly wage for an LPN in the New York City metropolitan area was $16.69.[24] Moreover, LPN programs do not provide college credits toward a degree or advanced standing for the next step in a health care career. She was not even sure that becoming a nurse, of any kind, would alleviate one of her major sources of frustration—the feeling of being undervalued. She felt this way even though she had been recently "multiskilled." One of the major outcomes of the hospital-union partnership and the new emphasis on training and education, examined in chapter 4, was the transformation of hospital nursing assistants like Marie into patient care technicians (PCTs). PCTs were trained to perform (but not interpret) a number of procedures in addition to their previous duties, primarily electrocardiograms (EKGs) and drawing blood (phlebotomy). Marie's PCT credential, however, did not fix the devaluation of the caring labor she enjoyed providing nor was it a step toward a better job. It expanded her workload while adding "technical" tasks she said were boring and repetitive.

As we will see, 1199 has addressed the working conditions and division of labor in hospitals only within the bounds allowed by partnership with management, an arena in which training is readily embraced as the remedy to a variety of workplace ills. On the other hand, the union has been confrontational and exceptionally successful when it comes to organizing. Originally a small local of mostly Jewish pharmacists and drugstore clerks, in the 1930s 1199 and its communist leaders emulated their labor counterparts in the radical Congress of Industrial Organizations (CIO) and committed to organizing the unorganized.[25] They started with those nearby—the drugstores' predominantly black porters and stockmen. As Leon Fink and Brian Greenberg explain in their meticulous history of Local 1199, the union had, by the mid-1950s, "all but exhausted its organizational potential in New York City drugstores," so leaders turned their attention to the underclass of workers in the city's private, nonprofit hospitals (known as "voluntary" hospitals), winning their first contract in 1958 at Montefiore Hospital in the Bronx. Prior to 1199's organizing and collective bargaining achievements, these workers—most of whom were black or Puerto Rican—had been essentially excluded from the postwar economic boom, their work regarded as a kind of philanthropy.

In the process, 1199 was able to surmount a feature of the 1947 Taft-Hartley Act, attached as an amendment by Congress under intensive lobbying by the American Hospital Association, which exempted nonprofit hospitals from provisions requiring employers to hold elections to determine whether workers wished to be represented by a union. Nonprofit hospitals argued that because they were charitable organizations, union demands for wage increases would undermine their ability to treat those who could not pay for hospital services. It was an irrational logic, one that pitted health care workers against a group of which they were a part, since they too lacked health insurance. In 1962, an 1199 strike forced then Governor Nelson Rockefeller to pass legislation that would include nonprofit hospitals under the State Labor Relations Act.

Within two decades, Local 1199 raised the living standards of largely immigrant and minority housekeepers, laundry workers, food service workers, and nurse's aides from abject poverty to something approaching the working class. Between 1958 and 1983 starting wages at the city's voluntary hospitals increased by 140 percent—adjusted for inflation—while the union also made gains in health and other benefits. Not all of these staggering wage increases can be credited to the union; some of it was made possible by increased government payments to hospitals and a rising minimum wage, but the extent of the increases would have been impossible without union pressure. Fink and Greenberg describe the "sense of release from the subsistence-oriented life-style of pre-union days" when a nurse's aide in 1977 said of her wages, simply, "now I'm able to go places."[26]

During the same period, 1199 consistently took progressive positions on larger social and political issues, associating with causes like world peace and civil rights—Dr. Martin Luther King praised it as his favorite union—a tradition Dennis Rivera continued. Yet Fink and Greenberg also note that a condition of the union's organizing success in New York City was its promise not to intervene in the affairs of hospitals. They depict the political path of 1199's first generation of leaders (who ruled the union well into the 1980s), noting in particular the eventual separation between their formative political ideals—radicalism rooted in communism and the original CIO—and their practical approach to day-to-day union affairs and strategy. So today too, when it comes to health care—at the level of policy, the decisions of hospital administrators, and the working conditions of its members—the union has been far less progressive and aggressive.

In its recent organizing efforts in Boston, when the union's overtures to nonunion institutions are rebuffed, the union will—as part of pressure campaigns—obtain and publicize "information about publicly funded grants and bond debt as a way of monitoring how a hospital spends money." In those circumstances, "advocating for quality care is about more than just improving health care jobs," explains 1199, "it also means workers are proactively ensuring that public dollars are being used in the best way possible to improve the health care system."[27] Yet its history in New York suggests 1199's role as a self-appointed fiscal watchdog and defender of quality care is an ad hoc organizing tactic, not a mission that affects its relationships with employers once organizing is achieved.

1199 has, of course, justifiably criticized the commonly espoused view that workers' wages are a major cause of rising health care costs, which has dominated health care policy debates in the United States for decades. While the costs of health care are to an extent a legitimate concern, U.S. health care is singularly expensive because it is an employment-based, largely privately financed health care system, in which there are layers upon layers of excessive administrative costs, untold regulatory costs and subsidies for controlling the inequities produced by "markets," cadres of managers and consultants charging by the hour to respond to the perpetual irrationalities on which their very existence depends, the highest pharmaceutical prices in the industrialized world, and few controls on whether clinical innovations respond to the health needs of Americans. These cost escalators have little to do with the wages of frontline health care workers, as 1199 recognizes. Nonetheless, the so-called pragmatic way in which 1199 uses its now considerable political might in the arena of health care policy has reinforced precisely those aspects of the U.S. health care system that siphon off resources and revenue that might otherwise go to workers' wages and patient care. Its strategies have even managed to reinforce, in the minds of many New Yorkers, the connection between its members' wages and skyrocketing costs, waste, and inefficiencies.

Unsurprisingly, frontline health care workers like Marie are the most insightful critics of what is wrong with how health care work is organized and care delivered, so before describing the training industry, the central topic of this book, I begin in chapter 1 with a detailed description of health care workers on the job. Health care is suffering from an acute shortage of workers. Talented, motivated, and even appropriately credentialed workers avoid or leave the field. The "workforce crisis" can be attributed to a mix of inadequate wages and poor working conditions. Although improved wages are a necessary step in retaining a talented health care workforce, without improved working conditions the commitment most health care workers feel toward their patients and their work will continue to be squandered and exploited. In addition to feeling overworked and underpaid, people in frontline health care jobs are told in a number of ways their work is not valuable and important. Understanding workers' complaints and what motivates them to enroll in training courses allows us to assess the relevance and usefulness of training programs to workers' goals and ambitions.

Chapter 2 briefly describes the health care policy context in which a billion-dollar industry for training health care workers emerged. The prospect of a more market-driven health care system and a greater role for managed care plans fueled the restructuring and reengineering movement that swept through hospitals in the 1990s. It also became the basis for high-stakes, secretive negotiations among New York's health care power brokers, out of which Dennis Rivera emerged with a massive industry to train his union's members.

Chapter 3 defines the scope of the new training industry as it emerged and took shape from 1996 to 2003—who was funded, what kinds of programs were offered, how it was justified as necessary, and what sorts of promises were made. Then chapters 4, 5, and 6 describe in detail three of the most heavily funded training programs in the period I conducted my research. These are multiskilling programs, in particular those designed to transform nursing assistants into PCTs; "soft skills" training in areas such as communication skills and customer service; and individualized upgrading programs that attempt to help workers create a career path out of the confusing array of occupations in the sub-baccalaureate health care labor market. We will see that these training programs do not address the key problems of health care work: inadequate staffing levels, expanding workloads, lack of material support, and unresponsive structures of authority. Instead, they focus on adjusting the worker to the situation. The training programs in New York City were established when unions, hospitals, and public officials expected massive changes in the health care sector as a result of deregulation and managed care. Characteristically, the response was programs to retrain workers for the "world of the future" rather than to reconsider the terms of employment in the present.

There were, in addition, significant differences between what was expected under managed care and market principles and how pro-market reforms actually unfolded in New York's exceptional political environment. Many of the changes—widespread hospital closings, greater competition for patients and payers, a growing role for commercial insurers, fundamental changes in the nature of health care work—that supposedly necessitated new training did not transpire, or at least were not as drastic as expected. The training industry, however, continued to expand even when the problems it was supposed to solve did not materialize.

Chapter 7 takes a closer look at the different rationales for this industry in order to better understand why the industry persists, even though it fails to solve the basic problems frontline health care workers face. All parties have distinct, overlapping but not entirely compatible interests in the training industry. Employers seek to create a flexible (multiskilled or cross-trained) labor force, decrease turnover, reduce costs, promote conflict resolution skills among workers, and mollify discontent. Labor unions seek to avoid layoffs, retrain workers threatened with displacement, and—as important—promote attachment to the union by offering learning as a benefit and a route to advancement, which functions as an alternative to improving conditions at workers' present jobs. Colleges and universities seek a lucrative market among adults who are perpetually in school, rather than young students who complete credential or degree programs and leave school for work. Private trainers and consultants seek a vast new market for their proprietary seminars and workshops.

Yet, the training and education programs I analyze had consequences that were often inconsistent with such interests. Multiskilling, in the case of PCTs, did not reduce employers' costs nor did it unquestionably prevent layoffs. Individual upgrading creates opportunities for only a few, and even for them advancement does not always result from their efforts. 1199 may find that training and education programs do not necessarily secure worker loyalty to the union (or hospitals), and that education as a benefit might in fact become a barrier to a fairer and more equitable education system. The $1.3 billion in training funds did indeed open up a vast new market, but the industry cannot be adequately understood in merely cynical terms as a grab for more state subsidies by hospitals and unions or as a payoff they received from politicians in exchange for certain concessions. In fact, one of the main reasons the industry commands continued financial and emotional investment is because those involved recognize that health care workers are in fundamental ways devalued, even if training programs can do little about it (and some training programs even exacerbate the difficult working conditions many frontline health care providers face).

The final two chapters of the book critically examine 1199's role in the training industry for allied health care workers. Chapter 8 explores why 1199 made training and education such a pivotal part of its strategy and how the union's decision to frame its relationship with New York City's voluntary hospitals as that of a "common cause" created a number of strategic dilemmas when it came to the lives and working conditions of the rank and file. Chapter 9 is a historically grounded speculation on what the creation of education as a benefit may portend for the future of education and, indeed, daily life for many Americans. Labor's embrace of employment-based education benefits may have perverse consequences for the collective security of the working class as a whole and the strength of American Labor, as did its embrace of employment-based health care following World War II. 1199 is a labor union that has been, and continues to be, a pivotal force in improving the lives of health care workers. Unfortunately, it has also, at times, placed its own institutional interests above those of its members, not to mention those of a reinvigorated labor movement or the working class as a whole.

I have drawn on several qualitative research projects to compose an account of what the training and education industry for allied health care workers is, and what political (perhaps even ethical) dilemmas it poses. The evidence in the book is drawn from several research projects in which I was involved from 1999 to 2003, each of which examined work in health care, life in the sub-baccalaureate labor market, and the genesis and significance of a health care workforce training industry, albeit from different angles. First was a study of occupational change in three subacute care facilities (essentially a level of care between that of an acute care unit and a nursing home), with the aim of identifying where workers might need training. Second was an evaluation of a communication skills training program at a midsize teaching hospital in the center of one of the city's poorest neighborhoods.[28] The third study focused directly on individual workers and the emergence of the industry to train them, for which I conducted in-depth interviews and observed several sessions of two additional training seminars—a customer service training program at a public hospital and an in-service on communication at one of the city's largest home health care agencies.

All the studies used qualitative research methods, primarily observations or fieldwork and interviews. For the subacute care study, I conducted observations at three subacute care units from September 1999 to February 2000, for about ten to twelve hours each week. Subacute care units are "step-down" facilities from hospitals, used for short-term rehabilitation and skilled nursing care. Two of the units were located within acute care hospitals, the third was part of a freestanding rehabilitation facility. For the evaluation of a communication skills training program, the research team of which I was a part observed seven 8-hour sessions of the training program, conducted semistructured follow-up interviews with twenty-one staff members (of whom I personally interviewed six), and conducted follow-up observations of staff and their interactions on six different hospital units. The focus of our interviews and observations were nursing assistants (PCTs at that hospital) and unit clerks. In addition, I attended several meetings of the hospital education committee and interviewed two consultants hired by the hospital to run training, including the communication skills instructor.

These two studies, and the conversations I had with health care workers as well as union and hospital officials during them, drew my attention to the extent of restructuring in New York City's hospitals as well as the prevalence of training and education programs. As I carried out fieldwork in health care settings, I was struck by the extent to which workers were exposed to training and education programs. On the job, nursing assistants were constantly being pulled into in-service training or continuing education seminars, where they learned how to operate a new electronic scale, heard about the benefits of a new pain medication, were "reminded" of hospital policies, or were exhorted to treat patients like clients. Flyers regularly appeared on the units from 1199 or hospital management announcing courses that workers could take on their own time, such as a course in computer skills or Spanish. Many health care workers were in more formal programs of study after hours and often tried to persuade their coworkers to enroll as well.

This constant exposure to training and education results in part from the fact that health care occupations are heavily-regulated, and advancement in the industry always requires a new credential and therefore a new set of courses. Unlike many other industries, there are few opportunities for promotion and advancement internal to the organizations in which health care providers work. A number of health care workers reported being stuck on a training treadmill, circulating through training or educational programs that were poorly run and organized and that often trained them for jobs no better in terms of wages and chances for upward mobility. Some workers I spoke with were on their way to better jobs, but their journey of years of exhausting days, as they worked full-time, attended school, and cared for their families, was a long and arduous one. It was troubling that the time and effort it took to just get by seemed to have been normalized. Moreover, there was always the risk that at the end of their long trek, the job category for which they trained might be downsized. These "better" jobs had themselves often replaced positions for more educated (and costly) workers who had just been restructured out of the hospital.

My conversations with health care workers convinced me that in-depth interviews would be necessary to capture the range of learning experiences that an allied health care worker might encounter. For this research, between 2002 and 2003 I interviewed seventeen allied health care workers about their educational, occupational, and personal histories, as well as twenty-one people involved in the planning and implementation of the training industry. The workers I interviewed were predominantly women ranging in age from twenty-one to fifty-five years, and the majority were black or Hispanic, reflecting the racial and gender segregation in this segment of the labor market. Consistent with immigration patterns to New York City, many of the workers were born in Caribbean countries. The extent of these workers' involvement in health care was great; many had moved through several different health care occupations, a large number beginning their health care careers as nursing assistants in nursing homes and home care agencies. Many also described the various other jobs they had held before finding stability in health care, doing retail sales work, domestic work, or office and clerical work. The trainers and health care workforce planners I interviewed were affiliated with labor unions, community-based training programs, college and universities, and health care organizations, and some worked as independent contractors.

This collection of evidence means there are some gaps in the story that follows. For instance, the workers I interviewed in depth are not the same people I observed in the studies of subacute care and communication skills (with the exception of Marie). The questions I asked, formally and informally, of workers during these studies varied, reflecting the different aims of each. Nonetheless, all of the research projects with which I was involved were focused on the working lives of frontline health care workers: how they felt about and perceived their jobs and working conditions, what they aspired to do, and what they had experienced in the past that had helped or hindered their ability to achieve their goals. Education and training emerged as a main theme in the stories they told about themselves and, indeed, had become a central part of their daily life in terms of the time and money they devoted to training and education programs of one sort or another.

The interviews and observations I conducted and describe in the pages that follow were not of a representative sample, either of allied health care workers, trainers and educators, training programs, or work settings. An 1199 staff member remarked:

> It's very difficult to generalize about the training industry, because I think you'd have to do such a detailed study of all of these different organizations to really look at to what extent are they market driven, or what extent are they mission driven, and what extent are they really providing outcomes that have an impact. So I think ... it's such a broad area. Even though we're just talking about training and health care, it's still very big.

His assessment is surely correct. It is very difficult to generalize about the training industry for health care workers in New York City, let alone for other industries in New York City or for training in other regions. However, this book does not evaluate narrow and immediate outcomes of these training programs so much as describe them and their social significance. I do comment on the effects and consequences of some of the training programs, but in a broader context than the term *outcomes* usually suggests. Indeed, in some cases considering the broader context makes clear the impact of such programs can only be very limited, so that if evaluations of the programs are to show success they must focus only on narrow measures, such as the numbers of people trained (though many in the training industry were not interested in evaluations of any sort). For some issues, differences in the types of training matter very much; the difference between tuition assistance programs for college degrees and noncredit classes not linked to specific jobs matter very much for individual mobility. For other issues, however, I explain why differences between training programs might not matter at all. For instance, I observed relatively few instances of the soft skills training programs to which tens of thousands of New York City health care workers were sent, but it is still possible to assess the larger political and social forces at work and comment on whether programs I did not observe could be expected to have meaningfully different consequences.

Furthermore, this approach does not constitute "generalization" in the statistical sense the term is often used. My approach is closer to that of Richard Sennett and Jonathan Cobb in their interviews with working-class men in Boston thirty years ago: "The only way we can generalize is to turn the matter around and ask what is representative or characteristic of American society in its impact on the people interviewed. It is not so much as a replication of other workers that their lives ought to bear a larger witness, but as focused points of human experience that can teach something about a more general problem of denial and frustration built into the social order."[29] Likewise, I ask how more general changes and problems in our society—changes in the economy and labor market, the organization of health care, the values and priorities of our culture—impact people with whom I spoke and the training programs I observed. These are focused points of human experience, no less important if they are not "representative." These focused points of experience, moreover, feed back into more general changes in our society, potentially reinforcing or altering them.

The experiences of those I interviewed, the characteristics of the training and work settings I observed, and the story of how this training industry came to be, teach something about denial and frustration built into the social order too. Perhaps even more important, they teach about the humor and creativity with which allied health care workers face it.

1

The Pull and Perils of
Health Care Work

When I met Veronica, a fifty-five-year-old nursing assistant and immigrant from Trinidad, she had been attending school in the evenings and on weekends for close to ten years, while working full-time and taking care of her family. First she spent two years attending a preparatory course offered by 1199 (more precisely, the joint labor-management Training and Upgrading Fund, described in chapter 3) for the general equivalency diploma (GED) exam, so she could obtain her U.S. high-school degree, and passed the exam on her third attempt. Then she enrolled in another union program, one that helps participants prepare for the entrance examination established for all four-year CUNY colleges, and passed the exam on the first try. As of 2002, Veronica had completed four college courses, for which her tuition was reimbursed by the union. Veronica first worked as a nursing assistant at a nursing home, but when we spoke was working in a hospital, where she was surprised to find she felt "more like a servant":

> Yeah, I figured if you get into the hospital I could become an LPN [licensed practical nurse] or something. I always wanted a job that means—you

know, it's something, but as a nursing assistant you don't get no respect—
I mean you get treated—it should be an important job, because you take
care of people, you listen to their problems, you console them, and yet you
get treated as if you're nobody.

Veronica started to say that she always wanted a job that "means" something, like a licensed practical nurse, but she corrected herself, reminded
herself (and me) that her job as a nursing assistant does mean something,
the problem is that it is not treated as an important job and those who do
it are not treated with respect. Nonetheless, she had begun to think of the
work of licensed or registered nurses as more meaningful in comparison to
her own. Her sense that her work was not valued motivated her to continue
with school and strive for something more.

Not feeling valued or respected is a common experience among allied
health care workers and particularly resented. My observations of health
care workers on the job, especially nursing assistants, suggest many frontline caregivers and other allied health care workers are treated as if they
are nobody. Sometimes they are openly talked down to and treated with
disrespect by coworkers, but equally damaging are the more hidden and
pervasive ways their lack of worth is conveyed on the job, such as the organization of the spaces in which they work, the constraints on what they
can do and record as part of their jobs, and the choices of their employers
about when and how to cut costs (from the availability of toothpaste to
staffing levels).

Yet the same workers know their work is valuable and, more often than
not, take some satisfaction from it, even if they feel undervalued or that
their skills and abilities are underused. Winsome, another nursing assistant, spoke of the gifts and thanks she had received from patients and their
family members. Steve, a respiratory therapist who thought of the workers
and patients at the community hospital where he had worked since the
age of eighteen as one big family, could not understand why more people
do not go into health care given its rewards. They included the rewards of
trying to save a person's life, but also the more mundane:

When you go to a patient's bedside and you're taking care of them...and
they have a concern or they're upset about something because someone either said something to them or they had some sort of miscommunication,

you speak with them and just by listening—maybe two minutes, three minutes—it's amazing what results you get from the patient. It's like, wow, why doesn't everyone listen? It's really rewarding.

Marie, the patient care technician described in the introduction, likewise took satisfaction from the care she gives, even its least glamorous aspects:

> You know, to tell you the truth, I take satisfaction that, if somebody's dirty or whatever the case may be, that I'm the one that's cleaning them. The simple reason is because I know that certain people can't do it for themselves, and I know that if it's up to certain people [other staff] they'll leave it to the very last minute, till it's like a cake you can't take off. So I'd rather clean them, know it, and it's something that helps me, too, in the process.

As we will see, many frontline health care workers are conscientious and caring even while reminders of their apparent lack of worth are everywhere. The sheer vulnerability and need they see in patients each day undoubtedly drives these workers' sense of compassion and responsibility and makes it impossible for them to treat their work like any other job. But in addition, like most of us, these workers would take pride in doing any job well, as a matter of self-worth. Their attitude is indicative of just how central paid labor is to identity and well-being in America today.

These workers' unique responsibility, however—to provide care to those who in many instances have been abandoned by others—is also one that not all of these health care workers have chosen. Since health care provides some of the best jobs possible to workers without a college degree, many people working on the front lines of health care have been driven, even coerced, into this kind of work. People who work in health care have made choices and decisions about how they would live and work, of course, and many are interested in the kind of work undertaken in health care settings. Still, the range of occupational choices available to them is limited. The experience of allied health care workers in the labor market is in crucial respects similar to the experience of workers in any economic sector struggling to get by in the sub-baccalaureate labor market: Getting a job is rarely a matter of choice alone, and the job hardly ever a "vocation."

Together, these ingredients are a foolproof recipe, if not for outright exploitation, then for the disregard to which frontline health care workers are daily exposed. The contingencies of the labor market, the nature of the work they do, and the fact that they may feel tied down to their jobs because few better exist means health care workers are, like their patients, unusually vulnerable. They are vulnerable to the whims of managers and policy makers who make their jobs and work the focus of incessant adjustments. They are vulnerable to the continual assertion that their wages are the cause of rising health care costs. Some have even implied their wages are excessive, since providing care is ostensibly inherently rewarding and therefore corrupted by the motive of material gain. The idea that these workers lack skills, reinforced by the constant emphasis on the need for new training and upgrading programs, can likewise support the suspicion that such workers are paid too much.

In fact, these workers need better pay. Veronica, who was making $12.86 an hour, was tired of having to work sixteen-hour shifts to save enough money for a vacation. I asked her if it was the money that motivated her to become a nurse, and she said, "That's a big thing. Yeah, because I want to enjoy life. I want to go on vacation, I want to take trips too." I asked Winsome if she works with other nursing assistants who are content with what they do. "No, nobody. If you go and ask them, 'Are you content with what you're doing'? No! We're just doing this...for our bread." What if she were paid more, I asked? "Does the money have anything to do with it? In a way, of course. Because sometimes you have to do overtime just to make your ends meet."

Better pay is essential to the lives of these workers, but low pay is not the only cause of "feeling like nobody." These workers must continually remind themselves, and others, why their work is valuable and important. They are in a constant struggle with messages from their supervisors, their coworkers, and even their union that what they are doing is not good enough. Participating in education and training programs is a way, then, to feel that they are growing and moving toward something more rewarding, a feeling they did not get at work. Marie told me that when her neighbors see her in uniform and ask if she is a nurse, she tells them she is a "professional butt cleaner"—to, as Marie put it, remind herself of where she is and where she hopes to be. Steve was in school to become a physician assistant because he felt there was no room for growth as a respiratory therapist. Juan said about his job as a registrar, "I feel that I'm wasting here." As in Marie's situation, even a job not that far removed in terms of training or the type of work—the difference between a nursing assistant and licensed practical nurse is in many respects quite small—might seem to promise an entirely different experience or those things most of us crave: a decent wage, autonomy, respect—a modicum of freedom.

So, there are thousands of health care workers putting in eighteen-hour days of school and work in the pursuit of something more "meaningful"— even though caregiving is usually considered the epitome of meaningful work. The lure of a different job and the perceived need to spend one's days and nights studying for the credential for that job are displacements of the talents and energies of some of the most crucial members of our society, displacements created by a general failure to adequately value their work and foster the conditions in which they might feel something approaching fulfillment.

Getting In

Many people in the sub-baccalaureate labor market will eventually find themselves drawn into health care work. They are neither entirely pushed nor pulled into health care—they could end up in health care work because of lack of other options, a desire to be involved in providing care, the perceived security of a union job and stability of employment in health care, the referrals of friends and family doing similar work, or a combination of any of these. With hindsight, when health care workers were explaining to me in interviews why they went into health care, many said they did so because they wanted to take care of people, or, at least, they framed their past as a series of choices they had made to work in health care in particular. In fact, how they got into health care work was usually more complicated.

Compared to most other options in the sub-baccalaureate labor market, any job in a New York City hospital, even one not directly involved with patient care, offers a number of advantages. Therefore many of the health care workers I interviewed did not work, or did not begin by working, in occupations directly involved in patient care. Cesar, for instance, started working in health care as a security officer at a Bronx hospital shortly after finishing high school. He immigrated from the Dominican Republic in 1978 at the age of thirteen and spent a few years after high school going to college, first taking general liberal arts courses at a four-year City

University of New York (CUNY) and then a two-year CUNY college, without obtaining a credential or degree. At the two-year school, Cesar enrolled in a computer technology program—computers, he said, are his main interest, and there were two computers and a number of computer books in the living room of his Bronx apartment. He did not finish the computer program, however, in part because of difficulties paying the tuition and the costs and hassle of the long commute to another part of city. He had by then also obtained the unionized, full-time security job at the hospital, so he dropped out of college. His motivation for attending college waned because of the stability the job provided, but he was also unclear about the purpose of being in college and what its payoff might be. There was nothing in particular about working in a hospital that appealed to him: "I wasn't attracted to the health field, I don't know why," he said. "I'm a technical person," he added later in the interview. By the time we spoke, however, he had become an operating room technician (OR tech), a job specific to health care, through a union-sponsored training program. He had also trained at one point to become a pharmacy technician, discussed in chapter 6.

Linda, who became one of Cesar's colleagues as a security officer and then classmate in the OR tech training program, had a few partial starts in the sub-baccalaureate labor market before finding stable work. Linda was born in the housing projects of the Bronx and had her only child at the age of fifteen, but with her mother's support and encouragement, she finished high school and immediately started working as an educational assistant for the New York City Board of Education. For many decades such public-sector, paraprofessional jobs provided full-time, reasonably well-paid employment where the private sector failed to do so. Linda, however, was laid off after about eight years with the city and had to face the perils of the private sector. She stayed home with her daughter for a brief period and then went back into the labor market, first working part-time for two years as a dietary aide (someone who prepares and delivers patient meals) in a hospital. She was laid off again, however, during a round of cutbacks, and then worked at a dry-cleaners making $5.00 an hour. "It was a real shitty job," she said, but she needed it. One day the owner hired a new employee to do the same job for $4.50 an hour and fired Linda the next. "I was devastated and I went home and I remember being so crushed, because I worked from 7 a.m. to 7 p.m. six days a week. I didn't make any

money, but it was all the income I had." Luckily, a friend who was working as a hospital security sergeant invited her to lunch at his hospital and
introduced her to someone in human resources. Linda was hired on the
spot. After a year working per diem at $9.50 an hour, Linda became full-
time and a union member, earning $12 an hour plus benefits.

It was not uncommon for the people I interviewed to take jobs just because they were in a health care setting, even if the job was not closely
related to their interests or education and training, because of the stability of employment in health care, buttressed in New York City by their
unionized status. Linda, for instance, said she had long wanted to become
a nurse, even after she had worked in three different occupations in health
care settings. A representative of the training program at District Council 37,
the union that represents workers in the city's public hospitals, noted:

> Some people have even come in [to apply for a job] as nurses' aides but there
> was no job opening for nurses' aides; there was an opening for a clerk and
> they did have the skills and they just went for it, and they took the job be-
> cause there was a need and they had to have a job. Later they would tell
> me, during orientation, you know I'm really a nurses' aide and I'm a CNA
> [certified nursing assistant]... I find that a lot.

Indeed, Shirley, a forty-year-old registrar at another branch of the
Bronx hospital where Linda and Cesar worked, thought a more natural
occupation for her would have been a nursing assistant. She originally
took a three-month CNA course so that she could better care for her ailing
grandmother, and a physician and social worker at the hospital where she
took her grandmother to a seniors' program were so impressed by Shirley
they told her there was a part-time opening in the psychiatric department.
"It just so happened that the position that was open was a unit associate
position where I would be doing paperwork instead of actually working
with the patients. So, I guess God knew where to send me. It wasn't what
I wanted, because I was going to be a nurse's aide." By the time a nursing
assistant position became available, Shirley was making more money—
about $11 an hour—as a unit associate, the person who handles the day-to-
day paperwork and information flow on a hospital unit. When we spoke,
she had been upgraded, or multiskilled, to work as a registrar in the emergency department. Shirley identified herself as a caregiver—"grandmother

always said I brought home every sick cat in town...I always try to take care of somebody"—but never had a job in health care that entailed providing direct care. Nevertheless, she found just working in a hospital satisfied her urge to care for others. "Like I said, I enjoy helping people. I've always liked to be around where I feel like I'm needed and that I'm doing something worthwhile."

For African American women like Linda and Shirley, jobs in health care have long been an important source of employment, but particularly so in hospitals, where wages are much better than in nursing homes and home care.[1] In other respects, Linda and Shirley's experiences were unusual since many women, especially immigrants to New York City, are channeled into jobs that involve directly providing care, which are the most numerous. Grace, a thirty-one-year-old immigrant from Trinidad, was working as a dietary coordinator at a major academic medical center in Brooklyn when we spoke. In 1988, at the age of seventeen, she moved to New York with her mother, who had been traveling to the United States off and on since the 1970s to work "under the table" as a nanny, returning to Trinidad regularly while she waited to receive a work visa. Grace's mother was part of the international "nanny chain,"[2] in which women from developing countries around the world leave behind their own children to find work as caregivers in wealthy, industrialized nations. For such women, the knowledge that they can get work as nannies informs their decisions to immigrate (or take extended trips) to wealthy countries. They do not generally immigrate and then decide to become nannies.

Grace's first job in the United States, while finishing high school in the late 1980s, was as a cashier at a grocery store, making $3.35 per hour. After graduating, she took a vacation, and when she returned could not bring herself to return to it. She needed a job, though, and was not sure about college. "I wanted to go to college, but I didn't know what I wanted to do. So until I found out what I wanted to do, I wanted to get a job. My sister was working here [at the hospital] and I asked her if she can help me with getting a job, and so I ended up here." Many of the people I interviewed, immigrant and nonimmigrant, were drawn into health care work through the referrals of friends or family members already working in the area. Like her sister, Grace was hired as a dietary aide, preparing hospital food and patient trays, making $4.50 an hour. By the time we spoke, twelve years later, she had been promoted to diet coordinator and was making just under $14 an hour. She was a union member, but employed by the private company to which food services at the hospital had been subcontracted. Grace had not, however, avoided the work of providing direct care, inevitable for many women in the sub-baccalaureate labor market. To make ends meet over the years, Grace had also become a CNA and taken second jobs, first as a home health aide—what her mother also eventually did— and then as a nursing assistant at a nursing home.

Like Grace's mother, Veronica also left her family back home in Trinidad when she started traveling to and from the United States in the 1970s on a temporary basis to do "babysitting jobs." When she received her green card in 1986, she and her son moved permanently to the United States, leaving her husband behind for several years. She started working immediately as a live-in nanny, but "I wanted some freedom, I wanted something to do. She [her employer] sent me to do—she asked me if I wanted to learn icing? So I went and did a little crash course in baking and icing cake. But somehow I felt that I wanted something more." Veronica enrolled in a CNA course offered by the Red Cross that she saw listed in the newspaper, and became a home health aide, then a nursing assistant at a nursing home, and, when we spoke, was working as a nursing assistant at a hospital. When I asked her why she went into health care, she said, "that was the easiest way. What could I go into without having any qualification, except being a homemaker? I didn't want to go clean somebody's kitchen."

Patrice, from Ghana, came to the United States on a visitor's visa but could not travel back and forth to renew it, so she worked in the shadow labor market for illegal immigrants for much longer than Grace's mother and Veronica. "Actually I moved here because of a man, I was supposed to be married to him and I came. But it wasn't good. It didn't work out." When her visa expired, Patrice worked for a brief period at a fast-food restaurant and then took jobs as a nanny and domestic, eventually becoming a live-in for a family in the wealthy suburbs of Westchester County. It was not the work Patrice would have chosen, but it was work. She was paid cash, and her employers did not pay her social security for close to ten years. But they helped Patrice pay for the GED course she passed through correspondence, and Patrice became very attached to their two children. Patrice moved out when she married a man from Ghana, who had a green card and applied for one for Patrice, and with whom she had her own child. She continued working for the family in Westchester, but had begun to reduce her hours in the last few years before we spoke in order to go to college. She had just recently received her green card.

Wanda, also from Trinidad, had been a student nurse in her home country, so she enrolled immediately in a CNA course when she arrived in the United States, rather than becoming a nanny or housekeeper. She too became a home health aide and later obtained a job at a midsize hospital in Brooklyn. A licensed practical nurse (LPN) when we spoke, Wanda said she too saw the nursing assistant course advertised in the papers. "I didn't know what it was, but I said I'm going for that." Winsome, too, had worked in health care in her home country, Jamaica, as a dental assistant, and her mother was a nurse there, so when she obtained her work visa in the United States it seemed natural to work in health care. Working as a home health aide or CNA in a nursing home, though poorly paid and difficult work, is, as Veronica suggested, often better work than cleaning someone's house or taking care of their children. Unlike private domestic jobs, it is possible to get health care jobs in New York City that are legitimate—employers pay social security and often some benefits—even if wages are low. (Though there is a substantial shadow labor market for home health and personal care workers.) Employment in a nursing home or for a home care agency can furthermore be a stepping-stone into work in a hospital, where most employees are unionized in New York City and wages are substantially better.

As these stories show, getting into health care is scarcely a process that can be reduced to an efficient matching process between people's skills, abilities, and desires with occupations that fulfill them. It is a combination of accident, coercion, and gradual self-adjustment. Indeed, the same holds true for health care workers' attempts to improve their lives once they are in the door. A mismatch between paid labor and people's talents and desires should always be a cause for concern, though it hardly ever is—even though few working Americans are arguably doing jobs that allow them to fully express their abilities and potential. In the case of those who are paid to provide care, however, there is often a great deal of concern about how and why people entered caregiving work, often as part of an agenda to justify paying caregivers less. If they are coerced into doing such work, it is assumed they provide poor quality care and deserve little. If they are motivated by their intrinsic desires and the inherent rewards of the work, then they can be paid little. Raise their wages too high, it has been argued, and the quality of care might suffer. I will return to this issue in the conclusion, but entering health care work, especially at the sub-baccalaureate level, is a multifaceted process, which cannot be explained by individual choices and motives alone.

Getting By

The way many of these workers got into health care is typical in so far as many allied health care workers begin as nursing assistants, often in home care agencies or nursing homes. After registered nurses (RNs), nursing assistants are the second largest occupational group in New York City hospitals[3] (and the core of 1199's membership). These are the people who do the hands-on, "dirty work" of health care: feeding and bathing patients, dressing and "grooming" them, physically moving them or getting them up, straightening up and cleaning their living quarters, and doing what one ethnographer called "bowel work"[4]—documenting "intake" and "outtake" amounts (food and liquid consumed, urination amounts, and descriptions of bowel movements), changing adult diapers, cleaning patients after they have relieved themselves, in bed or on the toilet. In some settings, nursing assistants provide basic clinical care as well, such as changing bandages, applying skin ointments and salves, and taking and recording "vitals," including temperature, blood pressure, and blood glucose levels.

Nursing assistants' experiences on the job are crucial to understanding the "workforce crisis" in health care. National studies cite annual turnover rates among nursing assistants in nursing homes ranging from 45 to 105 percent[5]—astounding figures for a segment of the workforce entrusted to care for the elderly and disabled. The Bureau of Labor Statistics projects that between 2000 and 2010, an additional 1.2 million nursing aides, home health aides, and persons in similar occupations will be needed to cover the projected growth in long-term care positions and replace departing workers. This increase in demand is over half the year 2000 supply.[6] Yet nursing assistants' working conditions and needs have received less attention than that of nurses, even though there is a similar shortage of both.

Research on the nursing shortage, nonetheless, suggests that shortages of RNs can be attributed, in large part, to problems with working conditions and the way the jobs are valued (not just financially). In 2000, there were nearly 500,000 RNs not working in nursing and, of that number, around half were currently licensed RNs working in non-nursing occupations or unemployed RNs who were potentially available for work. RNs reported they had left the profession because of concern for safety in health care settings, an inability to practice at a professional level, and especially because they were able to obtain better salaries and more convenient hours in other jobs. Studies of the sources of nurses' job dissatisfaction show too that until basic issues with their working conditions are resolved, such as inadequate staffing levels, stagnant wages, inflexible hours, and lack of voice and respect, problems with retention will continue to undermine recruitment efforts. Indeed, the most common strategies to address the nursing shortage—including increasing spaces in nursing schools, public relations campaigns to attract nurses from poorer parts of the U.S. population, programs to import nurses from abroad, transferring some nursing tasks to lesser-trained staff, and implementing cosmetic changes to working conditions—will never be enough as long as nurses are so dissatisfied with their jobs.[7]

My observations show similar issues affect nursing assistants and other allied health care workers. From 1999 to 2001, I directly observed dozens of health care workers in New York City health care settings (see the introduction and appendix for details on these settings). These observations were usually focused on frontline staff—nursing assistants, patient care technicians (PCTs), housekeepers, and unit clerks. I typically "shadowed" a health care worker during their shift, asking them questions about their work, training, experiences and personal stories as I followed behind with a small notebook in which I jotted important phrases or observations that I would expand into descriptive field notes shortly afterward. In following a single worker, I would also go with them to other units on errands and had the chance to observe and informally interview staff in a wider range of occupations—social workers, nurse managers, registered nurses, licensed practical nurses, physician assistants, physical and occupational therapists, recreational therapists, and patient care coordinators (a sort of junior nurse administrator). I attended some patient care planning meetings and in-services, joined staff for breaks or meals, and observed some recreational events for patients. I had little contact with physicians, who were a transient bunch; they would stay on patient units only long enough to review some charts, write orders, and consult with a few nurses or patients.

Problems with working conditions affect the morale and well-being of health care providers in a number of ways, but the problem of understaffing is among the most visible and glaring. Nursing journals are full of testimonials and editorials about inadequate staffing; research has linked negative patient outcomes with lower nurse staffing levels,[8] and many states are engaged in heated policy debates about whether minimum nurse-to-patient staffing ratios should be legislated. Inadequate staffing is due in part to a shortage of people going into the nursing field, which in turn is due in part to "restructuring" policies implemented in the 1990s, under which nursing positions were cut and the job de-professionalized and made less attractive.

The subacute care units I observed, which offered an intermediate level of care between acute-care hospitals and nursing homes, staffed a higher proportion of nursing assistants to nurses than acute-care units. The day shift at a subacute care unit with thirty-seven beds was usually staffed with four or five nursing assistants and three nurses, of whom one might be a licensed practical nurse (LPN). These units were often full and the patient census stable because patients generally had longer lengths of stay than in hospitals, but the level of care the patients required varied widely. In a general hospital unit with thirty-eight beds, by contrast, during the day shift I typically counted four nurses on duty, at least one of which was often an LPN, one nursing assistant (or PCT), and one unit clerk. The actual number of patients was often less than the number of beds, but nurses frequently had eight patients and the nursing assistant would have to cover the entire unit.

The nature of short-staffing, however, is impossible to convey by aggregate counts of the number of patients and the number of staff, even accounting for the severity of the patients' illnesses and the type of unit. The rhythm of health care work is not steady; certain work must be done at specific times and there are always unpredictable events that can throw off someone's schedule or list of tasks. A nursing assistant in a subacute care unit might officially have to care for seven or eight patients, but the amount of care each patient requires—for instance, whether they could dress themselves—is not wholly predictable and is a major factor in whether a nursing assistant could get her work done. I do not know if the staffing levels I observed always matched what was officially scheduled or officially reported in hospital statistics, but it was clear that staffing levels were just enough to get by and maintaining them next to impossible.

Many times staffing levels were disrupted because someone called in sick, or a temporary or agency nurse with less knowledge of the unit had been called to fill in (if possible), or staff had been "floated" to other floors that were acutely short of staff. Sometimes a nurse who had been assigned to administrative duties might be required to provide patient care to cover a shortage, or nurses were held past their shift to do mandatory overtime. On one unit that officially scheduled three PCTs for thirty-two beds, it was not uncommon for only one PCT to be on the floor, perhaps because one PCT called in sick and the other PCT was escorting a patient to a specialty clinic for tests. Although official records of such units might suggest staffing levels are adequate (assuming three PCTs was enough to begin with), the most minor disruption to those staffing levels causes havoc. Staff members complained to me regularly about staffing levels—in interviews and during observations. (Though not one of the health workforce planners or trainers I interviewed, on the other hand, did—except on the occasions I brought it up.)

From my perspective, there were two major indicators that staffing levels were problematic for nursing assistants and other frontline workers: the seemingly incompatible pressures on health care workers to cut corners to get all their work done, on the one hand, and to "come out"—as workers called it—of their own job description to help their coworkers or patients, on the other. Cutting corners and coming out of description were officially forbidden but unofficially required in all the settings I observed, putting nursing assistants in particular under a form of constant dissonance and stress. As Thomas Gass has written in his vivid account of his work as a nursing assistant in a nursing home, "We are always in the wrong position, no matter what we do."[9]

A shortcut at one subacute unit I observed was the practice of "double diapering" patients, especially at night—putting more than one adult diaper on the patients. At a staff meeting, the nurse manager was unhappy with the nursing assistants for doing this, and said it was being done even with those patients who were continent. The nurse manager implied it was done out of laziness, so that the aides would not have to take as many patients to the bathroom. Several nursing assistants replied that some patients felt more secure with diapers on, even if continent, because even when the unit was fully staffed it might be some time before someone responded to their request to go to the bathroom. Indeed, during one of my observations on the floor, a nursing assistant, Ms. Roberts, checked on a patient at the end of her day shift and found she was wearing two diapers, one over the other. Ms. Roberts tried to persuade the patient to wear only one, saying she would get in trouble with the evening shift nurses. The patient told Ms. Roberts she was more comfortable with two diapers. Ms. Roberts eventually caved to her wishes—but not without making the patient promise to tell the evening shift that it was she who *wanted* two diapers and that Ms. Roberts was not responsible for it. From the perspective of management, the practice of putting diapers on continent patients or patients who just wanted the security was not consistent with patient care protocols. From the perspective of many staff, and evidently some patients, it was a necessity given the likelihood they would not be taken care of right away in the event of an accident.

Similarly, by working as a nursing aide at a nursing home, sociologist Steven Lopez learned that the only possible way for aides to complete "a.m. care" for their residents—getting them up, bathed, dressed, and prepared for breakfast in seventy-five minutes—was "through the use of prohibited shortcuts, by skipping steps, and by ignoring rules." Some of these skipped steps, such as rounds conducted at the beginning of shift to make sure each patient had been recently changed or toileted by night-shift staff, potentially compromised patient care. Lopez found that for aides to follow all the care rules, seventy-five minutes was only enough time to care for three residents. In fact, most of the aides had to perform a.m. care for between four and six residents (most aides were assigned nine or ten patients, but usually not all of them required a.m. care prior to breakfast). The nursing home was staffed favorably compared to the national average for nursing homes and very favorably compared to the state's minimum requirements, and yet it was still impossible for aides to do all that was required of them. Aides might not necessarily be so short of time later in the day, but the bureaucratic rules required that all patients were awake and fed by a specific time, and during those important early hours aides took a number of risks to meet these requirements.[10] Skipping some of the bureaucratically proscribed steps in providing care is inevitable, even when such steps are an important part of patient care.

Lopez also found that the same time everyone knew it was impossible to meet all the bureaucratic requirements, it was the aides who were held responsible for any negative consequences of skipping them, not managers or regulators who imposed impossible rules. When a physical therapy aide told Lopez ninety minutes into his shift that one of his resident's diapers had not been changed by the night shift, and was filled and the resident's slacks soaked through, Lopez reported it to his supervising nurse. The nurse, however, asked if he had done rounds and, even though she knew no one had time to do rounds, reminded him that without doing rounds he would be held responsible for what happened to the patient.[11]

As a result of understaffing, health care workers not only feel that they must cut corners on bureaucratically proscribed steps but also do things that are not technically allowed or part of their official job descriptions for the sake of patients and their coworkers. Gloria, a registrar working at a hospital outpatient clinic, said, "Sometimes all of us gotta come out of description." Judith, a unit clerk at the same hospital's inpatient facility, for instance, was allowed—and sought—a good deal of leeway in coming out of description because she was also in school to become an RN. She would tell patients about their medications and follow-up care before they were discharged, normally a nurse's responsibility. "That much they trust me on. They trust me on a lot of things too, because I'm reliable like that." A nursing assistant I observed liked the subacute unit where she worked because she sometimes had the chance to perform nursing duties, such as applying bandages (dressings) to wounds.

None of the settings I observed could have functioned without workers coming out of description. As Judith said, "I even told my manager that if I was to do only what a unit associate does, there'd be no peace on the floor." In part this is because it is impossible to account for or predict every possible need or contingency in health care work, but more often it is because those who run health care organizations simply take for granted that most workers will come out of description and make up for poor staffing levels and patterns, as when Spanish-speaking health care workers are called away from their regular responsibilities to translate between Spanish-speaking patients and non-Spanish-speaking staff.

The willingness of some staff to come out of description or do work they have not been explicitly assigned can cause friction with their co-workers who come out of description less willingly because they fear their performance will become the new standard—without added pay, respect, or autonomy. As Nancy Foner observed in her ethnography of a nursing home in New York City, such workers are "rate busters," and are disliked, as in any other workplace, because they undermine the collectively devised informal strategies to resist pressure from management to do endlessly more work.[12] Like Foner, I have observed sullen workers helping a patient who has not been assigned to them while making it all too clear to the patient that they are doing them a special, and rare, favor. I have watched patients wait to be taken to the bathroom until "their" nursing assistant can be told and find a moment to take them. This despite that several staff, who could take them and know they need to go, are available. Rate busters, by contrast, are sometimes the best health care workers, but their hard work is likely to be exploited. Like Lopez, Foner also did her research in a relatively well-staffed nursing home. Until the early 1990s, New York State also provided relatively generous Medicaid reimbursement rates for nursing home care. In the wake of restructuring, however, most health care workers today have trouble keeping up with the bare minimum of their duties, let alone have time for rate busting. "Coming out of description" is, in my observations, more often a means of scraping by, of helping a coworker who has fallen behind or a patient who has been kept waiting for an intolerably long period.

Restructuring—largely a means of cost cutting—was carried out across hospitals and other health facilities in New York in the mid-1990s, and it gave health care workers good reason to suspect that coming out of description would be exploited. Such reforms were intended to assign as much work as possible to the fewest, least well-paid workers while avoiding lawsuits or running afoul of administrative or state regulations. Administrators' decisions revealed that they felt frontline health care workers were largely to blame for excessive costs, through their wasteful habits and unproductive ways. When one hospital "upgraded" some unit clerks, including Gloria and Juan, to new positions as registrars in the hospital's outpatient clinics as part of a new "multiskilling" initiative, the registrars were expected to do some coding of patient illnesses and diagnoses—a job for which there were dedicated, and more highly paid, coders working in the hospital billing department. Juan at first came to an informal agreement with his supervisor that he would do additional coding for some of the clinics after his shifts, unpaid, in exchange for flexibility with his work hours. He began to suspect, however, that he was not getting the best end of the bargain. "Now," he said, "unless I'm getting compensated for it, I'm not going to do it," and noted, "at one time, we used to have coders, we used to send all our billing and encounter forms to a specific place and there were coders coding it." When the same hospital conducted a mandatory communication skills training course (described in chapter 5), the emphasis on improving teamwork seemed to some participants to have less to do with cooperation than pressuring employees to come out of description and compensate for shortages of staff and resources not of their making. When Gloria was a unit clerk, she had also objected to being sent away from her desk on errands—delivering blood samples, picking up medication at the pharmacy, getting a stretcher for a patient—drawing for support on a former supervisor who said the unit clerk is the last person who should leave the floor since they have to answer phones and relay all communications, some urgent. Nonetheless, Gloria was told to "do it and grieve [file a grievance] later, because you're refusing, that's insubordinating."

An administrator with DC37, the public hospital workers' union, described what happened to several unit clerks who became patient care associates (PCAs—the public hospitals' multiskilled nursing assistant position) as part of restructuring efforts:

> Once the clerk was trained as a PCA they wouldn't go back to doing clerk functions, they would do PCA functions. And sometimes the facilities feel like "okay, this person is really good on this computer and even though I know they were trained to do all these other pieces and components...we don't have a backfill [someone to fill in] for this area and since this person has the expertise...we're going to let her or him do it all day." And we can't allow that.

In effect, the hospital had an employee who was trained to do two different jobs—that of a clerk who handles paperwork and administrative duties and that of a nursing assistant who handles patient care—giving them more flexibility and control over their workers. The worker's objection might be that they should not be required to shift between radically different jobs with no notice and no additional compensation. Such shifts might also have negative consequences for the continuity of patient care. The union objected that such behavior made it impossible to gauge how much workers should be paid and suspected it was a way of devaluing these jobs—after all, no one would ask a doctor to fill in for a lawyer for the day. Moreover, to unions such behavior was an indicator that the hospitals sought not primarily to upgrade its workforce but to create conditions in which it could be more easily downsized by reducing its staff to a core of highly flexible multitaskers.

Given these types of experiences, it is not surprising that heath care workers begin to feel that if there is a logic that guides decisions about what particular workers can and cannot do, it does not revolve around patient care or patient needs. Even though Gloria had been told when she was a unit clerk that she was not to have patient contact, she noted dryly that she was supposed to evacuate the floor in the event of a fire. Even though she had once been reprimanded for giving patients their food trays because she had no medical training, she said she had also been asked to escort patients to their rooms when they arrived on the floor. What could she do if they collapsed, she asked, without any medical training? She had even been asked to explain do-not-resuscitate forms to patients—documents in which patients indicate whether they wish to be resuscitated in the event of cardiac arrest.

For many health care workers the sense that there are no real limits to their work leads to a justifiable fixation on their job descriptions, which they see as the only basis for being able to draw lines around what can be asked of them in a work environment bent on stretching out their responsibilities. When we spoke, Gloria said she had resolved to stay within her job description because the pressure to go out of her way or be a better "team player" had become, finally, intolerable. Gloria also felt it was her union's place to enforce her job description, saying, "sometimes we do things that we're not supposed to as a union member." Not surprisingly, hospital managers and administrators often accuse labor unions of standing in the way of creative change or fostering a mentality that is opposed to teamwork. One trainer, who began her health care career as a social worker, talked about a nonunion nursing home in which she worked in the 1980s:

> There was a very strong sense of family between everyone. Back then I would go up and make beds, I could come in at 12:00 and do in-services with them. We were all committed. When we were first opening and waiting for our first state survey all of us were painting the corners of the doors,

and it wasn't 'you can't do that and I can't do that.' The nonunion element really lended [sic] itself to that.

The trainer invoked a truism in antiunion business ideology by contrasting the idea of the workplace as a cooperative family to that of a unionized shop in which people bicker over responsibilities. Yet, this trainer also recognized that unions cannot necessarily be blamed for the apparent lack of team spirit on the shop floor. She added, "it was also a different time"—a time before the regulatory oversight of nursing homes in particular became both more rigorous and overbearing, before the staffing shortages and cost-cutting that made painting the corners of the doors all but impossible (even in preparation for a survey or inspection), and perhaps before the feeling among health care workers that they were unappreciated and overworked was so prevalent. A fixation on job descriptions seems as much a result of workers' experiences with exploitative managerial tactics as of the negative influence of uncooperative unions.

Many health care workers I talked to in fact voiced frustration that 1199 in particular did not police job descriptions more closely. 1199, on the contrary, cooperated with much of the multiskilling and restructuring programs of the 1990s. Juan said of his new, multiskilled position as a registrar that "there's no real specific job details that a registrar would have.... The way they word it [job descriptions] is real vague, so that any time stuff can be handed to you." Gloria said hospital administrators would use the term "related duties" in job descriptions—a catch-all phrase that makes jobs infinitely expandable. Union-endorsed "multiskilling" initiatives made it easier for employers to blur the lines between several occupations and create generic job descriptions.

Job descriptions, however, are not adequate protection for these workers. Even if labor unions were more aggressive in their enforcement of job descriptions, they would necessarily fail to draw limits around caregiving work or establish its worth and value. As lists of tasks, job descriptions are daily contradicted by the unpredictable nature of the work in health care and the indivisibility of providing care; they can never account for every aspect of the work or divide it into discrete responsibilities. Job descriptions that are categorical and abstract, rather than merely descriptive, likewise fail to solve the problem of seemingly limitless work—when too general, they can be endlessly reinterpreted to suit the interests of supervisors and managers (those "related duties"). The purpose of job descriptions arguably has never been to accurately depict work as it is actually carried out. Hospitals use them primarily to protect themselves from lawsuits and show conformity to regulations. The mentality required to avert lawsuits—in which job descriptions categorize and reduce care to a series of isolated tasks—is incompatible with the complexity of delivering care. In so far as unions attempt to police or create more precise job descriptions, they too participate in obscuring or trivializing the complexity of tasks and decisions that make up the core of caregiving work.[13]

In practice, caregiving work requires flexibility and adaptability, yet caregivers have little discretion in when to be flexible, and managers' views of when cutting corners is acceptable or coming out of description is required did not seem to be dictated by patient interests. As Gloria explained: "We all tend to stray from it [our job description]...the big problem in this hospital, in the management, is that management has this persona...that we should do everything or even go out of our way to get things done." Although Gloria's managers might interpret her refusal to go "out of her way" as a poor work ethic and lack of cooperative spirit, her attitude was the product of the continual experience of being in the wrong position— always required to come out of description but arbitrarily reprimanded for doing so.

Job descriptions, like bureaucratically established steps, can themselves pose risks to patients when they prevent health care providers from responding creatively and humanely to patient needs. As Tom Gass explained in detail:

> It is my experience that the regulations that filter down to the front lines are not always applied rationally, and that their cumulative weight adds to an already undoable list of job tasks. Everyone knows that we cannot perform all the tasks required of us in the prescribed manner, and that sometimes it is best not to apply a certain regulation, but no one is allowed to openly admit this obvious reality. Technically we are never given discretion in such matters, so in fact we are routinely in violation of what we are told we must do. We are always in the wrong position, no matter what we do. We are always coming up short.[14]

Like Lopez, Gass found that he had to skip some proscribed steps. But he also points out that health care workers are not only forced to skip some bureaucratically prescribed steps because of a lack of time, but they may also feel compelled to skip them in the best interests of patients.

Nursing assistants, clerks, and others who are the front line of care in many health care settings must use discretion—they must see beyond and between a list of tasks or rigid protocols—but they are more likely to be punished than rewarded for their initiative. Nancy Foner called these the "hidden injuries of bureaucracy." She showed that the patient needs health care workers cannot meet because of bureaucratic rules and irrational polices are often simple. One nursing assistant she observed, Ana, ordered new glovelike hand protectors for a resident on her own, when the nursing coordinator did not order them after several requests. The nursing coordinator then told Ana that she could not order supplies independently and said the gloves had to be returned—even though Ana, and another aide, argued that the patient's old gloves were inadequate protection against injury and uncomfortable for the resident. More than a month later, the resident was still using the old gloves. Moreover, the resident was partially comatose and not able to demand them herself.[15]

Indeed, the aspects of their working conditions that health care workers seem to find most aggravating, disrespectful, and personally draining on a day-to-day basis stem from seemingly straightforward and even trivial bureaucratic decisions, making the most basic supplies and resources they need to provide patient care unavailable or available inconsistently. This source of frustration is much less remarked on than that of understaffing, yet it was pervasive in the health care settings I observed and exacerbated by hospital administrators' misplaced fixations on how to reduce costs. During one of her shifts in the emergency room, Marie had to tell a patient who had been vomiting that the ER was out of toothpaste. She made do and gave the woman a lemon-scented glycerin toilette and a bowl of water instead. Marie's job also entailed stocking various supply cabinets, but she was not allowed a key to them. As I shadowed her, she once spent ten minutes trying to find out who had the only key to the supply cabinets so that she could get an adult diaper for a patient. The nursing assistants at one subacute care facility complained that the hospital had stopped carrying ice cream suitable for diabetics. Michael Opoku, a nursing assistant from Ghana whom I followed for several shifts, remarked while helping a male patient shave in the shower and standing in an inch of water in the large, cold stall, that the hospital razor blades were useless, purchased at ten for ninety-nine cents. One nurse, sitting at the nurses' station writing notes in patient charts, said to those around her, "How can we work without scissors?"

The equipment that health care workers regularly use can be finicky, if it can be found at all: a blood pressure machine with a leak in the tubing to the cuff (which Marie covered with her finger but feared was affecting her readings), or for which the ball used to inflate the cuff is missing, or which has to be plugged in in every room because its battery is dead; or a Hoyer lift (an electronically controlled sling used to move immobile patients) that is too narrow to be of use for the heaviest patients on the floor or that can suddenly decompress, lowering the patient abruptly and without warning. At one subacute care unit, one of the two showers was broken, and the other had no hot water for two days. In this case, nursing assistants either did not bathe their patients as scheduled or subjected them to a cold shower. There was no space allotted for nursing assistants to write in the patient charts that a shower was not given because there was no hot water, only that a shower was "offered but not given"—a notation likely to draw unwanted attention from facility administrators or regulators, who require patients to take regular showers and would immediately suspect that nursing assistants were not making their "offer" firmly enough or somehow trying to avoid the work of giving them. When the problem came up in a staff meeting, the nurse manager said that it was up to the nurses, not nursing assistants, to document any special circumstances about why the shower was not given, but in any case she did not want it recorded in the patient charts that there was no hot water on the floor. As Timothy Diamond aptly entitled one chapter of his account of working as a nursing assistant: "If it's not charted, it didn't happen."[16]

These things, most not immediately threatening to the safety of patients, are nonetheless important to health care workers because they are the things that can make patients feel better when so much else is going wrong; they can have a disproportionate effect on how patients perceive the care they receive. Encountered on a day-to-day basis, such shortages of supplies or resources for patient care make staff and patients feel frustrated. And these are the staff who are most likely to bear the emotional consequences of patient dissatisfaction.

On a general medical unit at one hospital, the spiffiest piece of equipment on the floor was an automated supply cabinet. About six feet high and fifteen feet long, it nearly filled a narrow room behind the nurses' station. Enough space remained for a few lockers, into which staff stuffed their bags and coats at the beginning of each shift, and a plastic chair. The supplies in the humming cabinet—everything from toothbrushes, bandages, washing trays—were located in separate drawers that popped open after staff members entered their personal pin number and the amount of the supply they intended to withdraw (or return) on an electronic touchpad. The drawers had transparent fronts and were illuminated by a bluish-white lights, allowing staff members to see into them and giving the room a cool, sterile glow.

Undoubtedly the cabinet enabled "increased inventory accuracy" and "improved accuracy of patient billing," as the website for a manufacturer of such cabinets advertises. It was not clear, however, how the cabinet would "allow staff to focus on patient care." The nursing assistants I observed, who used this cabinet dozens of times during each shift, felt it slowed them down to have to report every single item they used. Ms. Jones, the unit clerk, was relieved that her pin number for the cabinet did not work—it was not a normal part of her job to use medical supplies and not having a functional pin number made it possible both to avoid dealing with the cabinet and reduced the possibility that she might be asked to come out of her job description to help the nursing assistants.

For the administrators, a bit of staff annoyance was perhaps acceptable given the savings from "lost" inventory. But the cabinet's effects on the staff went beyond annoyance. It conveyed a message to the staff that the hospital administration's main concern was not with the conditions of their work or patient care, but with monitoring untrustworthy employees. The only other computerized equipment on the floor was a terminal on the nursing station, which was used only by physicians and a few nurses to check lab test results, and an automated dispensing machine for narcotics in a locked room near the station, used only by nurses.

Everything else was based on old-fashioned technology. Communication between floors or units of the hospital happened either by phone or documents sent via pneumatic tubes. Much of Ms. Jones' shift was spent making phone calls (especially to schedule tests and procedures for patients), passing along or filing orders and documents, and writing by hand in various log books. It seemed that every bit of information on the floor went through Ms. Jones, and every bit had to be recorded by hand in several places. In addition to editing the census sheet several times a shift and compiling charts for patients new to the unit, Ms. Jones would handwrite the names and addresses of admits and discharges into a separate green, hardcover log book. Patient charts in fat three-ring binders, supposed to be stored in alphabetical order on rolling metal carts, were more often strewn across the nursing desk by the staff who consulted them, apparently none of whom felt it was part of their job to keep the charts neatly stored. Ms. Jones was already engaged in an explicit battle to get staff, mostly doctors, to return patient ID cards to their proper place after using them, arguing it was neither part of her job nor did she have time to straighten up after everyone on the floor; she was not about to volunteer to put back patient charts.

Even by health care industry standards, this hospital lagged behind in the use of information technology. There was no computerized patient census, so that security guards at the information desk in the main lobby had no up-to-date way to tell family members or visitors where patients were in the hospital. (But Linda, who had been a security guard there, commented wryly that this was probably for the best, since in her experience it was not uncommon in the hospital's rough, urban neighborhood for people to walk in claiming to know a specific patient in the hospital in order to steal things from their room.) In 2001, the year I did my fieldwork in this hospital, U.S. health care providers spent $20 billion on information technology, less than one-third of which was spent for hospital clinical (treatment-related) systems. Much of the spending went instead to upgrading and maintaining financial systems, such as billing.[17] Indeed, the major piece of information technology in development at the hospital was a billing system, paid for from the "infrastructure" piece of the federal grant that was also funding multiskilling and communication skills training programs.

The fact that the same level of security was applied to everyday, commonly used supplies as it was to narcotics and that one of the first pieces of automated technology invested in was a cabinet to monitor staff use of toothbrushes and bandages, rather than electronic patient records or an electronic admitting and discharge system or even an electronic system for scheduling tests and procedures, reinforced the feeling on the unit that patient care was not the hospital's main concern. "It's as if they think we're eating it up here," Monique, an RN called out to no one in particular one evening, frustrated that the pharmacy had not yet sent medication she had ordered and that her medication cart was so sparingly stocked she didn't even have extra Tylenol to give patients.

Neither, it seemed, was the well-being of staff a primary concern. The giant supply cabinet was located in the room that staff had formerly used for breaks. There was a conference room on the floor, but it had been commandeered by the physicians who often closed the door, making the room off limits. Some of the staff would still eat a quick snack next to the ominous supply cabinet, but otherwise they had to go to the hospital cafeteria in the basement, which one nursing assistant dismissed as a "cubby." But taking a long enough break to travel to and from the cafeteria and eat something was hardly feasible in any case. As Ms. Jones said, most of them chose not to take breaks at all, let alone their full breaks, because it just meant they would have to stay past their shift to finish all their work. Both the hospital cafeteria and the small café on the main floor of the hospital (the more pleasant eatery, with higher prices and table-service, frequented more by patient family members and physicians) closed at 8 p.m. anyway, leaving those on the night shift with no place for a break or to buy food.

For staff of the subacute care unit at the rehabilitation facility, there was a better employee break room in the basement, but no cafeteria at all. The hospital used to have food service for staff, but it took 1 percent out of their paychecks and served them the same food as the patients. Not surprisingly, the staff were less than enthusiastic about this "benefit." The café on the main floor was pleasant enough, but after a few days I could see why the staff did not want to linger there on their breaks—it was used by everyone: patients who were well enough, family members, supervisors, administrators, doctors, and visitors. It was not a space where staff could let down their guard and have a genuine break. The day shift nurse manager on the unit allowed staff to take their lunch breaks together in the patient lounge areas, where they could watch a bit of the afternoon soap operas on TV and chat, but the night shift nurse manager did not allow staff to eat or spend time in the patient lounge or dining room unless they were working with a patient.

Though using the patient dining area or lounge was a way to find a moment to take a break, it does not remedy one of the most difficult aspects of health care work—the lack of time and space for privacy and momentary respite. When they are on the job, nursing assistants, nurses, unit clerks—any employee without an office and who works directly with patients on the floor—are constantly exposed to the requests and glances of anyone who passes through—patients, family members, supervisors, coworkers. Managing the various types of exchanges, prioritizing the requests that they sometimes entail, and focusing on the regular set of tasks to be accomplished requires not only skill, but tremendous patience. More than once I saw patience break down, when staff became irritated with one another or irritated with no one in particular.

For patients, too, physical conditions at these hospitals are difficult. At one hospital's twenty-storey building used for offices and outpatient clinics, I waited with patients and staff for over five minutes for one of the two elevators serving the highly trafficked building. At the ophthalmology clinic where I was headed to do an interview, there were thirty patients and family members crowded in the waiting room, some of whom had to stand because there were not enough chairs. For a room full of people who had been waiting a long time for appointments, I was surprised to sense only resignation.

Finally, there is the issue of the physical safety of health care workers. Health care work is a high-risk occupation in well-known ways. There is the risk of infection to which health care workers are exposed, from HIV of course, but also from other dangerous and more easily transmissible diseases, such as drug-resistant tuberculosis and hepatitis. There is the risk of physical injuries, especially back injuries, for many caregivers who spend their days stooping to lift and maneuver patients. But in addition, many health care workers, especially nursing staff left alone on patient units through the night, felt that reduced staffing levels personally endangered them. One hospital where I conducted fieldwork had been in the news recently because a nurse was attacked by a visitor—the day before the Joint Commission on the Accreditation of Healthcare Organizations (JCAHO) was due to visit the hospital. "It was in all the newspapers," a worker there said. "Oh my God did heads roll that week!" Although heads may have rolled that week, workers in the hospital felt a pervasive lack of security. Melanie, a young unit clerk, said that it was difficult to get security to come and clear out friends or family members who stayed beyond visiting hours. "Nobody wants to leave. And when we try to tell the patient it's time for them to go, they get loud, they don't want to leave." I asked her if she felt safe working at night. "Not really, because there's not really security walking around. This exit out here is dark, there's no security there. Security is kept downstairs by the emergency room—there's no one walking the floors or on each of the floors."

There are risks in working with patients and their families, who are unknown, often emotionally distressed, and sometimes volatile. Many descriptions of health care work discuss caregiving as if it is a process involving only tenderness and sympathy, and when instances of abuse or mistreatment are mentioned, it is usually abuse committed by health care workers. I was always struck by just how difficult patients and family members could be, sometimes crossing over into what could be called abuse or mistreatment. One young nursing home aide in a training class told her classmates about a patient who liked to throw his dirty diapers at aides. Another male patient on a floor I observed was known for purposely farting in the nurses' faces whenever they lifted his legs to change a bandage on his tailbone. Each morning the nurses and assistants crossed their fingers and hoped they would not be assigned to care for him. When Wanda first started as an LPN in the emergency room of the Brooklyn hospital where she had worked for many years, she was "scared—because there used to be shouting and cursing, I was scared. But we always have to be on the lookout for these people, always." A patient kicked Linda in the knee when she was a security officer. The injury kept her out of work and required several surgeries. "It happened so fast, and nobody realized that it would be that detrimental. It changed my whole life," she said. "It wasn't until I felt like I might get seriously hurt, not be able to work, or get killed in here, that I decided it was time that I had to get out."

The physical aspects of the facilities and neighborhoods where many New York City health care providers work can also be dangerous, especially in areas with disproportionately high rates of poverty and crime. Marie's first job as a hospital nursing assistant was on the night shift at a long-term care facility in the notorious South Bronx. Her mother "said that was a rough area to go into at night, which was true. It was real rough." Even though she was making only just over $10.00 an hour at the time, Marie took a taxi to and from work to avoid walking in the neighborhood at night. One nurse, talking about the asthma epidemic in many New York City neighborhoods, noted it was related to the unsanitary conditions of many neighborhoods, including those of her hospital. "When you go to the car park at night," she told me half-jokingly, "you'll see dancing rats—rats as big as cats."

Despite all of these sources of injury in caregiving work, health care organizations can still rely on the fact that many of these workers will still show up for work. In New York City this is especially so because unionized health care jobs are relatively secure and well-paid in the context of the service sector. And regardless of how they got into health care, whether they "chose" it, the emotional elements of caring for others also exerts strong pressure to always do more. Despite her recent resolution to stick to her job description, Gloria continued to do a number of tasks—seemingly trivial except to the patients she helped—out of her description:

> Even if the [nursing assistant] is gone to lunch…I still give ice to patients if they need it.…I don't just say "well I'm too busy." I just go ahead and give it to them because I have a father who has cancer and I would like that when my father is treated, you know. I just hate that. I don't want nobody mistreating my father.

Though unit clerks were to have no patient contact, Gloria pointed out the obvious: If they cannot find a nurse or a nursing assistant, patients inevitably call or approach the nursing desk where the clerks work:

> I will sit there and the patient needs a bed pan and the nurse is occupied, and the nursing attendant or whatever, and I know how it feels as a person. For me, being a person kicks in. You know how holding your urine, what that is like. You need to go. I get up, and I put on a glove and I hand them a bedpan.

Marie, too, said she often does things outside her job description.

> Sometimes I feel like I overextend myself, and not because—I guess you could say I do it because I want to. Because if a person can't get up from bed and they need a family member to be called, they'll say, "oh, well let the social worker know." I feel, to put them at ease, yeah, I'll do it.

As she more simply stated, "I'm a human being, I know what that feels like."

Although Marie explained the pull to respond to patient needs humanely and creatively as a product of being "human," most direct caregivers are women, and caregiving is still largely perceived as a task that comes naturally to the second sex—a perception caregivers themselves may share. Deborah Stone found in her interviews with, and observations of, home care workers that they face a constant moral burden: "They cannot give enough to satisfy the needs they think people have or the care they think people deserve." "Virtually all" the direct care providers with whom Stone spoke visited clients on their days off. In an era of cost cutting and increasing rules about what care can and should be provided, home care agencies have become "caregiving bureaucracies," Stone argues, which are "betting that the caregivers will dip into the well of their own humanity to offset the budget constraints and stifling rulebooks."[18]

In the health care workplace, and even the private space of home and family, caring is a complex activity, one that does not always come naturally and one that often takes great effort to carry out. Not all moments of caregiving are filled with mutual warmth or free of pain, but they are nonetheless emotional and require skill and effort. Caregiving isn't always about doing what patients request. When I was shadowing an energetic aide, Jean, at a subacute care unit, she passed a patient dozing in her wheelchair in the hall and told her it was time to go to the bathroom. It was unnecessary, the patient objected, because she had not eaten anything. Jean insisted and pushed the patient into the bathroom, predicting, "now I will hear some yelling." Standing around the corner (to give the patient some privacy), I heard the sound of a long stream of urination, and the patient call out to me, "she knows me."

Michael Opoku told me that when he first started his job there were times he had to vomit from the "dirty work," the cleaning and bathing, that he does. As I watched him work, Michael said several times that it was not an easy job. Angela Michaels, an immigrant from St. Kitts in the Caribbean, who had been working as a nursing assistant for only five months, told me that when she first started she was so physically exhausted each day she didn't know if she would make it. As part of her work in the emergency room, Marie sometimes had to clean and wrap the bodies of the deceased. She did not know this would be part of her job when she was transferred from another unit, and she found it emotionally draining.

One of the most difficult emotional aspects of health care work is that health care workers are very far "downstream" from whatever it is that brought patients to the hospital or health care facility. In many instances, health care workers cannot ultimately do anything; they cannot compensate for the cruelties of life, some of which are the direct result of this particular society's choices about whose lives count and whose do not. Marie worked overtime one day doing "one-to-ones": sitting with patients who need constant monitoring. The people she sat with had all tried to commit suicide: one was a woman whose young infant had recently died; another was a woman who just cried for hours and wouldn't say why; and another was a young, gay, Hispanic man who was first beaten up by thugs, then the police, and later tried to jump off a bridge. Marie, clearly a very kind person whom I both interviewed and observed for several shifts, was still grieving her grandmother's death from breast cancer and could not seem to help but feel some of these patients' pain. Her eyes watered when doing an EKG test on an older woman with a cyst on her breast. "It is hard," she said to me. "It's hard sometimes dealing with it, because if you're looking at the pain—you're not experiencing it to the same extent that they are—but it does take a toll."

Kwame, a nursing assistant from Guyana, said that one of the most difficult aspects of the work is that some patients do not appreciate anything the aides do. Nursing assistants can understand why patients are upset or difficult, however. Ms. Roberts, a nursing assistant, told me that many patients are angry when they arrive on the unit, and she tries to see that it is the disease that makes them angry, not anything she has done. She tries to use a sense of humor, even though it does not always work.

Winsome, whose eyes began to water when she described how a patient's family member had called the administration and accused her of hitting a patient, was at her wit's end. Recalling the event, she said,

> If you see trouble, darling, are you going to walk into trouble? ... I am forty-two years old and I see trouble, am I stupid enough to walk into it and treat that person badly? I have a son to send to school, nine years old, my other son is getting his associate's [degree] this year, and am I going to jeopardize that? The little money I'm getting? I can't even pay my rent.

"There are so many people—patients—writing me and thanking me," she went on. "Patients buy, like the family member, they went to the Body Shop and bought me gifts, so many gifts I can't tell you. And then a few petty people write you up. That doesn't really make sense to me." Winsome was taking prep classes for the CUNY entrance exam because she was desperate to do something other than be a nursing assistant. "I just feel [I have] to go on because I don't feel—I don't know the standard right now, what they really want." Because of the incident, her supervisor sent her to a communication class. "When my supervisor was giving me this thing I said 'I'm so glad I'm doing something else so that I can get the hell out of here.' That's what I said."

Dealing with the seemingly unfair reactions and disrespect of one's coworkers and supervisors is in many ways more difficult than dealing with upset patients. As Felicia, a unit clerk explained, the latter are, after all, "sick." Or, at least their comments can be ascribed to their sickness. When Melanie, a young unit clerk, once had a run-in with a doctor, the doctor "said she was a doctor here for four years and I don't know what it means to be a doctor because I'm not one. You know? Like putting me down as if I could never be one. That hurt." When Marie's grandmother was very ill and about to be taken off a ventilator so she could die, Marie spoke to a supervisor about potentially leaving her shift to be with her grandmother. Though Marie was entitled to three days off after the death of a grandparent, the supervisor gave her a hard time, brusquely asking her, "How long do you anticipate that's going to take?" To be paid for her time off, Marie had to bring in a death certificate for her grandmother. These workers give a tremendous amount to their jobs and patients, but feel that no one is concerned about them.

Still, ultimately more important to most of them was that the emotional and caring work they do for patients is not rewarded. Timothy Diamond found by working as a nursing assistant, as did Deborah Stone by interviewing home care workers, that activities such as sitting and talking to patients are actively discouraged. There is not enough time for talking and it is not a billable task. Such activities are not only discouraged, but, as Diamond says, "written out of the job," erased in all the official charts and documents that represent what counts and what is valued in health care settings.[19]

When these health care workers are not given the time and resources they need to care for others, one of the insidious and inadvertent results is that the quality of the care they provide not only suffers, but so too does their own understanding of what good caregiving is and their willingness to go out of their way. When I was shadowing Ms. Roberts, we went into a room where a petite, older woman, who had recently had one of her legs amputated, sat in her wheelchair looking depressed. As soon as Ms. Roberts asked her what was the matter, the patient started to cry. "I didn't really want to come here," she said, undoubtedly recognizing that for some patients the sub-acute care unit is the last step before a nursing home. Roberts consoled her just enough to get the tears to stop, but then had to move on. A patient Kwame liked very much became angry when Kwame would not let him shower alone. Kwame knew the patient dearly wanted to take a leisurely, hot shower, but he could not do so unsupervised. How much time could he possibly give someone when he had eight patients to care for, Kwame asked me rhetorically. Steve, who spoke eloquently about the rewards of providing care and listening to patients at the beginning of this chapter, also noted that he could do this in only two or three minutes—a sign both of how much basic human courtesy is missing in many health care settings and how little patients and health care providers have come to expect.

The core of what nursing assistants are supposed to do is provide care. Indeed, everyone who works in a health care setting, even unit clerks and security officers, face the emotional and physical needs of patients every day. No matter how many technical or clinical tasks nursing assistants are required to do, the most consistent part of their job is that they have to physically and emotionally manage people. It is the part of the job for which they receive the least training and the least respect. The labor associated with caregiving is invisible—not reflected in job descriptions, supported by administrators, taught in training, or rewarded in pay.

Getting Out

When I spoke to Winsome, the nursing assistant from Jamaica, she was visibly stressed and tired. She was enrolled in the same GED-prep program Veronica had completed, and we met in an empty classroom at 1199's midtown Manhattan training center during the brief break between her day shift at a hospital and her evening class. Describing her managers and bosses, she said, "It's like their patients are special, but you the worker are not really special. Why do you think this place [the 1199 training center] is full of nurses' assistants trying to get elsewhere?"

Because of all the problems cited above, many allied health care workers I spoke to were hoping to move up or out of their current positions; they were taking classes part-time for a new degree or credential, or planning to do so. Hallway talk frequently turned to the question of which were the most promising health care occupations, in terms of the balance among pay, working conditions, and the credentials needed to gain entry. Facing workplace dangers, understaffing, a lack of resources, inadequate wages, and simple disrespect, many health care workers decided they "had to get out." A common exit strategy, particularly for nursing assistants, was to try to enter one of the many proliferating technical or paraprofessional occupations in health care. Although these occupations were still in health care settings, with its dangers and stresses, it was practically impossible to leave health care altogether since health care provides many of the best jobs in the sub-baccalaureate labor market. So, the allied health care workers I interviewed sought new positions in units or settings that they thought might be less stressful, give them more autonomy, or make them feel more valued and—hopefully—pay more.

Cesar, Linda, and Daniel became operating room technicians (known as "OR techs" or "surg techs"), assistants in the operating room who, among other responsibilities, clean and sterilize instruments, prepare particular instruments according to the type of surgery and surgeon's preferences, maintain a "sterile field" throughout the procedure, pass instruments to the surgeons, suction the surgical field, or cut suture materials or apply dressings as directed by the surgeon. Though the preparation for the occupation is not standardized, OR techs typically go through one year of training (six months didactic, six months clinical), for which they obtain a certificate and then can opt to take a credentialing exam. Most OR tech training programs are not for college credit, and college is not a prerequisite for the program. OR tech responsibilities are tasks once performed by nurses and even physicians.

Steve was studying to become a physician assistant (PA), a program that typically entails twenty-five to twenty-seven months of school. Most PA programs require two years of college for admittance, including specific science courses, and clinical experience. Many programs now require a bachelor's degree. Like advanced practice nurses (nurse practitioners), PAs in most states can prescribe medications and perform a range of clinical duties, but they work explicitly under the license of a supervising physician. In one subacute care facility I observed, the PA was the glue that held the place together. Physicians rotated through the floor for only brief periods of time, and most changes to medication or treatment orders requested by the nursing staff were handled by the full-time PA. While in school, Steve was working in another paraprofessional occupation, as a respiratory therapist, who installs and monitors breathing treatments—ventilators, oxygen tanks—and can also develop care plans for patients with respiratory problems. Steve expected to make at least $70,000 a year as a PA.[20]

Juan had completed his training to work as a physical therapy assistant (PTA), and Grace was about to complete hers. PTAs are typically trained in specialized associate's degree programs at community colleges. In 2001 in the New York metropolitan area, their average hourly wage was $20.48.[21] Juan maintained his full-time job as a registrar while he worked overtime and per diem as a PTA to supplement his income. He said he was paid $27 an hour to work as a PTA for a health care staffing agency, and reckoned if he did that full-time he could bring in over $50,000 a year. The staffing agency, however, provided no benefits and did not deduct taxes from his earnings.

Shirley, like Juan, had recently been "upgraded" from the position of unit clerk to a new "multiskilled" position as a registrar and was actively seeking a credential in the high-demand (given the irrational way health care is financed in the United States), though poorly defined, field of hospital coding and billing—an area to which she was exposed when the hospital initially required registrars to take over some basic billing and coding tasks. Patrice, Isabel, and Milagros were in school to become nuclear medicine technologists (NMTs). NMTs, who administer radioactive drugs and use a camera to monitor the tissues and organs in which the drugs localize, are typically trained in one-year programs, which are in some cases integrated with an associate's or bachelor's degree program. A math teacher at a CUNY two-year college encouraged Patrice to consider the NMT program when he saw she had changed her major three times. "If my professor hadn't said nuclear medicine I would have never known something like this existed," she said.

Michelle and Elena were working as ophthalmic medical technologists, who may assist ophthalmologists with a fairly open-ended range of tasks—performing diagnostic tests, obtaining medical histories, instructing patients, maintaining surgical instruments, and assisting with ophthalmic surgery. Unlike some other allied health care occupations, there is a hierarchy among a number of occupations that assist ophthalmologists: from assistant, to technician, to technologist, with the last usually requiring two years of schooling.

Some people were interested in these occupations because the anticipated wages were good in relation to the required investment in training
and education and in comparison to other options in the sub-baccalaureate
labor market. Daniel, who was an instructor at a hospital-based surgical
technician training program, said OR techs in New York City could expect to start at between $37,000 and $41,000 a year after completing the
one-year certificate. "It's awesome, awesome," he said. "I tell the guys [his
students], you don't know how lucky you are! One year you're going to
come out of here and making that kind of money. I'd be doing back flips if
that was the case. There's people out there with master's degrees in social
work who are making $20,000 a year." Indeed, the OR tech program had
one of the best starting salaries in relation to initial training of the various
programs in which people were enrolled. Linda, however, said she was
making only $28,000 a year to start as an OR tech at her Bronx hospital—
less money than she had been making as a security officer because in the
latter job she could work overtime. And like many of these occupations,
the OR tech is not the first step in a career ladder; there are collectively
bargained wage increases, but little chance of promotion or advancement
without returning to school for a new credential.

Sometimes, the workers I interviewed did not know exactly what they
could expect to be paid from the job for which they were training. This
indicated both that the quality of counseling and information they received
was poor and that their desire to do something—anything other than what
they were doing—meant that money was not their central concern. Possibly they also found it necessary to proceed on the basis of hope rather than
face the breadth of irrationalities and uncertainties in the labor market.
Isabel said her brother, a doctor in Texas, told her nuclear medicine technologists make $100,000 a year in San Antonio. Milagros, her classmate,
said their instructor promised she could expect to make about $70,000 a
year. Patrice was under the impression she would make about $40,000 a
year in New York City. Patrice had the most realistic view: In 1998, the annual starting salary of a nuclear medicine technologist in a New York City
hospital ranged from $29,250 to $46,490.[22]

The most obvious route into the working class in health care would seem
to be to become a registered nurse (RN)—they make a livable wage and
there is a great demand for them. In 2005, the *New York Times* featured on
its website the picture of an African American woman above the headline

"Angela Whitaker's Climb"—enough information to correctly guess that Angela had become an RN and that she had once been on public assistance.[23] But becoming an RN, as the article made clear, by no means guarantees security: nurses have relatively high salaries, but they have stagnated. Real wages for RNs (adjusted for inflation) were identical in 2000 and 1990.[24] Working conditions are grueling and in many places deteriorating. Unless RNs have a bachelor's or master's degree, their opportunities for upward mobility in their careers are also limited. It is also still largely considered feminine work: Almost 95 percent of RNs nationally are women.[25]

Though many nursing assistants and some unit clerks I interviewed hoped to become RNs (often seeing the LPN position as an intermediary step), many others—after working alongside nurses—did not see this as a promising career path. Some of their perceptions of nursing work support the argument that the nursing shortage is, at bottom, due to problems with working conditions. Marie, who "always wanted to be a nurse," said she had doubts about becoming a nurse because she felt they take a lot of verbal abuse from their superiors. She had also watched the nurses she worked with grow disillusioned because of their dissatisfaction with the treatment of patients and problems with staffing levels. After spending time as a volunteer at a hospital, Isabel felt that nurses were a "slave" to the doctor. She hoped as a nuclear medicine technologist she would have more independence. Isabel was also concerned about the sheer physical work involved in nursing, through moving and lifting patients. Michelle, an ophthalmic technician, saw the "whole divide between doctors and nurses" as a disincentive to enter the profession. Steve, in school to be a PA, felt that nurses (except nurse practitioners) didn't have the kind of autonomy to make diagnosis and treatment decisions he might as a PA. "The nurses...take orders from a doctor and then from there they just dispense [medications], instead of actually diagnosing and treating," he said. Shirley said she wanted to be a nurse "until I started with working nurses...I found out they do more paper care than patient care." Like Shirley, I had also observed nurses spending what seemed to be the bulk of their shifts—and more—sitting at the nursing station writing in patient charts or filling out data forms.

Finally, some people I interviewed, especially those who had worked as nursing assistants, had a negative view of nursing because they felt that many nurses treated them with disrespect or refused to come out of their own job descriptions to help them, especially with bodily care. Ms. Fink, a nursing assistant in a subacute care unit, said that nursing assistants, not the nurses, assess a patient's skin integrity when they are admitted because they are the ones who "roll" patients to clean their whole bodies (that is, their behinds). "When are nurses ever going to roll them?" Ms. Fink asked rhetorically. After Veronica said that as a nursing assistant, "you get treated as if you're nobody," she added, "especially by the nurses." When pressed to name a concrete goal for going to school, Veronica said she wanted to get an associate's degree in nursing, but her feelings about the profession were ambivalent. For some nursing assistants, working with nurses had raised questions about the values and perspectives of the profession.

This brief survey of what these workers hoped to do suggests some of the challenges to creating a career—if by that we mean an occupational trajectory that offers increased opportunities for autonomy, respect, and better wages—in the health care labor market. Many jobs do not themselves prepare workers for a better job; every job change in health care requires training and a new credential, taking courses and classes that do not necessarily build toward a degree or even provide college credit. These problems are examined more closely in chapter 6.

Instead of improving their working conditions and valuing the work that allied health care workers do, unions and employers in New York City have made continuing participation in supplemental education and training a necessary condition of getting ahead—or, in many cases, of merely getting by. As Shoshanna Zuboff has said, "learning has become a new kind of labor."[26] And training and education programs have been positioned not only as a way for health care workers to move into better jobs—in which presumably they will find the respect and meaning they seek—but also as a response to problems with how health care is delivered and work organized. As I will show, training and education are inadequate responses to all of these problems. This raises the question of why has so much been invested in creating new training and education programs rather than directly wrestling with the larger organizational, structural, and political factors shaping health care work. To answer that question, it is necessary to understand the political context that made New York's health workforce training and education industry possible.

2

Restructuring the New York Way

In the mid-1990s, health policy analysts proclaimed the U.S. hospital was an "institution...being shaken at its core foundations." An influential 1995 report by the Pew Health Professions Commission predicted the closure of "as many as half of the nation's hospitals and loss of perhaps 60% of hospital beds" and the "massive expansion of primary care in ambulatory and community settings." Surviving hospitals would be those that merged with other hospitals or health systems and expanded into non–acute care services such as home care and outpatient clinics. The health policy analysts saw a silver lining, suggesting that amid the rubble, competition and restructuring would forge a new breed of hospital, capable of providing an "integrated, clinical continuum of care" and "cost, quality, and outcome data for purposes of accountability" never before possible. The Pew Commission recommended hospitals "rightsize" the workforce and predicted a looming *surplus* of 100,000 to 150,000 physicians and 200,000 to 300,000 nurses. It advocated the "consolidation of many of the over 200 allied health professions into multi-skilled professionals" and the "fundamental alteration of the health professional schools."[1] Such predictions were grounded in the assumption that managed care would play an increasing role in U.S. health care, and, less probably, that it would produce radical changes in the health care system.

Classic fee-for-service insurance, now nearly moribund, pays for health care services on an arm's-length, indemnity basis and plays little role in shaping how health care services are delivered. Managed care plans, by contrast, play roles in both the financing and delivery of services. They attempt to reduce the gap between how care is delivered and how it is paid for, through tactics such as limiting patient access to physicians and hospitals contracted with the health plan, controlling access to specialists through primary care physicians, making providers share in the financial risk of caring for patients, and reviewing physicians' clinical decisions. Some of the first managed care plans were health maintenance organizations (HMOs), which often employ medical staff directly, own their own clinics and hospitals, and were conceived as more effective ways of regulating health care services and limiting the professional power and market forces that foster costly, high-tech care at the expense of more basic and essential preventive services. Today, however, many managed care plans have been reduced largely to vehicles for cutting costs, limiting access to care, and introducing greater competition and market mechanisms into the health care system.

A comprehensive study of health care in the San Francisco Bay area showed that "the era of managerial control and market mechanisms" began there in 1983, when the federal Medicare program, the single largest payer for health care services in the United States, adopted a defining feature of managed care health plans—it began to pay hospitals flat rates for treating patients based on their diagnosis, rather than the services they actually used. By the mid-1990s, in New York too, "general business ideologies and practices—for example, an emphasis on product lines, cost centers, and strategic planning" became "widely accepted as normal ways of thinking about conducting healthcare."[2] In 1994 employer health care costs declined for the first time in a decade,[3] a decline many assumed was a result of managed care and market forces.

Therefore, when Governor George Pataki, a Republican devoted to cutting budgets and taxes, took office in January 1995, he quickly took steps to accelerate the expansion of managed care and market mechanisms in

New York's health care sector. The two main reforms he initiated were the deregulation of payment rates to hospitals and the mandatory enrollment of Medicaid recipients—the government health care program for the indigent and poor—into managed care plans, which would manage and coordinate care and be reimbursed by the state. In terms of deregulation, the New York State legislature passed the Health Care Reform Act (HCRA) in 1996, which ended state-regulated rate-setting for hospitals beginning in 1997 and thereby required hospitals to bargain with insurers, including the growing number of commercial managed care plans, for payment rates instead. This, it was hoped, would force hospitals to compete for favorable contracts with insurers and restructure their operations to provide the best services at the lowest cost.

In terms of the Medicaid program, the largest single expenditure in the state budget, the general expectation was that managed care would generate substantial savings by reducing the state's administrative costs and by entrusting patients to health plans with expertise in providing the most cost-effective care and the muscle to force health providers and organizations to reform their services. It was hoped managed care plans, which in theory emphasize the use of primary care physicians, ambulatory clinics, and preventive health care programs, would curtail the overuse and misuse of the most costly and scarce medical resources as well as redirect the health care system's resources away from acute care. For instance, many New Yorkers use costly hospital emergency rooms as their first point of contact with the health care system, even for non-emergencies. It was expected that managed care plans would create more appropriate "medical homes" for patients, such as in doctor's offices and clinics, and give them access to providers who normally did not serve Medicaid patients. Furthermore, the Medicaid program traditionally reimbursed providers by paying a fee for every service they provided, while managed care plans would reimburse providers at prenegotiated flat rates per patient or diagnosis, so that providers would no longer have an incentive to provide as many services as possible. Because Medicaid is the largest source of payments for many New York City hospitals, this change in financing mechanisms alone was expected to have widespread effects on the way care was delivered.[4]

Medicaid, created with Medicare by the 1965 Social Security Act, is jointly administered and financed by the federal government and individual states. Under 1991 legislation, Medicaid recipients in New York had already been encouraged to voluntarily enroll in managed care plans, and although less than a fifth of those eligible for Medicaid had done so by 1995, the experiment was deemed—on the basis of little evidence—a success. In 1995, Pataki initiated talks with the federal government to allow the state to make enrollment in managed care plans mandatory. New York City's newly elected Republican mayor, Rudolph Giuliani, who saw savings to the Medicaid program potentially generated by managed care as a quick source of funds to cover the city's 1994 budget shortfall, also supported the governor's efforts to dramatically expand the Medicaid managed care program.[5] In July 1997, the federal government gave the state permission—a waiver—to make enrollment in managed care plans mandatory for 2.4 million of the state's 3.1 million Medicaid recipients, as it had already done in twelve other states.[6]

Hospital leaders and administrators in New York claimed that such policy changes required drastic action at the organizational level, and turned to then-popular managerial theories such as "reengineering" and "restructuring" for guidance. Reengineering was an adaptation of private-sector strategies, and restructuring, which emphasized "patient-focused care," was attributed to Lakeland Regional Medical Center in Florida and private consultants from the firm Booz Allen Hamilton.[7] The terms were not always used clearly or distinctly, however, and their associated reforms often blurred in practice. For instance, when Mount Sinai hospital in New York City undertook a "reengineering" initiative, team leaders took a fieldtrip to Lakeland Regional Medical Center.[8]

The influence of such theories was not limited to the United States; health care restructuring became a widespread phenomenon in the health systems of Canada and Western Europe as well.[9] Not only had the political climate made such managerial theories more acceptable, it had also reinvigorated a faction of health care policy makers and administrators who felt health care organizations should be operated more like profit-driven businesses. The pro-market and pro-business messages were especially influential when they came from the Joint Commission on the Accreditation of Healthcare Organizations (JCAHO), which accredits hospitals and, in the 1990s, rewarded those who appeared to be introducing changes consistent with total quality management (TQM) and continuous quality improvement (CQI) processes, adapted from Japanese automobile companies. JCAHO mandated that by 1994 all hospitals must have in place a

CQI program.[10] In the mid-1990s, analogies between health care and business therefore became ubiquitous in New York City, and one could not talk to an administrator or read a health services trade journal without encountering terms like process, teamwork, customer service, and value-added. Such managerial theories enabled hospital administrators to appear invested in meaningful change, while largely proving to be a pretext for cost-cutting measures that they had probably long wanted to implement but for which there had never been such an ideal economic and political environment. Hospitals in New York City immediately began to threaten layoffs—beginning with nurses. In 1996, a *New York Times* headline read: "Once in big demand, nurses are targets for hospital cuts."[11]

At the same time that hospital administrators were talking the language of reforms and even implementing some of them, they fought with considerable success to maintain their privileged position in the health care sector, with key support from 1199. Under both HCRA and Medicaid managed care reforms, hospitals joined with 1199 to persuade lawmakers to secure important concessions. In terms of HCRA, the state had historically set payment rates high enough to compensate hospitals for services for which they could not bill health insurers and other payers, such as training physicians and providing so-called charity care to the uninsured. As a result of 1199 and hospital lobbying, the legislation therefore established several pools of money external to the state's budget for such services, funded through taxes on insurers and some health care services, including a new permanent fund of more than $1 billion a year for graduate medical education and an expansion of an existing pool to cover charity care.[12] In terms of the Medicaid managed care program, as a result of negotiations between union president Dennis Rivera, president of the Greater New York Hospital Association (GNYHA) Kenneth Raske, and then vice president Al Gore, the federal government agreed to provide $1.25 billion dollars in "transitional aid" to help hospitals and workers implement the changes market forces would ostensibly require, funded from anticipated savings generated by the program.[13] This aid, called in unwieldy bureaucratic fashion the Community Health Care Conversion Demonstration Project (CHCCDP), was largely intended to finance "infrastructure" reforms, especially the expansion of primary care services and what was vaguely termed "managed care readiness." 1199 lobbied for this money to go entirely to voluntary hospitals (where its members worked), but after facing considerable criticism, consented to making CHCCDP funds available to the city's public hospital system, the Health and Hospitals Corporation (HHC).[14] According to the final terms of the deal, hospitals would be eligible for the aid only if 20 percent or more of their annual admissions were Medicaid, self-pay[15] (i.e., uninsured), or indigent patients, and the amount of aid was to be pro-rated according to the percent of admissions from these patients.

These set-asides were also the foundation of a publicly funded health workforce training industry. Voluntary hospitals in New York City agreed—at Rivera's request—that at least a quarter of the federal waiver grant money, about $300 million, would be used specifically for health care workforce training.[16] In addition, HCRA established a pool of over $100 million in new funds for worker retraining, known as the Health Care Worker Retraining Initiative (HWRI), which was expanded by renewals of the legislation in 2000 and 2002. By 2005, total HWRI grants reached close to $500 million. Furthermore, these programs supplemented several other types of grants for health care workforce training programs. The state continued its already existing Rate Adjustment Program, which provided increased Medicaid reimbursement rates to private hospitals that used the extra funds to recruit and retrain nonsupervisory health care workers—totaling $82.5 million in grants from 1996 to 2005.[17] From about 2001–2004 the state also provided over $100 million dollars in health care workforce training grants to target individuals receiving Temporary Assistance to Needy Families (TANF), the federal welfare program, to expedite the reduction of state welfare rolls by moving recipients into health care jobs.[18] The workforce system in New York also included a number of other federal and state programs, such as the Workforce Investment Act, which did not focus solely on health care but often funded training for health occupations.[19]

Though it is impossible to describe and assess all of the programs funded by these training grants—in part because the information simply is not available to do so—I will argue the bulk of the training programs have not touched those problems in health care that have the greatest impact on working conditions, the lives of health care workers, and the quality of patient care. Moreover, the faith that the introduction of competition and market-based negotiations would revolutionize the health care system, or even make it less costly (access and quality arguably never drove the policy agenda), was never well-founded. The "reforms" to which training programs were supposedly a response never took the comprehensive and radical character many expected.

There certainly have been some significant changes in the way health care is delivered in the United States in the era of managerial control and market mechanisms. The number of hospitals in the United States fell gradually but steadily between 1980 and 2003, as did the number of hospital beds. These declines were associated with a decrease in inpatient utilization, particularly in the length of stay in hospitals.[20] Hospitals have also expanded into nonacute services. By 2003, 64 percent of hospitals offered home health services, 45 percent offered skilled nursing facility services, and 57 percent offered hospice care. The number of outpatient surgeries performed increased sixfold from 1980 to 2003, and the rate of outpatient visits doubled. In 1980, outpatient revenues accounted for only 13 percent of hospital gross revenues, by 2003 they accounted for 35 percent.[21] National health expenditures likewise shifted away from hospital care and toward services such as outpatient care, long-term care, and prescription drugs.[22]

These national trends were evident in New York State, where the number of hospital beds per 1,000 persons declined in the 1990s, as did the average length of stay in hospitals. Some hospitals in New York used the federal waiver (CHCCDP) infrastructure grants to set up outpatient clinics, a reform sought not only by managed care enthusiasts but also by community health advocates. But beyond that, the extent to which New York's health care system was reformed is highly debatable—even the effect of primary care clinics has been arguably limited. New York continues to have a much higher than average number of hospital beds and a much longer than average length of stay than hospitals nationally.[23] In addition, managed care never achieved the same market penetration in New York State as in other places. The percent of the state's population enrolled in HMOs declined from 34 percent to 27.1 percent between 2000 and 2004, while in California, which has the highest HMO enrollment rate in the nation, the percent declined from 54.1 percent to 47.8 percent. In the New York City metropolitan area, the estimated HMO penetration is even lower, estimated at 27.6 percent in 2002.[24] New York City's health care sector is also unusual because it is dominated by large, academic medical centers that draw patients and doctors-in-training from around the world; inpatient revenues there still accounted for 77 percent of total patient revenues in 1999.[25]

One heavily reported result of the new policy environment was a flurry of hospital mergers beginning in 1997. By 2002, three-quarters of the city's forty-two private hospitals had joined one of four "networks," each centered on one or two major teaching hospitals. Although these so-called mergers reportedly produced some administrative savings (though no data to prove this was made available), they were mostly "hastily arranged marriages of convenience driven by the need to strengthen bargaining leverage against insurers, increase market share, and achieve modest cost reductions." Moreover, "other goals such as clinical integration and elimination of excess capacity were considered off limits because of the power of hospital medical leadership, boards of trustees, unions, and other special-interest groups."[26] Such mergers did little to create an integrated, clinical continuum of care promised by managed care. In addition, few hospitals closed, despite the Pew report's predictions. Only seven small hospitals closed in the boroughs of New York City between 1996 and 2003, of which only three had over 100 beds (none had over 300).[27]

National aggregate employment figures from the period also show that workforce downsizing never occurred in health care to the extent predicted. Restructuring did entail selected layoffs and a significant reshuffling of the division of labor in hospitals, which negatively affected morale and patient care (examined more closely below and in chapter 4). Nonetheless, the number of full-time equivalent employees working in hospitals nationally grew between 1980 and 2003, even during the 1990s when massive layoffs were predicted.[28] When examining the number of employees per patient admission, the number of people working in hospitals changed very little from 1980 to 2003 nationwide. Currently, the number of full-time equivalent employees per patient are about the same as they were in 1980.[29] In New York City, total employment in hospitals did decline by 5 percent between 1990 and 2000, but all of this decrease occurred in public hospitals. Employment at voluntary hospitals, in which 1199 represents most paraprofessional workers, increased slightly. Employment in other health care settings, such as offices, clinics, and home health care grew much more rapidly, but hospitals still employed 52 percent of all health care employees in New York City in 2000.[30]

Policy analysts' predictions of (or better, wishes for) seismic change were rooted in the recognition of actual inefficiencies, irrationalities, and waste in the health care system. However, they failed to make a realistic accounting of the fragmentation of the health care system, the *realpolitik* of health care policy, and the inherent limitations of market-based reforms when it comes to a public good like health care. Less understandably, they failed to account for changes in demographics (a rapidly aging population) and historical trends that have shown nothing but a consistent escalation in demands for health care.[31]

Inducing change in a fragmented system of public and private payers, all of whom seek to impose different financial incentives and rules on a diverse range of public and private providers, requires larger-scale action and planning than merely offering a few carrots for greater competition. In 2003, a multiyear assessment of New York's Medicaid managed care program concluded tepidly, "the premise of managed care—that new financial incentives would bring fundamental change to the delivery system—has been difficult to achieve."[32] Perhaps indicative that these reforms were guided by ideology more than concern for patients, the Medicaid managed care program tracks little to no data on members' use of services or the type of contact they have with the health care system—a substantial barrier to assessing the success or failure of the program. Nonetheless, the limited data available suggests that Medicaid recipients in managed care plans were no less likely to use the emergency room as their first point of contact with the medical system.[33] It is more definitively known that the Medicaid managed care program failed to create an "integrated, clinical continuum of care for a defined population" and a "medical home" for recipients, through which they would have access to a primary care provider and continuity in their contacts with the health care system. Medicaid eligibility is often episodic and short-term, so that managed care plans understandably have difficulty sustaining contact with members, and the continual turnover of enrollees entails more paperwork and administrative steps. The biggest barrier to this continuity, however, has to do with how Medicaid and welfare eligibility are handled in New York: Welfare recipients are often discouraged from claiming benefits, including Medicaid, and there are no computer systems to continue coverage for those who are dropped from the cash-benefits welfare program but nonetheless remain Medicaid eligible—such individuals were involuntarily disenrolled from their Medicaid plan.[34] The state's fragmented bureaucracy for administering Medicaid and minimal reporting requirements also means its ability to influence managed care plans in the program is limited. The state has similarly been reluctant to regulate providers such as doctors and hospitals. It has yet to release promised data allowing consumers to compare the quality of hospitals, for instance.

Nonetheless, even if there existed the political will and capacity to more effectively regulate and monitor health plans and providers, individual managed care plans in turn have a limited ability to impact the behavior of providers. Even if all Medicaid recipients were enrolled in managed care plans, any plan's Medicaid members would still be a minority of the patients with whom any given provider interacted. It is difficult for individual plans representing only a few of a provider's patients to demand that providers change their behavior (becoming more oriented toward prevention, for instance), or that they supply plans with detailed data on their practices, or compete with one another to better serve plan members. If the entire U.S. population was covered by managed care plans, they would still—as fragmented, individual plans competing with one another—be in a poor position to create wholesale change in the health care system. Managed care plans in New York City also have to contend with a rotating workforce of physicians-in-training in hospitals, so that they cannot build long-term relationships with many providers there. Competition for Medicaid patients among managed care plans has, in sum, failed to produce both a continuum of care and the "cost, quality, and outcome data" for accountability that even community and patient-advocacy groups thought might be a benefit of the reforms, regardless of their skepticism of the effectiveness of competition in health care.

Pro-market policy analysts are likely to attribute the failures of such reforms to program adjustments that served politically influential special interests and often contradicted and undermined the principles of competition. Indeed, a number of mechanisms, in addition to the federal and state set-asides and aid, were created to protect acute care hospitals, in particular, from the effects of competition. As part of the federal waiver negotiations, Rivera and Raske helped to obtain a provision that would favor the assignment of Medicaid patients to provider-sponsored health plans,[35] most of which were "sponsored" by—at least partially owned by—hospitals. In addition, the Pataki administration's draconian bidding process implemented in 1995 for Medicaid contracts caused the major commercial plans in the state to abandon the Medicaid population.[36] As of January 2003, therefore, more than two of every three of the city's Medicaid managed care enrollees were in provider-sponsored plans. Only five of the seventeen plans covering Medicaid enrollees were commercial HMOs.[37]

There are, unsurprisingly, tensions between such managed care plans and their sponsors (hospitals). Research has shown that "safety-net" managed care plans (those formed by sponsors who traditionally serve a high number of Medicaid patients) have attempted to manage and shape the care provided by their sponsoring organizations, for instance by creating disease management programs and using some of the tools of managed care such as reviewing specialty referrals. Most plans have also contracted with physicians and providers that are not affiliated with or owned by their sponsors. Still, the plans' efforts to remain independent can meet resistance from sponsoring providers. The chair of the board in most of these plans is an employee or board member of a sponsoring organization (usually a hospital), and employees or board members of sponsoring organizations control the health plan. Such board members can prevent the health plan from contracting with providers who offer services at a lower cost than sponsor organizations or from negotiating lower reimbursement rates with competing providers (undermining competition over payment rates that was intended to save Medicaid money). Most plans have also found that many techniques for managed care cost more than they save, and they have faced barriers to getting the necessary information from providers for improving the way care is delivered. Sponsoring organizations may also use the plan to direct patients to settings and facilities they control, rather than potentially more appropriate settings, which may be competing clinics or facilities, such as community health centers.[38] A substantial portion of ambulatory care in New York City is in fact delivered through hospital outpatient departments, not community-based clinics and doctors' offices that community advocates argued were more accessible and less costly.[39] (Commercial managed care plans, by contrast, are more likely to rely on clinics and doctors' offices as the initial point of contact for members.) Finally, when patients with Medicaid are required to enroll in managed care plans and most of those plans are sponsored by providers, they do not often have an expanded choice of health care plans, since a provider-sponsored plan may be the only plan that includes the hospital and doctors in their neighborhood. They also do not have access to the wider range of providers that commercial plans might offer. All of this raises questions about the necessity and wisdom of shifting Medicaid recipients into managed care plans.

In any case, a major result of these reforms was that hospitals in New York City are now both health care providers *and* insurers, for better or worse.

In New York, political support for pro-market reform was tempered by the recognition that health care is a major producer of jobs and wealth in the regional and state economy. New York politicians and policy makers have therefore long been tolerant of inefficiencies and irrationalities. The Greater New York Hospital Association estimated that in 1996, the academic medical infrastructure—comprising teaching hospitals, medical schools, graduate medical education in other hospitals, and research funded by the National Institutes of Health—produced 459,000 jobs in the state through direct employment and spending. The majority of those jobs were in the New York City region. Moreover, the academic medical infrastructure spent over $43.13 billion annually in the state, over half of which came from out-of-state sources, such as federal funding.[40] This made health care a primary producer of new revenue in addition to jobs, rather than simply a cost center. Reforms that entail any kind of contraction of health care services and employment are potentially devastating to the region's economy, not to mention the careers of elected officials. Those that predicted massive change to the health care system in the wake of the pro-market reforms underestimated the political and economic value of health care as usual.

In addition, attempts to bring managed care and market mechanisms into New York's health care system, such as those contained in HCRA and the federal waiver programs, became the basis for the expansion of the state's role, and public investment in, health care—albeit channeled through private groups and organizations. This paradox—that the government's periodic efforts to decrease its role in health care and increase that of private markets have only further entrenched it in the financing and delivery of care—has been at the core of health policy since 1965, when the federal government became the largest single purchaser of health care and was drawn into a regulatory role it has tried, in vain, to shed ever since.[41] As we have seen, in New York, "reform" was achieved only on the condition that the state and federal government create various extrabudgetary pools to subsidize the health care system, among them pools to retrain the workforce.

Government regulation and intervention in the health care system is not simply unnecessary interference with market processes, however; it is in many instances necessary to compensate for the gaps and inequities in the private health care market and ensure that services are accessible to the population as a whole. The largest HCRA pools, for "charity care," were an attempt to help hospitals provide care to New Yorkers whom the private and public insurance systems have failed to cover. Elderly and disabled Medicaid recipients were generally excluded from the managed care program because it was feared the greater complexity of care they require could not be provided by managed care plans. (These are also the most costly-to-serve Medicaid recipients, so that the possible impact of managed care on overall Medicaid program costs was limited from the outset.)[42] This policy mirrors the larger system of health care financing as a whole, in which the private insurance market covers the most healthy and least costly Americans and is even permitted to cherry-pick enrollees in many states, while the government is left covering care for everyone else. The most remarkable feature of discourses about the need for markets and competition in health care is their ability to persevere in the face of a growing public role in health care and increasing evidence that markets are an inefficient, costly, and unjust method of allocating health care. Even if Medicaid recipients were enrolled predominantly in commercial managed care plans, there are, as we have seen, real limits to such plans' ability to influence those who provide health care services. The assumption that market-based reforms would introduce efficiencies and reduce the costs of health care—if given the chance to operate without constraints and interference—is dubious at best.

Even though the pro-market reforms at the level of financing and insurance coverage did not create radical change in the way health care services in New York are delivered (by hospitals, physicians, and other providers), some hospitals did embrace organizational reform under the rubric of re-engineering and restructuring. At the prestigious academic medical center Mount Sinai, for instance, reengineering began in 1993, and by 1999, physician and CEO John Rowe estimated that $10 million had been invested in the process. Of that, $1 million went to consultants[43] and $5 million to training.[44] But the major outcome of the hospital's years of reform were a series of highly publicized layoffs—often recommended and legitimized by its consultants. In 1999, Rowe "boasted" that Mount Sinai was one of the lowest-cost major medical centers in New York City, but by the fall of 2001, a year after he left to head the giant insurance company Aetna, the hospital was reporting significant operating losses[45] and the biggest outcome of its once-heralded merger with New York University Medical

Center was $700 million dollars in joint debt.[46] The hospital also endured a public examination of the quality of its care after several patients in its live liver donor program died. A lengthy *New York Times* investigation of Mount Sinai's troubles found there were larger problems at the hospital stemming from repeated staffing cuts. The article reported, "the medical staff is being stretched thin. Physicians say they are working far harder, in some cases for less money; some have left. Morale has suffered badly; patient satisfaction is down." But the article made only one reference to the so-called ancillary personnel who had in fact borne the brunt of layoffs and blame over the years, saying that "layoffs of housekeepers have left parts of the hospital visibly dirtier."[47] The *New York Times* investigators concluded that Mount Sinai's leaders were as responsible for the hospital's problems as external forces such as changes to reimbursements or the burden of providing care to the un- and underinsured.

The hospitals and health care facilities where I spent the most time were not academic medical centers. It might be therefore surmised that the workers I observed were sheltered from some of the more drastic restructuring initiatives, which only more "cutting-edge" institutions may have felt the competitive pressure to adopt. One of the subacute care units I observed was located within an academic medical center, but the subacute care unit was not among its high-prestige services. The hospital in which I was part of the communication skills training evaluation team and which plays a large role in this book was a midsize teaching hospital, but had no affiliated medical school. Nonetheless, the subacute care unit in the academic medical center had created new multiskilled positions in keeping with reengineering practices, and the hospital where I observed communication skills training was the recipient of among the largest grants to train and upgrade hospital workers, since the funding formula for the CHCCDP program favored hospitals with a greater proportion of patients on Medicaid and without health insurance. It also received among the largest federal grants for infrastructure, which it used in part to open satellite clinics throughout its inner-city catchment area, becoming a sort of poster-institution for efforts to shift care away from acute care hospitals and emergency departments into primary care and ambulatory clinics. Such an institution was uniquely able to implement restructuring.

Although hospitals and health care facilities across the city doubtless reacted to the new policy environment differently, the reforms they did undertake were often less drastic than reengineering in theory required, and aimed at their most vulnerable employees. Reengineering reforms at Mount Sinai, like other hospitals, were ultimately about cost cutting. Cost cutting meant laying off staff (or threatening to lay them off as a point of leverage over wages and hours) and cutting corners on materials and supplies. It was a common administrative response to the admonition to become competitive. If the institutions where I carried out fieldwork are not typical, the processes they underwent and pressures they faced were. In New York City, the simultaneous emphasis on reengineering and managed care was debilitating to frontline workers; the former emphasized getting rid of middle managers and laying off staff, while the latter continuously created more paperwork and an increasingly complex administrative environment. The new, multiskilled allied health care workforce therefore had to contend with decreasing resources and increasing responsibilities, most of which took them away from the bedside.

"Reform" exacerbated rather than remedied what were widely recognized as the key problems in health care work: its labor-intensive nature; the fundamental contradiction between the hierarchical division of health care professions and the indivisibility of caregiving to patients; and the social and economic undervaluation of caregiving work. Perhaps this explains why such reforms were so rarely evaluated. A 1998 study of twelve New York City hospitals found that "none of the hospitals is attempting a comprehensive evaluation of the impact of redesign on quality of care and patient outcomes."[48] The problem was not unique to New York. The authors of a study of restructuring in hospitals nationwide commented dryly, "the initial reengineering principles counseled managers to become leaders and leave storekeeping behind. Perhaps this mandate explains the almost complete lack of tracking outcome measurements the authors found with reengineering projects."[49]

A large portion of the training grants in New York went toward soft skills training and multiskilling initiatives, which were largely means of expanding the workload of the least-trained workers and suggesting problems in the workplace could be surmounted with the right attitude. Even when substantial organizational and systemic reform was nonexistent, the *idea* of a revolution, the expectation that fiscal reforms would introduce a marketlike environment in health care, coupled with the availability of substantial training grants to prepare allied health care workers, meant that the ideology of the market and competition played a central role in the training and education programs developed across the city for those workers.

The public discourse of the mid-1990s presented market-based reforms as inevitable and became the basis for a realignment of political and economic actors with an interest in the fate of health care. In that realignment, 1199 consolidated its position as one of the most powerful labor unions in the country. But the consequences of restructuring and reengineering were mostly borne by those in the health care workforce who make up the bulk of 1199's membership, those with the least power and control—nursing and allied health care workers. Training and education became a point at which inordinate pressure was exerted to improve the health care system. It was as if improvements were to start from the bottom, from training allied and paraprofessional health care workers. Other aspects of health care service delivery that needed change—a fractured system of patient care; organizational dysfunction; the disproportional and, from the perspective of medical needs, irrational emphasis on acute care rather than preventive, community-based services—were addressed with much less vigor than the jobs and attitudes of allied health care workers.

3

THE PROMISE OF TRAINING

In a 2002 report on training and workforce development in New York City, the Center for an Urban Future, a public policy group, observed, "accessing training dollars has been a competitive tussle amongst over 150 nonprofits, community colleges, private universities, unions and for-profit trainers."[1] Nowhere were the potential rewards of winning the tussle greater than in health care, in which state officials claimed they had invested nearly $1.3 billion between 1996 and 2005 for training, retraining, and retaining the workforce, including $800 million from the Health Care Reform Act (HCRA) and Community Health Care Conversion Demonstration Project (CHCCDP) programs described in chapter 2.[2] The Center also noted that by the late 1990s, "critics began to charge that training funds were less an engine of economic development for the city than a jobs program for the training industry itself. Often, the data backed them up."[3]

The training funds now support a cottage industry of trainers, educators, and consultants specializing in the health care sector, who make broad promises to justify their role. H*Works Consulting, a group that received major contracts, tells employers on its website that its consultants will avoid the pitfalls of a hospital staff that has not been "enfranchised" and thus "reverts to old habits." Their approach "fosters staff ownership, permanent change and permanent results" and, in deference to the concern with costs above all, a "targeted approach to gaining control of labor costs and creating the workforce to support the future." TechLeaders Consulting, another major contractor, advertises courses in coding and billing, cultural competence and diversity, computer literacy, and "other customized courses all of which will help a company enhance its bottom line."

Neither unions, state health officials, or hospitals have provided an accounting, even schematic, of how the $1.3 billion in health workforce training grants have been spent, let alone a detailed description of the content of training programs under each category and their impact on health care workers and hospitals. The state and federal grants were not accompanied by expectations of meaningful evaluations. The state has released some reports that include very rough categories of spending, the totals allotted to each (with no breakdown by individual institution), and the number of participants who were either targeted by or completed programs, but even those are not available for all of the grant programs.

Nevertheless, it has been possible to assemble enough information to describe scope and emphasis of the training industry as it took shape from 1996 to 2003. In addition to the skeletal reports that are available (from the state, hospitals, and unions), I was able to obtain copies of reports thirty voluntary hospitals filed with the state in the spring 2003 about how they used, or planned to use, the first three installments of CHCCDP training funding.[4] (Those installments—called "cycles"—were released in mid-1999 and early 2001; there is no information at this writing on how the final two cycles of the CHCCDP grants for training, about $120 million of the $300 million total, were spent.) The reports included the titles of training programs, amount spent on each, numbers of participants, and the trainers hired. I have additionally examined state press releases and news and media stories for indications of how these training grants were used. I was also a researcher for an evaluation of a soft skills training program in New York City (the only such evaluation during the period under consideration of which I am aware) and observed several other soft skills training courses. Together with my fieldwork in health care facilities and in-depth interviews conducted with trainers, hospital administrators, and union representatives, as well as with workers themselves, a number of details about the training industry emerge.

At the center of the industry are 1199's labor-management training trusts, which are officially distinct from the union itself and administered jointly by labor and management representatives, but managed on a daily basis by the union. These trusts, known as "Funds," received among the largest federal and state training grants (in addition to their core revenue from collective bargaining agreements). 1199 first negotiated a Training and Upgrading Fund for its workers in 1969, financed by employer contributions as a percentage of gross payroll (today, 0.5%). In its first two decades, the Fund was largely a passive entity, providing limited tuition reimbursement to union members who took university or college courses on their own. In the early 1990s, however, training benefits became a major stake in the collective bargaining process. The 1992 contract with the League of Voluntary Hospitals, the bargaining group representing most New York City private hospitals, established a Job Security Fund to assist laid-off members by providing them with training and placement services and supplemental health and unemployment benefits. A 1994 Memorandum of Agreement, which extended the 1992 contract for three years, established a Planning and Placement Fund to develop labor-management committees, provide employment services, and conduct research on health workforce issues. The Memorandum also combined these two new Funds with the Training and Upgrading Fund into a single entity, the joint labor-management Employment, Training and Job Security Program (ETJSP).[5]

The Funds' revenues quickly expanded well beyond that collected from employers. As mentioned, the CHCCDP grants were allocated in five installments, or "cycles," of 20 percent each, of which three had been released by 2001, when I was conducting my research. Of the $180 million designated to be spent on training and education programs in the first three cycles, over $100 million went to voluntary hospitals (or networks) in the New York City area, in which 1199 members worked. (Over $65 million went to public hospitals in New York City.) Although labor unions could not be direct recipients of CHCCDP grants, 1199 Funds did receive some revenue from them and played a central role in managing and coordinating the grants at New York City voluntary hospitals. In particular, the state required hospitals to have labor union endorsement of their use of the CHCCDP training dollars, and 1199 provided such endorsements only on the condition that hospitals sign a contract making the Training and Upgrading Fund the grants administrator—and therefore the recipient of a percentage of the funds for administrative costs[6]—and that each hospital set up a labor-management committee to determine how funds would be used. In the end, the Training and Upgrading Fund received the CHCCDP training funds from the state and distributed them to the hospitals after submitting the hospitals' work plans to the State for approval. In addition, the Fund coordinated the hospitals' progress reports to the state and maintained a database of universities, colleges, schools, and consulting firms who could run training programs—called "vendors"— organized according to the area of training in which they specialize. To be in this database was essential for any entity breaking into the newly expanded market of training health care workers. The Training and Upgrading Fund even drew up contracts with vendors on the behalf of hospitals. Finally, the Fund also arranged with hospitals to keep any CHCCDP training funds they did not spend for its own training programs. Hospitals and other organizations whose staff were not 1199ers received CHCCDP grants directly.

Under the 1996 and 2000 Health Care Worker Retraining Initiative (HWRI) programs, various joint labor-management Funds of 1199 directly received over $29 million dollars of the $70 million in total grants (released in 1997, 1998, and early 2000). In the same period, public hospitals, the Health and Hospitals Corporation (HHC), received (as a network, rather than by individual hospitals) over $8.4 million,[7] but the public hospital workers' union, DC37, did not receive direct funds and had much less say in how those funds were spent than 1199. Other HWRI grants were provided directly to individual health care organizations outside both the League and HHC, including hospitals, medical centers, health systems, primary care providers, home care agencies, nursing homes, and human services agencies. Grants were also made to some medical schools and nursing schools as well as some trade and industry associations, such as the Greater New York Hospital Foundation, the philanthropic arm of the Greater New York Hospital Association, and the Home Care Council of New York City.

Grant recipients turned to and cultivated a group of specialists and consultants who could advise them how best to use their grants and, above all, serve as contractors to run specific programs. Some grant recipients, particularly large hospitals and 1199 Funds, used internal staff to plan, implement, and even teach training courses, but they also paid contractors, including educational organizations and independent consultants, to do much of the work. The Consortium for Worker Education, a training organization co-established in 1985 by a number of city labor unions, was a central training vendor. In 2004 alone, the Training and Upgrading Fund paid the Consortium over $2 million for training services.[8] Under the 1996 and 2000 HWRI programs, the Consortium was also a grant recipient, receiving close to $6 million dollars. The consultant who taught the communication skills course I describe in chapter 5 was, according to hospital CHCCDP reports, one of the most frequently hired vendors for that type of training.

The availability of funds to train health care workers hastened the entry of cash-strapped colleges and universities into the contract- and vocational-training market. In 2004, the Training and Upgrading Fund contracted training services to the Helene Fuld School of Nursing ($855,052), St. John's University ($332,498), Long Island University ($503,344), and City University of New York (CUNY) colleges including Lehman College ($548,825), Borough of Manhattan Community College ($449,300), and the College of Staten Island ($368,363), among others. In addition, 1199 paid tuition individually for many of its members enrolled in colleges and universities, particularly at CUNY. Some colleges and universities also received direct grants. Under HWRI, private, nonprofit colleges such as Mercy College and Touro College received $776,435 and $1,167,650, respectively; public colleges such as Kingsborough Community College, a CUNY campus, received $224,550.

All of the college and university officials I interviewed for this study said they offered or were developing contract courses, many of which did not provide college credits or degrees. A CUNY dean indicated his college "relies a lot" on contract courses, especially with 1199: "They're programs that have grown." In 2003, close to 24,000 students received skills training at CUNY through direct contracts with employers, including hospitals and other health care facilities.[9] The relationship between CUNY and 1199 is of particular importance for workers in the city's sub-baccalaureate labor market, who are disproportionately people of color, and who rely on the health care sector and 1199 for stable, decent jobs. A 2003 report found that over 45,000 of 1199's members had attended CUNY at some time. 1199 members attending CUNY were furthermore more likely to be women, older, and attending part-time than CUNY students as a whole. In addition, over three-quarters of 1199 members enrolled in CUNY undergraduate programs in 2001–2002 were black or Latino.[10]

In 2002, CUNY cooperated with 1199 to open a center in the Bronx focusing on work-related training. With $3 million in state grants, several stories of a former department store building in the Bronx were turned into a training facility shared by CUNY and 1199.[11] CUNY's half of the space, called "CUNY on the Concourse" draws on the academic and administrative resources of three CUNY colleges in the Bronx (Lehman College, Hostos Community College, and Bronx Community College). It is expected to become a self-supporting fiscal entity, with revenues to be shared by the three colleges. It advertises itself as a one-stop consulting firm, which can design contract courses for businesses in a number of industries, but does not itself offer degrees (students who seek degrees must transfer to a CUNY college).

Because of CUNY's pivotal role in the lives of working New Yorkers, especially those in the sub-baccalaureate labor market, it is important to recognize the extent to which CUNY officials came to see, like their counterparts in the worlds of private, for-profit consulting and education, training health care workers as a new market. As an administrator at one of the colleges affiliated with CUNY on the Concourse remarked, in response to the suggestion that health care workforce dollars were the object of a competitive tussle:

> I'm really trying to do away with the notion of competition and figure out how we can work collaboratively to really corner the health career training market in the Bronx. I don't think about the sense of competition, because we do well and we have good programs and there's more than enough for everybody.

Although he didn't think in terms of competition, this was because there was such a large influx of funds, apparently more than enough for everybody. Nevertheless, he thought of health care training as a "market" and one he could "corner" in collaboration with other CUNY colleges. Cornering the market in the case of CUNY on the Concourse required, quite literally, occupying a high-profile corner of the city landscape. CUNY on the Concourse sits at the intersection of Grand Concourse and Fordham Road, a transportation and commercial hub, where a subway line and several bus lines converge and the flow of traffic and people promises both CUNY and 1199 greater visibility. An official at CUNY on the Concourse drew an analogy between adult education and shopping, describing how the school's location meant it could attract students who just happened by, who would presumably react to a new training or skills program as they would a new pair of shoes in a shop window.

Just half a mile from CUNY on the Concourse is Monroe College, a small, for-profit college that has also stepped into the health career training market. The college targets a slightly different group of "shoppers," with its higher tuition (approximately $6,000 per semester) and degree-granting programs. It is attempting to corner the market in the Bronx for nonclinical allied health care occupations, such as clerical staff in medical offices and health information technicians. It has also branched into contract training. The office of the college's director of health sciences was cluttered with college paraphernalia: posters, stickers, mugs, pennants. "I'm a really aggressive marketer, personally," he said. The college prides itself on a more personal, less bureaucratic approach to its students than CUNY. He too commented on the physical nature of his school as a means of drawing in students: "It is different here. It is a very customer-service type college and things are just much different here. It's clean, every room is white and washed and painted and vacuumed. It's amazing, it's such a pleasure really."

Like hospital administrators under the influence of reengineering gurus, these college administrators adopted an outlook in which the people they serve are consumers shopping for a product, who they can please by offering better customer service and pleasant spaces. In education as in health care, the influence of market forces and privatization, along with the decline in public support, can be readily seen.

But what is being sold? What does this new cadre of health workforce trainers and educators do? The primary rationale for the new training funds was that health care workers lacked the skills that market-driven, efficient health care organizations would require. Governor Pataki's 1997 press release on the first round of HCRA grants said they would "help New York's health care workers adapt and prosper in today's rapidly changing health care industry," mentioning in particular the anticipated shift from inpatient to outpatient care and the growing role of managed care.[12] At least initially, then, the programs on which training grants were spent were always framed in terms of the necessary skills they would provide the workforce in a market-driven health care sector.

Early HWRI funds, those allocated under the original version of HCRA in 1996, were largely spent on multiskilling programs, an idea taken directly from consultants and how-to books advocating reengineering and restructuring. The Training and Upgrading Fund indicated it would spend the $7.3 million it received in 1997 under the HWRI to train 1,833 "patient care associates" in fifteen hospitals.[13] Also known as "patient care technicians" or "nurse techs," these were nursing assistants trained primarily to draw blood (phlebotomy) and perform EKGs, in addition to their regular duties. The network of Catholic Medical Centers in Manhattan likewise spent its HWRI funds to train "300 nurses, phlebotomists, and EKG technicians, who were at risk of losing their jobs, as patient care associates." Another hospital in upstate New York retrained clerical workers as "clerical associates." The 1199 ETJSP received a grant to train 300 employees at risk of losing their jobs as "financial assistants."[14] The Training and Upgrading Fund also earmarked $7.8 million in further HWRI grants, received in the spring of 1998, for the creation of multiskilled positions such as business associates, x-ray support associates, and medical billing and coding associates.[15] A number of hospitals hired the Consortium to train nursing assistants as patient care technicians, and the Consortium also developed programs for operating room technicians (OR techs) and medical assistants. After the nursing shortage became apparent in the late 1990s, training future nurses apparently became a major focus of colleges. Well over half the training grants released under the renewal of HCRA in 2002 were contracted to be spent on training new nurses, both RNs and LPNs.[16]

According to the CHCCDP reports filed by thirty voluntary hospitals, the single largest category of spending under these grants, in terms of dollars spent, was on "soft skills" training: programs in customer service, communication skills, team building, and conflict management. There were reportedly 43,464 training "encounters" in customer service in voluntary and public hospitals in the first CHCCDP cycle alone.[17] A Training and Upgrading Fund internal Executive Directors Report on the use of the first cycle of CHCCDP grants by New York City voluntary hospitals indicated that 21,239 workers "were served" in 207 programs and that the most frequently offered training program was customer service training, offered in nineteen hospitals.[18] According to a Consortium staffer, the Consortium used at least some of its own HWRI grants to train 35,000 workers in the city's public hospitals in customer service, though it subcontracted for the curriculum to a private consulting firm. Indeed, private consultants and firms were the most common vendor for soft skills courses, although some colleges and universities also sought to offer such training. They offered courses in areas such as leadership training, team building, conflict resolution, customer service, communication skills, and cultural diversity. In 2004 alone, the union's Training and Upgrading Fund paid private consultants such as The Training Group (just over $1.2 million), H*Works Consulting ($866,106), TechLeaders Consulting ($483,375), and Stuart Levine and Associates ($448,742), among others.

Another important way health care workforce training grants were spent was on programs to assist individual health care workers improve their skills and education and move into supposedly better jobs, especially in shortage areas. Colleges and universities were usually best suited to offering this type of training, since some of the jobs required credentials and degrees and many required clinical and technical training. CHCCDP grant recipients (mostly hospitals) hired colleges and universities to offer programs, some for college credit but many not, for positions such as pharmacy technicians, respiratory technicians, and radiology technicians. The most commonly funded technician program was for OR techs, which did not entail obtaining a degree and was commonly subcontracted to the Consortium for Worker Education. The Training and Upgrading Fund's internal report stated that fifteen voluntary hospitals created OR tech training programs in the first cycle of CHCCDP funding. Both Cesar and Linda, whom I interviewed for this project, became OR techs, and chapter 6 describes their experiences as well as those of other workers who participated in individual upgrading programs funded by the various grants. 1199 also supported individual workers through tuition assistance programs.

In the next three chapters, I focus on cross-training or multiskilling, soft skills training in areas such as customer service and communication skills, and individual upgrading programs, which were, aside from computer skills, the most heavily funded areas of training. According to the CHCCDP reports filed by thirty voluntary hospitals, the single largest training expenditure was over half a million dollars by one hospital for "computer literacy," also contracted to the Consortium. Unlike the other areas of training examined in this book, in the case of computer skills there was a close connection between the way hospitals were spending the "infrastructure" portion of the CHCCDP grants and the training portion, since much of the infrastructure funds were spent on computers and new billing software. One CUNY college had been hired to train hospital employees in their new billing software program, and even established a direct fiber optic connection to the hospital to do so. The urgency assigned to this area was not surprising—hospitals in the United States (like other providers) find it is often difficult to accurately bill and secure payments in the labyrinth of private and public payers for health care. As TechLeaders Consulting says of its medical coding and billing program, "Rapidly changing health insurance plans and the need to provide current and accurate insurance claims can either invigorate or threaten the existence of your healthcare facility or practice. Having employees who are knowledgeable and up-to-date in providing necessary expertise in medical billing, coding and documentation will insure that claims get paid in full, the first time they are submitted—and that translates into positive cash flow."

People with whom I spoke noted such training was not in general computer skills or conceptual issues that might provide health care workers with the skills for better jobs in other sectors. Rather it focused on narrow issues related to specific software programs. Although such training might have been urgently needed, there is also an underlying irrationality in the fact that much of the federal and state grants were spent on billing systems and training workers to use them. In a health care system with fewer payers and less "competition" for patients, such as in Canada, much less money and time needs to be spent on billing and recouping funds. In the United States, there are different rules that hospitals and physicians must follow for every payer, which can be government programs, private insurers, or individuals.[19] For institutions that are at the same time constantly claiming, with some justification, that government reimbursement rates for the clinical and therapeutic services they provide are inadequate, it should be more disturbing that the government can free up millions of dollars to help them *cope* with inadequate payments and fractured health care coverage by investing in computer systems and software.

As the enumeration of how training funds from 1996 to 2003 were spent suggests, much of the training promised to provide health care workers with the skills that would enable them to survive and thrive in a market-driven health care sector and rapidly shifting labor market. It would create a "workforce to support the future." Consultants in the training industry claimed that the nature of work in health care facilities is that of continual transformation, requiring even the most junior workers to be capable of working autonomously and handling responsibility. Those in the health care workforce training industry did not seem worried that their funding might one day dry up. As an official at the Consortium said:

> There's always going to be a need for training and upgrading and there will be other [training] monies available as time goes on because we understand that the economic development of the workforce depends on constantly being upgraded in order to have any kind of job security. That's the future, really, of employment in this city and in this country, because things are changing so fast. Technology forces people out of jobs and hopefully unions help to direct employers to retain their employees by upgrading and training them.

This claim—that jobs are constantly changing and health care workers must constantly upgrade their skills—is widely taken at face value. It is also a claim repeated by managers and employers in almost every industry and has been a means of shifting responsibility for the declining quality of U.S. jobs onto individual workers for decades. As we will see, a good deal of evidence supports skepticism of this "skills gap" argument, both in terms of health care in New York City but also in the economy as whole. Such evidence also calls into question the Center for an Urban Future's taken-for-granted assumption that training is an engine of economic development. And in any case, since "economic development" has never meant improvements in the living conditions and standards for everyone, my concern is with whether these specific training dollars, and the programs they supported, improved the lives of allied health care workers and the conditions of their work.

The programs I have studied, far from having "permanent results," had little impact on the conditions of health care work that create frustration and a sense of being undervalued among allied health care workers. Much of the most heavily funded training was oriented either toward cutting costs or getting workers to adapt to its effects, even if it did not always achieve those goals. Furthermore, such programs continued to be funded and rarely evaluated even after it became clear the effects of "market" reforms and competition would be less revolutionary than anticipated. The idea of rapid changes in health care due to market forces and a consequent skills-gap retained political and intuitive appeal, but could not be the only rationale for this industry if it was to be sustained. The rationales for this training shifted, so that stakeholders in the industry could continually position the training as important and useful even as the necessity of much of the training was called into question. So, what else did the training industry promise? Moreover, why do those individuals in the training industry—certainly those whose livelihoods depend on it, but also many workers who participate in it—seem to value it so highly, almost in complete disregard for the industry's outcomes, apparent in the almost total lack of evaluations?

One important, alternative rationale that seemed to emerge alongside the industry was that training could address something less tangible and more serious than a lack of skills—the value and meaning gap. Such a rationale positioned training as necessary no matter the state of the health care sector or labor market. As a 2002 report by the American Hospital Association Commission on Workforce for Hospitals and Health Systems, titled "In Our Hands: How Hospital Leaders Can Build a Thriving Workforce," argued, fostering meaningful work is the first key to solving the "workforce crisis" in health care.

> People enter health careers to make a difference in the lives of others. But hospital work is also demanding, hard, and exacting, requiring skill, focus, and attention to detail. As the demands on each caregiver and support workers have increased, the work has become less meaningful and more tedious.[20]

A number of troubling assumptions appear in this comment and report. Nonetheless, it identifies a real issue, one that would become central to the rationale for a training industry—that it might reinvest health care work (and even health care workers' lives) with meaning. Trainers running a wide variety of programs said they hoped to provide workers with self-esteem and validation often denied them. They hoped to reengage and reenergize the health care workforce and produce greater job satisfaction, better attitudes, and enhanced productivity.

Some critics might see such a goal—to provide self-esteem and self-worth—as a rationalization of their programs invented once the need for skills training in response to restructuring became a less plausible justification. After all, if such rationales are accurate, there is potentially no end to the "need" for more training and education. In that way, there is a glaring contradiction between policy makers' stated intention of using training as a means of encouraging a more efficient health care system and the desire of those in the industry to continually expand their role. The goal of any industry is to continually expand its market and the need for its products; the workforce training industry is no different. This puts the industry at odds with state actors' goal of containing costs—both in health care and education. State grants were provided for training programs that would ostensibly prepare workers for specific roles in a leaner, more competitive health care system, yet they have spun off another branch of the health care jobs machine.

Consider the following comment by the administrator at Monroe College, who suggested that the industry is creating a need for itself as much as responding to external demands:

> One of the things that I started doing about two years ago was continuing education…We felt there was a big market for that. Health care is probably one of those industries that no matter what you do, what level of your education, continuing education is so important. So what we started doing initially was just biomedical science, maybe a terminology class, maybe an anatomy class. Then we branched off into coding, into coding and finance classes at hospitals and I guess about six months ago we decided we wanted to hit a new market so we looked at the people who are registrars and we wrote a curriculum for them and I have to actually tell clients "we can't fit you in for another year."

The administrator evoked the need for continual education—"lifelong learning," as it is called by many—and its particular importance in the health care sector. Equally interesting, however, was his suggestion that he does not merely respond to the to the demands of employers and ever-changing jobs, but is "hitting" and creating new "markets," developing curricula that "clients" perhaps never realized they needed.

Nonetheless, the conclusion that workforce dollars are merely a "jobs program for the training industry itself" is quite far from an adequate depiction of this industry and its significance. First, the industry includes an array of programs, which serve different purposes and cannot all be lumped together (although the industry and state have not done themselves any favors by refusing to collect and release quality information on the impact of training programs). Second, the idea that the training programs provide workers with self-esteem touches on real problems with health care work, which individual trainers may indeed be trying to solve even if the structural position of the training industry makes that impossible. Furthermore, and more sociologically, "needs," even if invented to expand a market, can nonetheless be internalized and deeply felt, so that arguing there is no real "need" for this industry, that the premises on which it are built are merely manipulative and false rationalizations, is not only paternalistic but fails to provide an account of this industry that helps us understand it, and, more important, figure out what we can do to make it better. I too am concerned with whether these training programs are useful and effective in very concrete ways, but their persistence suggests that we must also look to them to learn about the changing role of training and education in American life more generally, a role that may be unrelated to the specific outcomes and skills acquired. The role of this training and education industry in the lives of those it employs and serves, as well as in the larger social and political context, is more complicated than either critics or advocates of the industry suggest.

4

Too Skilled to Care

Multiskilling

In 1996, the *New York Times* reported that city hospitals were hiring nursing technicians to do some of the work of registered nurses, including taking temperatures and electrocardiograms (EKGs). Nurses worried "that the technicians, who may have as little as a few weeks of training, are not always up to their new tasks," and 1,500 nurses at Columbia-Presbyterian Medical Center went on a one-day strike in July to protest the changes. Another hospital, St. Luke's-Roosevelt, had reportedly laid off more than 100 nurses in the previous two years and the Greater New York Hospital Association reported a decline of 1,316 nursing jobs, 3 percent of the total, in the New York area from February 1995 to February 1996. In addition, the *Times* reported that St. Luke's had dismissed all of its phlebotomists—specialized technicians who draw blood for tests—as of July 1, and the hospital's remaining nurses were drawing all patient blood.[1] If nurses were drawing blood, however, it was only because the new nursing technicians had not yet been trained to do so. The article identified what would be the single biggest impact of reengineering and restructuring in New York City hospitals: the "multiskilling" of hospital nursing assistants with the aim of laying off more specialized and highly trained personnel.

Issues of cross-training, job redesign, and the emergence of "nurse tech" positions had been mentioned in the pages of 1199's newsletter, *1199 News,* since 1994. The *Times* article, however, revealed that the experiments of a few managers in a few hospitals had become an industrywide trend. Though briefly resistant to and perhaps always skeptical of these types of job redesign, even as early as 1994 Dennis Rivera was telling union members, "we don't have the ability to stop restructuring of the health care industry. It's already well underway." Vice President Debby King agreed, "these changes are happening whether we like it or not."[2] By 1997, 1199 was a partner in the cross-training and multiskilling process, playing the pivotal role in securing training funds that made it possible to implement the process across the industry. In the union's eyes, multiskilling was no longer a management tactic to reduce jobs, but a potential vehicle for saving them. Although the process was thereby standardized and subject to a measure of union oversight, it was a move fraught with contradictions.

In almost all New York City voluntary hospitals, nursing assistants (nursing aides) are now known by the newly created title of patient care technician (PCT). They have also been called patient care associates (PCAs), and many people use the terms interchangeably, although sometimes they refer to slightly different jobs. PCTs continue to do the work they previously did as nursing assistants, most importantly the hands-on care of patients: helping them to eat, giving them baths, dressing them, changing linens, helping them walk and move. But PCTs have been additionally trained to perform EKGs, take and record "vitals" such as blood pressure, respiration, temperature, and blood-sugar levels, and draw blood (phlebotomy). In addition, in voluntary hospitals, nursing assistants became certified as part of the PCT training—a qualification that has been required for nursing assistants in nursing homes by state regulations since the late 1980s, but not in hospitals. New York State requires a minimum of 100 hours of classroom training for the certified nursing assistant (CNA) credential. 1199 was able to negotiate a nominal wage increase for PCTs in voluntary hospitals as part of the new job title. In public hospitals, nursing assistants were cross-trained into two different titles, the patient care associate (PCA), equivalent to the PCT in the private sector, and the PCT, a less-skilled position that allowed nursing assistants only to take vitals and transport patients. In public hospitals, neither title required the nursing assistants to become certified.

There were other types of multiskilling in New York City hospitals as well. One academic medical center in the Bronx created its own version of a patient care associate position by combining tasks that used to be separated between housekeeping, dietary, and nursing departments. The PCAs served food and helped patients eat but also cleaned their rooms, beds, and bathrooms between meals, and unlike traditional housekeepers or dietary aides, remained on a single unit all day. Union officials raised objections to the idea of workers cleaning bathrooms and serving meals, feeling it might raise issues of sanitation and infection, but the process went ahead. Multiskilling experiments also occurred in non-nursing, or non-direct care occupations. In some hospitals, unit clerks were made into "business associates" and trained in a wider array of office and clerical skills. For example, Shirley participated in a program to cross-train some unit clerks in a new computerized billing and admissions system, so that they could work as registrars in the ambulatory care clinics the hospital was opening (the clinics and training were paid for by federal waiver grants). As we saw earlier, some coding and billing tasks were initially "just thrown on" the new registrars as part of the hospital's efforts to fire more costly, specialized coders and devolve the work onto lesser-paid staff. But both the union and the registrars successfully resisted the imposition of coding responsibilities onto registrars. Upon completing the program, Shirley was assigned to the emergency department, for which she received a pay increase—negotiated by the union for the new job title—of about $3 per hour. (She was making about $15 an hour when we spoke.) This trend has been repeated throughout the health care sector. In some cases, the new positions were indeed new—not old positions that had been "multiskilled"—but which nonetheless served the same purpose. For instance, one of the most common training programs was for operating room technicians (OR techs), who were trained to do tasks once carried out by nurses.

Nurses in New York City were obviously concerned that such changes were merely excuses to reduce staffing levels or substitute less educated staff for those who were more educated or highly-trained. Nursing assistants themselves were also concerned. One former training executive from a hospital that received substantial training grants said, "in the beginning," there was "a lot of grumbling" among the staff when the new multiskilling programs for nursing assistants were announced. "There was a lot of feeling, 'oh, it just means the nurse is going to dump on us more,'" she reported.

Their concerns were justified. The former training executive said openly, "the nurses' aides became PCTs and that was a way of downsizing the number of phlebotomists and EKG technicians." PCTs were also used to contain the number of registered nurses (RNs) and shift the latter's work away from patient care. A 1997 survey of twelve New York City hospitals found the majority of those that had restructured their services reduced the number of RNs on general patient care units.[3] One official at the Consortium for Worker Education, which conducted much of the PCT training in New York City, reported having to continually fight hospitals' requests to train nursing assistants in skills, such as inserting catheters, that encroached further into the role of nurses. A DC37 official informed me that PCAs at one public hospital were suctioning tracheotomy wounds, the wisdom of which both union officials and the PCAs questioned. At another private hospital where I conducted fieldwork, PCTs in the maternity ward were conducting hearing tests on newborns, a job they said the nurses used to do and in which they had never been formally trained. Another hospital had nursing assistants doing ventilator care and ambulation, functions that "RNs used to do on the unit."[4]

Public justifications of such work redesign couched them in the terms and principles of restructuring and reengineering theories, which mandated that workers/employees be trained to perform multiple functions— called multiskilling and cross-training by each, respectively. For-profit consultants hired as gurus of reform insisted multiskilling and cross-training were not firstly means of cutting costs but means to improve patient care. J. Philip Lathrop, a self-proclaimed restructuring "proselytizer" and executive with the firm of Booz Allen Hamilton, pointed out in his book that a typical patient had contact with fifty-three different staff members, not including doctors, during a three- or four-day hospital stay, and that only 16 percent of personnel time in hospitals was devoted to the direct care of patients.[5] Cross-training or multiskilling was proposed as a way to reduce occupational specialization and create "patient-centered" care, but also to give workers more breadth of responsibility along with, at least in principle, more autonomy and decision-making power.

Nonetheless, many of the cases of reengineering described by management gurus Michael Hammer and James Champy in their best-selling book were successful in large part because they reduced "head counts"—an image that likens firing workers to sending them to the guillotine. Thus at Ford, reengineering came "close to eliminating the need for an accounts payable department altogether. In some parts of Ford...the head count in accounts payable is now just 5 percent of its former size."[6] Health care administrators must have found the promise of reduced labor costs even more appealing than many corporate CEOs, since labor accounts for over half, on average, of total hospital operating costs.[7]

In 1999, the vice president of reengineering initiatives at Mount Sinai, Patricia Garcia Sullivan, frankly reported, "in the beginning this was not fundamentally a patient-focused or a staff-satisfaction-focused initiative. This was a cost-cutting effort."[8] Despite her suggestion to the contrary, re-engineering never evolved into something else, neither at Mount Sinai nor most New York City hospitals. In a 1999 article about Mount Sinai's reengineering efforts, the director of organizational development said,

> Who is it that gets reengineered? For the most part, it's the lower-level peo-ple. And they perceive it as a hatchet job. It's about cutting the workforce, layoffs. Oh, I've seen people rise to positions that are glorious—people do now have new opportunities! But I think you'll find that overall morale is lower. People are very worried about healthcare these days.[9]

Moreover, Mount Sinai was unable to solve its financial problems by re-ducing headcounts. In the translation from management speak to hospi-tal practice, reengineering and multiskilling efforts undermined the goals of improved patient care, not to mention staff morale. They also had pro-found, and less remarked upon, consequences for the labor market and structures of opportunity for allied health care workers as a whole.

National and regional data on hospital staffing levels from the period show little change, but such aggregate data fail to capture significant shifts in how hospital staff were distributed and their work organized.[10] In terms of nursing, restructuring initiatives, which were widespread in the 1990s, promoted a less professional mix of staffing, in which patient-contact and hands-on care formerly done by RNs was assigned to nursing assistants or vocational nurses.[11] Nursing practice has long been based on hierarchi-cal teams of nurses and assistants, in which each member has specific and delimited responsibilities, called "team nursing." Indeed, many hospitals in the United States have never organized nursing any other way. But in the 1970s and 80s, some hospitals—especially large academic and teaching medical centers—abandoned team nursing and increased the ratio of RNs to less-trained nursing staff, under a model called "primary nursing." A higher proportion of RNs in those settings had bachelor's degrees, and they performed the full range of tasks associated with patient care. RNs in those settings tended to regard their way of work as more professional and safer for patients.[12] The shift was partly driven by economics and the supply of nurses, but for some institutions it was above all an attempt to improve patient care and nurse satisfaction.[13]

For RNs, the kind of nursing practice proposed by restructuring and reengineering in the 1990s was not merely another incarnation of team nursing because it was coupled with the multiskilling of nursing assistants. An article in a hospital administration journal pointed out that under team nursing, a caregiving team typically consisted of one RN, one or two licensed practical nurses (LPNs), and one or two nurse aides. In a reengineered environment, by contrast, the same team might consist of only one RN and one or two nonlicensed, multiskilled caregivers *and/or* LPNs, so that the team was typically less skilled on average and also had fewer people. Such teams were "based on the premise that non-RN caregivers, notably nonlicensed caregivers, can be trained to competently perform some of the tasks previously performed by RNs," with the "primary objective of eliminating unnecessary staffing costs, a form of nonvalue-added activities."[14]

At the level of the specific medical units, or work groups that directly care for patients, then, this change in nursing practice is evidence for the theory of "deskilling"—Harry Braverman's classic assertion that profit-driven organizations always attempt to divide complex work into a series of routine tasks for which the cheapest labor can be hired.[15] The creation of PCTs was not necessarily deskilling at the level of specific occupations: Nursing assistants' skills were ostensibly increased, and those nurses who kept their jobs were perhaps able to shift more routine tasks onto PCTs and, it might be argued, focus on those areas requiring more training and skill. In New York City, nurses in the mid-1990s were taking on new responsibilities related to case management and discharge planning.[16] National surveys of nurses suggested that under reengineered working conditions, the average staff nurse found herself responsible for more managerial and administrative tasks at the unit level—although this took time away from patient care.[17] Nonetheless, it is not indisputable that such administrative duties required more "skills" than direct patient care. Even if such changes did not deskill entire occupations, they raised serious issues for patients at the level of medical care units. As staff nurses became responsible for the increasing amount of paperwork generated by managed care and competition, patients became more dependent on multiskilled nursing assistants for their immediate care, who in turn found they spent as much time doing EKGs and taking "vitals" as providing hands-on care. Nurses, not surprisingly, had grave and legitimate concerns about whether nonlicensed caregivers such as nursing assistants could take over nursing tasks in a competent fashion, as did many nursing assistants themselves. And both groups questioned the idea that nurse contact with patients was a non-value-added activity.

Reengineering and restructuring consultants also advocated the "flattening" of the organization: getting rid of layers of nurse managers and administrators whose oversight functions were supposedly unnecessary to the actual delivery of the "product." The dismantling of senior ranks of nurse administrators was detrimental to morale in the nursing profession because it seemed to confirm the sense among nursing staff and administrators alike that their perspectives on organizational change and patient care counted for little.[18]

The former hospital training executive concluded, "by and large," the nursing assistants "were happy to get the training and happy to get the money." However, the new tasks PCTs took on were supplemental to their other responsibilities. For many, the PCT position seemed a means of broadbanding, of simply expanding their workload rather than giving them the tools to provide better care. Moreover, they felt pressure from the reductions in the number of nurses. Nursing assistants regularly said in interviews that they felt "dumped on" by nurses and disrespected by them. Doubtless increasingly stressed nurses assign as much work as possible to nursing assistants, even if they think it would be preferable and safer to do the work themselves, because of the lack of time and staff. In many hospitals where I conducted fieldwork, units were functioning with barely adequate staffing levels.

Multiskilling and restructuring boosters are quite clear that downsizing is possible only because they promise to squeeze more work out of those who remain. As Hammer and Champy claim in a moment of terminological hair-splitting: "downsizing and restructuring only mean doing less with less. Reengineering, by contrast, means doing *more* with less."[19] For many health care workers, both reengineering and restructuring meant doing more less well.

The consequences of multiskilling were also problematic at the level of the labor market, in addition to that of medical units and individual workloads. Most obviously, the companion to multiskilling some occupations was downsizing others that were better paid and trained. This tendency would seem to support Braverman's central claim that there is a tendency under capitalism toward the deskilling of the workforce as a whole (meaning the economy produces a growing proportion of routine jobs).[20] When, in the mid-90s, nurses were being laid-off and many thought there was a nursing surplus, the PCT position likely encouraged deskilling in the health care labor force, since the proportion of high-skill RNs declined in relation to lower-skill nursing assistant and PCT positions. However, labor market conditions changed swiftly, so that a widespread nursing shortage was evident a few years later. Upgraded PCTs, apparently, could not effectively substitute for nurses nor was the health workforce as a whole large enough to keep up with expanded demand. Therefore, if one analyzed the growth and distribution of occupations within health care in the nursing shortage era, it might not support the theory of deskilling at the level of the health care workforce. However, the data available to make this analysis would also not provide enough detail to warrant firm conclusions. There is no available aggregate data on the division of tasks and roles within health care occupations or by setting. For example, an overall growth in the proportion of nurses does not say much about what those nurses are doing, which can also vary considerably by setting. Furthermore, former staff nurses who are now case managers doing paperwork might be classified as upgraded when in reality their work has been degraded and routinized.

Regardless, 1199's approach—to endorse and even make multiskilling possible through the training funds it secured, while at the same time emphasizing the promise of career ladders in its communication with the rank and file—was paradoxical. The union was facilitating the removal of higher rungs in the health care job ladder while promising increased opportunities for upward mobility. Once the nursing shortage was evident in the late 1990s, nursing of course became a reliable career option for

1199ers. Still, in light of the nursing shortage, the union continued to support the development of other positions that might substitute for them, such as OR techs—positions with less room for mobility and less pay. The union's actions therefore conveyed that it was willing to sacrifice nurses, other higher-skill workers, and perhaps even the quality of care itself, for the benefit of its members.

Still, the benefit was dubious. For instance, some PCTs felt the certificate was a waste because it was not the basis for promotion into other health care occupations, nor did it provide advanced standing in other health career training programs (such as nursing). The certificate might make it easier for them to get work in nursing homes—which in the climate of looming hospital layoffs of the mid-1990s was undoubtedly part of 1199's rationale for folding the CNA certificate into the PCT training. However, such jobs did not pay as well as hospital jobs and would be a distinct step downward. Similarly, the credential is not transferable since hospitals outside of the New York City region do not necessarily have a similar job title.

One instructor who had been teaching 1199 members for years in the Training and Upgrading Fund's general education program, which helps union members prepare for college, reported:

> As part of the federal waiver deal, there's a lot of job training type stuff and a lot of this broad-banding, multiple-job…they all hate it, universally. It's more work, it's not that much more money, and it also doesn't solve, for them, their fundamental—what they can't necessarily articulate, but I think feel very deeply, which is their fundamental problem, which is that they don't have transportable skills. They don't have critical thinking abilities, they don't have developed understandings of the field in a way that would allow them to make good strategic decisions.

To him, becoming a PCT was not a "good strategic decision"—it was not a qualification that enabled a step up in a job ladder or career, which ultimately depended on acquiring a college degree. Furthermore, it was through a college education that workers could acquire truly marketable and life-changing "skills" like critical-thinking abilities. The PCT program was, in a sense, a detour away from these more important aspects of education.[21]

Just as problematic for the long-term position of the workers 1199 represents, multiskilling hastened the process of credential inflation, an increase in the training or credentials required for jobs that is unrelated to changes in the nature of those jobs and the abilities they require.[22] This process was already underway for nursing assistants. In 1970, only 9.1 percent of nursing aides working in New York City's health care industry had some college education; by 1990, 29.1 percent had.[23] Health care facilities favored nursing assistants with greater training and education not because fundamental changes in the nature of the work required them, however, but because of changes in the pool of workers available. Several trends affected the pool of workers for aide jobs in New York City: as unionization initially increased the wages and improved the working conditions of hospital aides in the 1970s, aide positions attracted better-qualified individuals with other options in the labor market. Hospitals also began to recruit nurses trained abroad, not all of whom could pass licensing exams to practice once they arrived. Many of these nurses became aides instead, raising the level of education and training of people in those jobs.[24] This made it possible for health facilities to hire increasingly well-educated aides while feeling little pressure to raise their wages or improve their working conditions. The PCT position continued the upward trend in the requirements for becoming a nursing aide, a trend with larger consequences for the types of workers the union represents. Positions in private hospitals are at the top of the ladder for nursing assistants and they are now increasingly difficult to obtain because nursing assistants must also be CNAs and trained in phlebotomy and EKGs.

Meanwhile, the core work that PCTs do—caring labor—remains the same. The original justification for the investment in health care training programs was that market-based reforms would substantially alter the organization of health care and its labor process, so the existing skills of workers would soon be inadequate. But the PCT position was not the product of significant change in the technological basis or nature of health care work. The new tasks that PCTs do, such as drawing blood or taking EKGs, has long been done in hospitals, just divided differently between occupations.

Moreover, as the bar for entry to the occupation has risen, nursing aides' wages have stagnated. Starting in the 1980s, the wages of nursing aides in comparison to other health care workers declined even as their educational levels increased: At private hospitals, the wage rate of aides in New York City declined from 0.86, in 1980, to 0.72, in 1990, of the income of all health care workers.[25] The stagnation occurred largely because the number of unionized and best-paid aide jobs—those in hospitals—became smaller relative to all aide jobs. In response to rising wage pressure from unions, employers and payers for health care services attempted, whenever possible, to shift the site of care away from hospitals into nonunionized settings, especially home care. Nursing aide jobs, the point of entry to the labor market for many immigrant women in New York City, are today more likely to be in the home care sector, where the wages and stability of hours are worse than in hospitals.[26] The movement toward managed care in the mid-1990s provided further support for their efforts.[27] Increased competition for the declining number of better jobs means there is little pressure for hospitals to raise wages to recruit workers; those raises they have provided, which have not kept pace with increases of pay for health care workers as a whole, have resulted from union pressure, not the increasing skills of the workers or complexity of their jobs. 1199's role in the multiskilling process ensured that at least the PCT position came with a raise.

People who work in health care settings—particularly hospitals—are to an extent an exception to the finding that people who provide caring labor are penalized financially. The appeal of a strategy that inflates credentials is clear: any occupation that can impose social and legal barriers around itself—through licensing, credentialing, unionization, or other practices of "social closure"—will positively impact earnings. Health care occupations are particularly likely to be regulated, with strict licensing and educational requirements, and in New York City these effects are magnified by unionization.[28] Still, the wages of those in such occupations are not a reflection of the value attached to the work they do, and as a long-term strategy for raising wages, social closure tends to increase forms of discrimination in the labor market and the barriers to well-paying jobs.

As Karen Brodkin Sacks' research on efforts to unionize employees of Duke Medical Center (in North Carolina) concluded in the 1980s, she found that many of Duke's paraprofessional service and technical workers had been "upgraded," by being moved into higher grades of their job titles when they obtained new credentials or certificates through formal schooling. Sacks reported that at Duke "there are more advanced everything: nurses, aides, food service workers, and secretaries." For some occupations (in that period, especially nurses), the expansion of "advanced" titles seemed to Sacks to be primarily vehicles to expand the workloads of those upgraded. At Duke, it also served to restrict the opportunities for those who were less able to obtain formal schooling—in essence working-class, mostly black, women who were particularly supportive of unionization and workplace militancy. Sacks concluded,

> These gains [for some workers] are undercut by restrictions on upward and lateral mobility that stem from demands for schooling in place of on-the-job training for many technical and nursing positions, and by the relative, and in some cases absolute, shrinkage of jobs in clerical, services, and technical classifications. The combined effect is to restrict real job and promotion opportunities for working-class people at Duke, even though the number of pay mini-grades and job titles seem to grow like cancer.[29]

1199 has tried to counter the same trends in New York by creating opportunities for more of its workers to access formal schooling (the limits of which are discussed more fully in chapter 6), thereby working to ensure its members can keep up with the credential inflation the union has itself encouraged.

It might seem that the only legitimate claim many workers have for increased wages are increased credentials or training. Endorsing upgrading has not been, however, the union's only strategy to improve the wages of its members. Above all, the union hopes to unionize nursing assistants and aides in the home care and nursing home sectors. If history is any guide, unionization will be essential to temper the increasing polarization of wages in the nursing assistant labor market and make it more difficult for hospitals to use the surfeit of underpaid nursing assistants in the labor market as reason not to raise wages and improve working conditions. Still, the PCT/multiskilling effort reinforced the idea that wage increases are warranted only through increased training and credentials. A preferable, if more difficult, strategy for obtaining wage increases and better working conditions for nursing assistants would focus on the idea that they deserve recognition (and a livable wage) for the work they already do. Nursing assistants (and the patients they care for) could undoubtedly benefit from some kinds of additional training, but a strategy that makes wage increases dependent on increases in "skills" and credentials fails to touch the basic problems that make health care workers undervalued and creates a barrier to a classwide agenda of social justice. A different fight for higher wages and better working conditions would focus on the systematic devaluation of caring labor.

Furthermore, there is reason to believe the new, reengineered division of labor compromises patient care and devalues caring labor. The EKG technicians and phlebotomists who were laid off did not have greater training or credentials than patient care technicians, but they were arguably more adept at their jobs because they practiced specific procedures more consistently. In one unit, I observed a PCT react with trepidation when asked to draw blood on a patient and eventually refuse to do it, protesting that the "three days" of training she had in phlebotomy was inadequate. There is no evidence that nursing assistants do the other, "nontechnical" aspects of their job better now that they have the PCT title and credential, but they are certainly pushed to do more with less. People who are better educated may provide better care, but it is not clear the limited skills training in the PCT upgrade constitutes an education or that better care can be provided at the same time as workloads are increased.[30] The recent nursing crisis would suggest that high workloads defeat the best education.[31] And their new skills largely entailed collecting and recording information—not understanding it. Nurses, by contrast, are taught to interpret many of the tests they carry out. When PCTs provide EKGs and measure other patient vital signs without knowing how to interpret them, another barrier is created between those gathering information about patients and those taking action based on that information; it introduces another opportunity for miscommunication and delay.

The PCT initiative also contributed to the devaluation of hands-on care work in health care settings. Veronica, who was a nursing assistant in a hospital that had not (yet) adopted the PCT job title, was envious:

> Where I work on the orthopedic floor we don't get to take blood pressures—we do temperatures, but we don't get to take blood pressures. We're just there, on that floor, to be like little handmaids, for nothing. Okay, my duties are to bathe the patients in the morning.... You help who needs to be fed, you help them, you open up their trays. You don't get to do technical stuff—you're like a maid.

Still, according to Marie, a PCT at another hospital, this "technical stuff" had become routine. Comparing her new position to being a nursing assistant, she said:

> You know it's pretty good now, it's way better than what I did before so I'm glad. But I'm just tired of doing EKGs and UCGs [urinary chorionic gonadotropin—a urine test]...I'm sick of it. It's boring, it's the same thing all the time, and I just don't want to deal with it anymore...If you're in triage you're testing like 20–25 urines a day. And you're doing vital signs....There's only so much I could do after I check somebody's urine, whether it's positive or negative. Or you know, I do an EKG: I type it in and let the machine do the rest of the work. You know, it's not challenging for me anymore.

The PCT training program suggested to nursing assistants that the way to earn more money and gain status was to have more "technical skills," such as performing EKGs. Yet the new tasks in which most PCTs were trained were routine; they did not entail an increase in autonomy or decision making to accompany their new responsibilities. After experiencing work as a PCT, Marie found that it did not excite or challenge her as she hoped it would. It likewise reinforced the predominant cultural perception that the kind of work that merits a raise and better status is technical work, not caregiving work. When Marie said she liked being a PCT "way better than what I did before" she was, I think, internalizing this devaluation. It was as if she felt obligated to acknowledge that her new job was better because it involved more than those tasks typically dismissed as natural or obvious—caregiving, but also tasks Veronica likened to being a maid. After all, it was Marie who described the satisfaction she gets from caring for others but also said when her neighbors ask her if she's a nurse, she tells them she's a "professional butt cleaner."

Veronica also attested to the rewards of providing hands-on care and interacting with patients. Even though Veronica was not (yet) a PCT, she preferred working in a nursing home to a hospital because in the nursing home she was more involved in patient care and had more autonomy:

> I was more fulfilled in the nursing home because I was doing something, hard work. The only way I wasn't fulfilled was economy-wise, in the nursing home. I was satisfied because I was helping people, but the money wasn't

there. In the hospital, although I get a little more money it's not satisfying at all because you don't feel like you're doing anything.

Veronica's comment suggests that many caregivers would be happy providing care if their working conditions and wages were better. Veronica and Marie both liked to provide care, but they could not help internalizing the idea that such work is not valued or important. The PCT "upgrade" seemed to be a vehicle for obtaining more respect and status, but the core work of nursing assistants remained unchanged and undervalued.

Multiskilling and restructuring initiatives are also based on troubling assumptions about workers themselves. In his book, Lathrop presents the case of an admitting clerk who had been cross-trained to handle a greater array of patient paperwork: "In her new job, she works carefully and well because if she does not, the patients will get hassled by their insurance companies and the hospital business office...She now has control over enough of the patient's paperwork that she herself can assure its accuracy and completeness. Furthermore, she feels an intense personal ownership of the work on the patient's behalf."[32] As if reading from Lathrop's script, Shirley described her new position as a registrar in the emergency department this way:

> With this job we're at the front window for everything that comes in so we really have to try to get the information right. It starts right here....I take it very seriously because if the hospital is going to get paid I have to get that insurance in right, I have to get that billing address right, get that name right. There are a lot of things that you really have to be aware of just getting the patient in initially.

Shirley knows that hospitals have real difficulties getting paid given the number of insurers they have to bill, each with their own rules of payment and coverage, to say nothing of the number of people hospitals serve who have no insurance whatsoever and cannot pay. She knows that her new job was created in order to make sure the hospital gets paid.

It is not difficult, in contrast to Lathrop's suggestion, to get health care workers to take their roles seriously, either toward the hospital or patients. Lathrop implies that such commitment was lacking until the admitting clerk was cross-trained. Shirley, however, expressed a strong commitment to patients and the work of the hospital, quite apart from her new position. She had in fact originally wanted to provide direct care to patients and had completed a CNA course to better care for her dying grandmother. She took a unit clerk position simply because it was available first.

Shirley's enthusiasm for her new job stemmed not from her greater sense of control and ownership of her work, but from the higher wages she received as a registrar and the possibility of mobility she perceived in the field of coding and billing. When registrars were, at first, asked to do coding and billing, she became aware of the tremendous demand in that area. On her own time, Shirley took a medical terminology class offered for free at her hospital because it was a prerequisite for classes to become a certified coder. She then enrolled in an entry-level billing and coding certificate class that met two evenings each week at CUNY's new training center in the Bronx, CUNY on the Concourse, during its first semester of operations. The billing and coding courses had gotten Shirley's "blood boiling." "I want that certificate...I found out I can make $100,000 a year after you get the three certifications."

She was not motivated by an increase in "control" supposedly inherent in her new, multiskilled job; neither as a clerk nor as a registrar does she have the kind of voice and autonomy many health care workers want—a say in how their job is organized, more discretion with their time, and support for making the best decisions for patients. That is a kind of control and autonomy that is granted only when managers and administrators recognize that the vast majority of health care workers take their roles and work seriously. Once she had received the highest level of coding certification, Shirley hoped she might be able to set up her own business and work from home, potentially even moving back to South Carolina, where she was raised. When we met, she was very excited by the possibilities. Shirley spoke genuinely about how much she liked providing care, and at the same time said every training or education program she enrolled in was "for the money." At that point in her life and at her wages, Shirley could not afford altruism.

Hammer and Champy argue that the reengineered workplace is based on "complex jobs for smart people, which raises the bar for entry into the workforce. Few simple, routine, unskilled jobs are to be found in a reengineered environment."[33] In health care, the bar for entry into the workforce has been raised by new, multiskilled job titles, but the nature of the work has not changed, nor in any profound way have the jobs. Arguably no job in health care (or perhaps, anywhere) is "unskilled"—the very categorization of work as "skilled" or "unskilled" typically fails to consider caregiving altogether. Marie suggested reengineering made her work more routine rather than less. Contrary to the vision of Hammer and Champy, multiskilling did not create "complex jobs," if by that they mean jobs requiring more independence and providing more voice and responsibility.

1199 officials, even if privately skeptical of multiskilling and at times resistant to it, publicly asserted that the training would provide workers with improved, more marketable skills and, at the very least, prevent layoffs. The union presented multiskilled positions as an upgrade rather than a mere work speed-up. The fact that Dennis Rivera could be largely credited with obtaining the workforce training money and that the labor-management Training and Upgrading Fund played a large role in administrating the funds potentially gave the union more leverage with the hospitals and a greater say in the reform process. Nonetheless, the former hospital training executive noted, "in effect, a lot of times it was the union and management facing together the worker," trying to persuade them that multiskilling was in their interest.

Did, however, multiskilling save jobs and minimize layoffs in New York City's private hospitals, as 1199 has claimed? This might, after all, compensate for the other troubling and contradictory effects of multiskilling (at least from the perspective of 1199ers). Employment growth in New York City hospitals did indeed slow markedly in the 1990s. From 1995 to 2004, employment in New York City private hospitals grew by only 1 percent, while total health care employment in the city grew by over 8 percent. In New York State, employment in health care as a whole grew by nearly 19 percent between 1990 and 2004 (while employment in all other sectors grew by only slightly over 2 percent).[34] There were net losses in New York City private hospital employment in 1996 and 1997, when employment declined by 4,095 jobs, or 2.6 percent of 1995 employment levels.[35] 1199 also reported layoffs of its members in every year from 1993 to 1998, totaling roughly 2,000 layoffs (but the union did not report which of its members were laid off).[36] The multiskilling of nursing assistants began in earnest in 1997.

As we know, the creation of PCTs made it possible for hospitals to lay off more specialized EKG and phlebotomy technicians and, at least for a year or two, nurses. When hospitals faced the nursing shortage at the end of the 1990s, multiskilled nursing assistants perhaps made it easier to cope with (and made it more difficult for nurses' unions to use the shortage as a point of leverage in bargaining for improved working conditions). But that does not mean nursing assistants would have been laid off had they not been multiskilled (nor is it clear how many were laid off prior to multiskilling). According to one hospital administrator I interviewed, the increase in salary nursing assistants received as PCTs actually increased her hospital's overall costs, failing to alleviate the financial pressures hospitals leaders claimed necessitated layoffs (and raising doubts about their claim of financial crisis). Furthermore, some hospitals, like Beth Israel, laid off nursing assistants even after they had been cross-trained. At Mount Sinai, reengineering did not prevent layoffs of frontline workers, but aided in them. Similarly, cross-training and multiskilling were undertaken at public hospitals (the Health and Hospitals Corporation), but were not adequate to stem the hemorrhaging of jobs there. Public hospital employment in New York City declined by 33.4 percent between 1990 and 2000.[37] Finally, by the time the multiskilling of nursing assistants was underway across the city, several other forces had dampened the supposed need for layoffs. 1199's lobbying efforts resulted in pools of public funding that offset the cuts hospitals anticipated as a result of pro-market policies. So, too, had 1199's political efforts temporarily dampened Governor Pataki's zeal for reform; when he was up for reelection in 1998, he even gained the union's "neutrality" in the race. National trends furthermore showed that managed care could not contain health care costs in any case, reducing some of the ideological force behind pro-market reforms.

To the extent layoffs were minimized in New York City in the mid-1990s, therefore, it seems more likely to be due to 1199's ability to secure a variety of public subsidies for private hospitals and, as important, obtain job security provisions in its contracts (see chapter 8). In addition, the union tacitly allowed most contraction in the hospital sector to occur in public hospitals, which were slashed dramatically by a mayor and governor who felt, largely on ideological grounds, that the state should have no direct role in providing care. Health and Hospitals Corporation (HHC) hospitals, however, provide close to a third of emergency room and clinic visits in the city and almost half of the "charity care" to those who are uninsured.[38] While HHC beds and jobs were cut, the proportion of charity care in the city provided by HHC did not decline. By 1999, HHC's burden of charity care costs to total costs was nearly four times that of most voluntary hospitals; its ratio of bad debt and charity care costs to total costs rose by 32 percent from 1995 to 1999.[39] Although some voluntary hospitals were, like HHC hospitals, just scraping by financially,[40] the politics of health care policy in New York favored voluntary, private hospitals, particularly those downstate hospitals where 1199 members work. In fact, the number of hospital beds in New York City hospitals was largely unchanged, and total hospital admissions increased in the period nursing assistants were being multiskilled, again raising doubts about whether hospitals had too many staff or could safely lay them off.[41] 1199 was able to achieve its goal of obtaining public financing for private hospitals, including the training of its workforce, but the union's strategy has been the target of considerable criticism among advocates for New York City's poor, who depend more heavily on the public hospital system, and among those who represent and advocate for health care workers other than those represented by 1199.

Finally, in addition to the problems multiskilling raised in terms of the opportunities for 1199's members and its limited nature as a tactic for improving their wages and working conditions, multiskilling had a negative impact on hospitals. A 2003 report commissioned by the 1199 Planning and Placement Fund found, during site visits to eleven hospitals nationwide that had undergone restructuring, that one of the most significant outcomes of restructuring was that morale was negatively impacted. "The restructuring often left deep and lasting emotional wounds in many hospitals," wrote the authors, among whom was someone who would know: Patricia Garcia Sullivan, retired from her position as head of reengineering at Mount Sinai (and now working in the University of Pennsylvania Health Care System).[42]

The report also found that many of the changes initiated in the 1990s— including multiskilling initiatives—had since been "reversed or significantly reworked."[43] It may seem that the potential negative consequences of reengineering could have only been known with hindsight—and therefore that 1199's only choice in the mid-1990s was to cooperate with and thereby try to mitigate the effects of restructuring. Perhaps the union gauged the political situation accurately and its decision not to meddle in hospital affairs more deeply was strategically sound. But there were reasons to be skeptical about reengineering and restructuring from the beginning, not just in hindsight. Most obviously were the reports and concerns of workers themselves.

The 1199 teacher who said the 1199ers he taught strongly disliked multiskilling, spoke derisively about 1199's support for such initiatives:

> [W]e have all this pent-up dissatisfaction, so people come lining up for these things [the PCT program] because the opportunities that they actually have are so limited. And we're going to plug them into these things and then we can write an evaluation of how we spent your money and say "look, 250 PCAs two years later when there were none two years ago." This is a tangible, countable, observable result... [but] we've done nothing to change the workplace that's tangible.

Multiskilling left untouched the problems on the job many health care workers face, when it did not make them worse by increasing workloads. It did not solve the problems in health care work discussed in chapter 1, such as shortage of supplies and resources, staffing problems, and a lack of respect.

The way hospitals spent the CHCCDP infrastructure grants—the grants designed to promote managed care readiness—suggests that there was little interest in the kind of organizational or workplace reform that might tangibly improve the daily lives of health care workers. Reengineering and restructuring gurus argued that reform required fundamental, organizationwide change in areas like management processes, operating policies and systems, compensation schemes, as well as the physical size and layout of various operations. Therefore, "reengineering... is an all-or-nothing proposition," an approach that "means starting all over, starting from scratch."[44] New York hospitals, however, used their infrastructure grants primarily to purchase and implement new billing and computer information systems and open ambulatory care clinics.[45] Such investments were made largely so hospitals could capture revenue lost in the labyrinth of billing and payment that is the U.S. health care system and expand their revenue base into areas of care that payers would presumably reward. Such investments did not affect the basic way health care work is organized; they may have required training in computer skills and certainly served as an excuse for cross-training and multiskilling of some jobs, but they were not part of an overhaul of health-care-as-usual in New York City. Organizational reform in New York City was, ultimately, reduced to a series of training seminars and "skills" programs aimed at the most powerless members of the health care workforce.

Dennis Rivera has characterized his strategy the same way restructuring and reengineering boosters do their own—as "pragmatic."[46] It is a label with tremendous emotional appeal in the U.S. context and is often used to make an insidious distinction between those who act on the basis of the resources they have and those who merely criticize and complain. Recall Lathrop's description of the newly empowered multiskilled unit clerk. He asserted that multiskilling was necessary because of the amount of paperwork in the health care system—so much paperwork that insurance companies and hospital business offices "harass" patients. Lathrop not only accepts this barrage of paperwork and treatment of patients as given, he legitimizes it and suggests that the solution lies with frontline health care workers taking ownership of their work. The transformation of the way health care in the United States is financed, on the other hand, is preemptively ruled out as impractical. As Lathrop establishes in the opening pages of his book, the latter is a "policy-level black hole" about which "there is precious little any one institution can do."[47]

The irony of multiskilling programs is health care workers have always been multiskilled because of the nature of their work. For patients to receive adequate care, health care workers must (and do) cross the boundaries of their job descriptions. From the perspective of health care workers, multiskilling is nothing new: They have long been asked to take on extra responsibilities and have often responded to a patient's need when it wasn't part of their official duties. The receipt of a new, multiskilled job description by no means ends the need for health care workers to help each other and patients in new ways, particularly in conditions of inadequate resources and staffing. Multiskilling programs merely attempt to exploit this good will.

Like the teacher above, I saw in my observations of health care settings a good deal of "pent-up dissatisfaction" among the health care workers, dissatisfaction that is exacerbated by continual refusals to address what they consider to be the most frustrating aspects of their work. Signs of this dissatisfaction emerged even more clearly in soft skills training courses. Irrespective of the goals of such courses, they often became spaces in which health care workers could collectively vent and discuss their frustrations—activities for which they have very little time back on the shop floor.

5

"It All Comes Down to You"

Self-Help and Soft Skills

When millions of dollars for training the health care workforce became available in the late 1990s, tens of thousands of New York City hospital workers were sent to training classes in such areas as customer service, communication skills, team building and teamwork, cultural diversity, conflict resolution, and leadership training. These "soft skills" courses were among the most heavily funded areas of training and, like multiskilling courses, presented as necessary preparation for the world of market-driven, competitive health care. In the courses I observed, health care workers were asked to compare their hospitals to Microsoft, McDonald's, Disneyland, and Singapore Airlines, and themselves to Donald Trump and Bill Gates. Patients became "customers" or "clients" and clinical services "product lines." Private consultants, some new to the world of training altogether and others possessing proprietary training packages they had long offered to private businesses, created presentations tailored for health care. As one said, health care was an "untapped market."

Much of this training was built on two questionable premises: that health care is like other businesses and that soft skills training for frontline health care workers is an effective response to changes and difficulties health care organizations face. The weaknesses of these premises were vividly exposed in the training courses themselves, which I observed in 2001–2002 in three settings: a communication skills program at a midsize private hospital, a "retreat" on teamwork and customer service for employees of a public hospital, and in-services at one of the city's largest (and recently unionized) home health care agencies. I also interviewed trainers and officials at these organizations, as well as independent training consultants working in the area of soft skills. In the courses, instructors encouraged the participants to think of their employers as businesses and themselves as salespeople. They sought to teach soft skills for the hard realities of a market-driven health care sector. They consistently posited that individual workers were responsible for producing the cooperation necessary for improving care. As the communication skills instructor succinctly put it, "the most fertile area for greater control lies within the self."

The participants' reactions to such advice, though, pointed to the complex and social nature of the problems they faced, of which instructors themselves were sometimes aware or participants forced them to confront. Just as the instructors' messages were similar, so were the dilemmas they faced. They carried out their training seminars in the absence of a larger plan to improve the conditions of health care work. In fact, training programs arguably became the only, and therefore inevitably inadequate, response to the pressures and stresses frontline workers faced.

The conversations, interactions, and exchanges that took place in the courses themselves were not scripted, and it was in these moments that the problems health care workers face and the limits of training were evident. There were tensions between what instructors wanted to teach and what participants needed and between the expectations of those who implemented training programs and their effects. From the perspective of almost any stakeholder in the process, one might argue soft skills training programs were a dismal failure. Yet they were and continue to be highly funded, and many participants enjoyed them. Indeed, the conversations that arose during the training itself not only show the limits of this kind of training but also indicate why so much was invested—emotionally and financially—in it.

The communication skills class[1] began like a self-help or personal development seminar. At 8:00 a.m. sharp in a windowless room adjacent to the hospital's training department, the instructor opened with a section on the "essentials for success." She encouraged participants to assess their present situation and think concretely about their futures and aspirations. She handed out various self-assessment forms; some asked participants to "think about where you are now" and whether they were "satisfied with your personal life progress." Some contained questions aimed at encouraging participants to make more concrete plans for their future, asking, "are your underlying values clear and sharp in your mind?" and "are you as successful as you can be?" The instructor stressed that participants should write their goals down, since what is written down is "more real." And she warned, "failure to plan is a plan to fail."

As she discussed various pathways to success, the possibility of varying definitions of success, and the idea that success is a process rather than a destination, the instructor's idea of success seemed broad. Yet while the first hour or so of the class used generic and generous concepts and the instructor sought to "empower" course participants to make the changes they desired in their lives, she began to gradually build to a more specific point: One of the most critical skills to being successful was "effective self-management."

The instructor had already positioned herself as a role model of success by describing her own career and achievements. Many of the course participants seemed to like and admire her. Charismatic and herself an immigrant and woman of color, the instructor began her career as a nurse, eventually becoming a high-ranking nurse administrator before retiring to form her own consulting firm. When the instructor listed her own multiple degrees (a registered nurse degree, two master's degrees, and a doctorate) as evidence of her success, the students in one class spontaneously applauded.

The instructor insisted that one indicator of her success was the flexible character of her work as a consultant and discretion in managing her time. So when it came to self-management, she asked the class, "do I have more time than you do?" One participant, unsure of the answer but aware the instructor had one in mind already, replied rather tentatively, "maybe." "No," replied the instructor, "we're all given the same amount of time—twenty-four hours a day, seven days a week. It's a matter of maximizing time efficiently and effectively."

The instructor then began what would be a difficult process throughout the two-day course—applying reasonable but generic principles to the specific, daily process of providing health care. Although she defined self-management broadly as "the process of maximizing individual time and talents to achieve worthwhile goals based on a sound value system," she then argued more specifically that if health care workers wanted to be successful, they needed to manage their seven and a half hour shifts well, finding a way to get all their work done. This meant they needed to find a way to *give themselves* enough time. If they were standing around and chatting during their shifts, she said, they were not managing themselves well and giving cues that they needed to be managed. For the instructor, if the course participants felt they were being too closely supervised, they should ask themselves in what ways their behavior might be eliciting that supervision.

The course then turned to a discussion of the necessary attitude to be successful (though the disposition workers should adopt was conveyed repeatedly during the course). Participants were told to be assertive (as opposed to aggressive), receptive (rather than defensive), and proactive (rather than reactive). The instructor said that by acting confidently others would have confidence in them, that they should project a positive attitude, and that they should be lifelong learners always open to new ideas. They should take risks, not procrastinate, practice self-discipline, and laugh often. One handout encouraged them to be "big thinkers" rather than "petty thinkers," by talking about the positive qualities of their friends, company, and competition, believing in expansion (rather than retrenchment), looking for ways to help others, setting goals high, and ignoring errors of little consequence rather than magnifying them. Indeed, by the time the instructor moved on to the next section of the course in the afternoon, "the power of attitudes and professionalism," she had already made what would be its central point: Many of the problems and challenges the workers faced could be traced back to themselves—a negative attitude, an inability to manage how others perceived them, a lack of professionalism, and ineffective time management strategies.

The instructor also seemed to take seriously what J. Philip Lathrop, in his managerial guide to restructuring, called the "real training challenge": "to change the way people act and the way they *think*."[2] Explaining why it can be so difficult to change the way one thinks, the communication skills instructor drew a distinction between the conscious and unconscious (or subconscious) mind. The conscious mind, she said, is one's conscience, the ability to know right from wrong, or "will power." The unconscious or subconscious mind was, by contrast, one's "personal slave": its sole concern is the individual, and it is responsible for creating and reinforcing one's own personal (and highly subjective and unreliable) reality. The instructor pointed out that the unconscious mind is likely to be deceptive, so she stressed the importance of "counting to ten" and taking a reflective moment in order to question the basis of one's emotions before translating them into action/reaction. This, the instructor noted, is necessary because people often misperceive events or see conflict where there is none. Her message was that control lies in the ability of the conscious mind to will positive thoughts against its deceptive alter—the quintessential "power of positive thinking."

In this area, and in several others, the instructor was influenced by David McNally's best-selling self-help book, *Even Eagles Need a Push.* According to McNally, "those who learn to soar have the courage to take a *positive* attitude toward life." He, however, ascribes a slightly different role to the subconscious, arguing the subconscious is a powerful force that can materially create the goal that we have set for ourselves, even if we cannot consciously imagine how we will ever attain it. "To grasp the importance of this believing without an apparent *how* is to understand that the mind attracts the physical representation of that which it holds as an image. It works by subconsciously guiding you into the correct actions to bring out the manifestation of your vision."[3]

The most time-consuming section of the communication skills course was on anger management, which took up over half of the second day. The instructor focused on how participants should handle their own feelings of anger. Her primary message was that they should not "stuff" anger inside or escalate it, but rather acknowledge and reveal feelings of anger with "respect and calm." The instructor readily acknowledged that anger could be justified by some of their working conditions or the abusive behavior of colleagues and managers, nonetheless it was the workers' responsibilities to manage and diffuse the situation. She described how differing levels of anger required different reactions. Her root message was that it was never appropriate to *express* one's anger, though it might be unavoidable on occasion to feel anger. Staff should deal with anger (whether theirs or others') by confronting others in a calm and reasonable way.

The instructor's most persuasive argument for why the workers should avoid situations of anger or take responsibility for diffusing them (no matter who was at fault) appeared to be that anger could be dangerous to one's health. There are a number of physical effects of anger, she pointed out, including raising levels of blood sugar and increasing the risk of diabetes. In the home care in-services I observed, one instructor similarly cautioned aides not to get worked up about a miscommunication with a patient or nurse or take it personally because their blood pressure might go up and endanger their health. The home-care instructor said she had seen two aides in her classes with high blood pressure from their work, and she had sent one of them straight to the emergency room. This focus on the physical effects of anger not only appealed to the workers' desire to protect their own well-being but also to their training as health care workers. When I spoke to participants after the communication skills course, biophysical aspects of stress and anger were among the most well-retained themes.

The one-day customer-service retreat at the public hospital focused more on team building, but the instructor of that course also emphasized the value of positive thinking and argued the participants needed to consider how they, themselves, produced any discontent or unhappiness they might feel on the job. Only then could they remedy their job-related problems. For one exercise, she had participants write an advertisement for the unit. Explaining the exercise later in an interview, she said, "the reason we want them to do advertising is for them to think positive." Like the communication skills instructor, she emphasized the importance of loyalty to one's organization and argued that criticizing where you work is like criticizing yourself. She was also herself a manager in the hospital's nursing department.

To develop teamwork, the retreat instructor used interactive activities and exercises inspired by what she had learned when she worked at a private hospital that hired a major consulting firm to reengineer its operations. Restricted by a more limited budget than at her earlier job, she relied on nonproprietary games and exercises to accomplish similar objectives. So, the participants played Pictionary and did an exercise that involved assembling a helicopter out of Legos. For the latter, we (I participated in this case) were broken into teams and had to assemble a helicopter exactly like the model the instructor's assistant kept at the front of the room and out of view. Only one team member at a time was allowed to go to the front of the room and look at the model. Team members, therefore, had to communicate with each other precisely how to build the helicopter. Pictionary was played in the usual way: We were again divided into teams and each team had to identify a word or concept based on one of the team member's drawing of it. The instructor explained that these games served to unite team members with a common goal—"to win." After the helicopter exercise, she pointed out that by working as a team we ignored the "levels" (i.e., job titles) between us and united in a single task.

The day-long in-services at the home care agency were taught by agency staff and designed in part to address workers who had been written up for specific infractions. In the sessions I attended, the instructors spent part of the day going over nurses' write-ups of particular aides with the whole class (although not all of the workers attending had write-ups and those that did were sometimes surprised to find out about them). A good deal of in-class discussion then focused on not only the agency's policies and procedures, but how to communicate with patients and supervising nurses so as to avoid either violating policies and procedures or (and not exactly the same thing) getting in trouble. One of the instructors was a tall, pretty, Jamaican woman and former aide to whom the agency (in its pre-unionized days, she emphasized) gave a scholarship to become a nurse. Although she never criticized the agency's policies and procedures, she often showed understanding and sympathy for the aides even while maintaining a maternal and authoritative demeanor. She seemed to possess an endless supply of aphorisms, which she aptly applied and the participants enjoyed: "Don't fight fire with fire." "Dot your I's and cross your T's." "You can't catch a fly with vinegar, you have to use honey." "When in Rome, do as the Romans."

The other instructor, too, was a former aide and nurse who offered similar advice, saying for instance that aides should never get angry with a supervisor—"your grass has to be green"—if they want to have any chance of being taken seriously. She seemed to identify with the aides more personally, however, especially with the ways in which they might be treated dismissively. When she first became an instructor, she told the class, supervisors at the agency continued to talk down to her because they didn't know she had been promoted. They mistook her for "just an aide."

Much to everyone's aggravation, however, the second instructor showed a videotape of a seminar on communication skills at the end of the very long training day, rather than excuse the aides early. The videotape,

presented by "Drs. Rick and Rick,"[4] featured a number of skits intended
to be stimulating, but which largely fell flat and struck me as disingenuous.
In one skit, Rick and Rick demonstrated how to "state your intent." In it,
a female (white) secretary told her male (white) boss that she had done
an analysis of her time and determined the two hours a week she spent
getting coffee were not a good use of it. First, they enacted the skit in the
"wrong" way, in which the secretary was "passive-aggressive" and said,
"I'd like you to look at this report which shows how you are mismanaging
my time." Then, they reenacted the scenario to show how the interaction
could have been improved. In the second version, the secretary said, "Do
you have a moment? I know you are quite busy. I want to start off by saying that I want to be the most efficient secretary that you've ever had, and
make this the most efficient unit this company has ever had. Therefore,
I have prepared this analysis of the use of my time which I thought you
could look at." The boss looked at it and immediately declared, "Oh my!
I can't have you spend all this time getting coffee, I'll get it myself." Rick
and Rick pointed out that in the second version the secretary spoke her intent. One has to wonder, however, if her intent was to be the best secretary
ever, or merely not to deliver coffee. Moreover, surely the most plausible
outcome would have been that the boss, deciding his own time was most
valuable, continued to ask his secretary to get his coffee or passed the time-
consuming task on to someone even less well paid and with less bargaining
leverage than she.

Sometimes it was clear the participants admired and liked their instructors. In follow-up interviews with participants in the communication
skills training, many described how much they enjoyed the course. Many
agreed that the instructor was, as one PCT put it, "humorous and engaging." Another said of the communication skills class, "I enjoyed it—I really
did. It's always good to get to know more and learn. I was really very glad
to be there." Some things stuck with them. One unit clerk who attended
the communication skills class said some months afterward that when she
feels angry she remembers to take ten deep breaths or try to express her
anger positively, as she learned in the course. Another said she told her husband about what she had learned and tried to apply the principles to her
personal life.

Even if participants retained some of the lessons, were they applicable to
situations they encountered on the job? At times, the questions participants

raised in the courses indicated they were skeptical of their relevance to the specific problems they faced at work. At other times, the staying power of such courses was undermined when the instructors' advice was vague or even inconsistent, a position in which the communication skills instructor in particular found herself on a number of occasions, because of her curriculum but also because of the questions to which participants pushed her to respond.

For instance, when the communication skills instructor told participants that it was their responsibility to "give themselves enough time" during their shifts and fully commit to their seven and a half hours of work, one participant immediately raised the problem of "shorting" (understaffing on the hospital floors). This is perhaps the most pressing concern of many health care workers. How, the participant wondered, would it be possible to solve the problem of not having enough time when the hospital didn't provide enough staff?

In another session, a recreational therapist named Carmen asked, "What if we don't have supplies? I use my time and dollars to buy supplies!" The instructor initially replied with a formulaic answer: Carmen's behavior was sending a "negative" message: "You're more than ready to blame management, but usually you're asking to be managed." Carmen pushed the issue. If she does not buy supplies on her own, she insisted, the job does not get done: "How can we have a grooming [special events in which patients dress up and do their hair or makeup] without grooming supplies? What should we do, twiddle our thumbs?" Perhaps because she was an external consultant and not a manager within the hospital, the communication skills trainer was clearly sympathetic to the difficulties many participants described. Even though her course was more didactic than the customer service retreat, she was also more open to interruptions and feedback from the participants. However, these interruptions, like that with Carmen, pushed her into awkward situations, and she occasionally seemed disappointed that the participants were so regularly raising objections and pointing out the limitations of her formulas. In the end, the instructor said to Carmen, "Yes, twiddle your thumbs. That's your choice—behavior that is rewarded is repeated."

So, the instructor initially contended that by complaining about the lack of supplies rather than making the most out what was available, Carmen was "asking to be managed." Yet she also acknowledged that there just might not be enough supplies to do her work and if Carmen started to regularly buy her own then such behavior would be rewarded and expected. Carmen would be, in that way, contributing to her own exploitation. The instructor was, in a sense, advocating a work slow-down. However, she would never promote open protest or complaint since it would be inconsistent with her ideas about the correct attitude and loyalty to the hospital. Nor would she openly criticize management for failing to provide needed supplies since she had been hired to defuse discontent, not fuel it. She was stuck. The issue was the same with staffing. How was it possible to "give themselves time" during their shift if there simply weren't enough staff to do the work, no matter how efficiently they worked?

Much of the tension in her course stemmed from the nature of the work itself—to provide patient care. A work slow-down in health care could have troubling consequences for people who are sick and vulnerable. Indeed, in the sections on professionalism and teamwork the instructor told the participants they must do whatever necessary to ensure good patient care. She also expressed her disapproval of nursing assistants or nurses who took their jobs for the salary and stability rather than because of a commitment to serve. But in Carmen's situation, the instructor was suggesting that Carmen compromise her standard of good patient care because she recognized that it was unfair of the hospital to depend on its workers to provide needed supplies. Carmen felt pressure to buy her own supplies because it was she who had to interact with patients and face the emotional consequences of not being able to provide the best possible care. This was evidently a common feeling. One of the instructors in the home care agency repeatedly reminded the aides, "We have to use our judgment. Don't let your compassion take precedence."

Gloria, a unit clerk, enjoyed the communication skills class but said:

> I understand it [the section of the course on anger management], but sometimes it can't happen. It just can't…Sometimes we have patients' relatives that come in, and okay, they meet the patient in a mess [they have wet or soiled themselves]. But maybe that happened right just before you came in. And then we're understaffed. So, if that nurse is taking care of this patient, or just finished taking care of one patient, that patient will have to wait. You have come in how many days and not met the patient in that situation? It's not something that's willful. It's not because we *want* to isolate that patient.

For Gloria, the lack of time and poor staffing meant it is inevitable that patients will at some moments receive less than optimal care, no matter how hard the staff work. This is not something the staff enjoy and not something that can be remedied by a communication skills course.

Some tensions also arose in the course when the instructor's emphasis on doing whatever is necessary to provide good care collided with the strictly enforced differences in power and responsibilities among occupations in health care organizations. For instance, the instructor told the participants they should never "pass the buck." In the section on anger management, the instructor described a hypothetical situation in which a nurse asks a PCT to send a fax. The PCT reports the fax machine is broken, so the nurse calls "Joe" in the facilities department who says he'll take care of it. The next day the fax machine is still broken, so the PCT gets angry at the nurse, who gets angry at Joe, who gets angry at the technician he sent to do the job, who gets angry at another supervisor who pulled him away from repairing the fax machine. For the instructor, no one in this chain of events took responsibility for making sure the fax machine was fixed. This set off a chain of angry interactions. The examples the PCTs in the class raised, however, were more complicated because they related to patient care and safety rather than fax machines. For instance, they wanted to know how to respond when a nurse became angry at them for mentioning something that the nurse should have done but had not, such as ordering a medication.

Workers in health care must adhere to a hierarchical employment structure and strict job descriptions established by professional organizations, state regulations, and, in this case, reinforced by collective bargaining agreements. The communications skills course sections on anger management and teamwork failed to systematically consider the differences in power among those who work together in health care. After advocating the need to work together as a team to provide the best care, the instructor also said teamwork might have to be sacrificed in some instances to do so. All workers, she argued, should take responsibility for the medical well-being of patients, even if it meant confronting and perhaps alienating a coworker. The instructor told one unit clerk that she was obligated to go over the head of a nurse or doctor if she noticed they forgot to follow through on a medical order that the unit clerk had given them. The clerk—Judith, who was also a nursing student—retorted that she had been reprimanded, not rewarded, for correcting a nurse's recording error regarding a patient's medication.

The bulk of the participants in the course were frontline staff, and several expressed reservations about whether they could or should confront someone in a superior position about a conflict or go over their heads to make a decision in the best interests of the patient. The course did not offer a considered framework for how staff might have to adjust their response to anger according to the relative power of the persons involved or what teamwork meant in a strict hierarchy. After all, some people have the power to discipline, to shame, to dismiss, while others do not. Physicians did not take the course. Some nurse managers took a one-day version of the course, but they suggested to the instructor their own anger and mistakes were not the problem, rather their concern was how to deal with the anger of physicians or "old-timer" nurses and nursing assistants whom they felt had intractable attitude problems.

When the communication skills instructor was pulled back from the shibboleths of self-help into the world of actual health care work, she had to acknowledge the participants' concerns. Even though she told workers never to pass the buck, she also urged them, as with Carmen, to "know where your responsibility begins and ends." Implicitly acknowledging the pressure for them to do more and more work and continually come out of description (and the risk of being reprimanded for doing so), she could not seem to reconcile this with her messages about the need to do whatever possible to provide good care, nor could she define the boundaries of good care and caregiving work.

Ultimately, the instructor's injunction not to pass the buck and be willing to take greater responsibility seemed to participants to be just another way to pressure them to "come out of description" because of shortages of staff or resources. Staff, particularly lower-level staff, were not only officially required to adhere to their job descriptions and roles, many also saw them as their best protection against being overworked and exploited. For them, both the call for teamwork and the idea it would need to be sacrificed in some instances seemed to be ways of asking them to come out of their job descriptions and take responsibility for problems not of their making. Moreover, teamwork was a loaded term since they could not imagine that nurses and doctors would start changing bedpans or coming out of *their* job descriptions.

Finally, in the course section on essentials for success, the instructor indicated that it was not necessarily a good idea to trust one's coworkers, which seemed to undermine the possibility of teamwork altogether. She used a handout that asked participants to indicate whether their coworkers knew about their future goals and plans. Rather than encouraging participants to share their goals and dreams, as might have been anticipated, the instructor said it was not always a good idea to tell coworkers about your plans. She, herself, had not told her coworkers when she was working on her doctorate. The section included a PowerPoint slide with the title "Learn to Swim with Sharks." The need to trust, and cooperate with, coworkers was therefore juxtaposed, without commentary, with the message that one must vigilantly guard against coworkers—the vicious sharks.

The communication skills instructor was trying to make the best out of a difficult situation. It was never in her (or other trainers') power to change those things that would really make these health care workers' lives and patients' experience better, and yet they sincerely wanted to improve those things. In a session in which most of the participants were PCTs, the instructor at several moments acknowledged problems peculiar to their position, such as being referred to as "just a PCT" and having their opinions dismissed by nurses and doctors. In solidarity, she said that PCTs rather than nurses now provide most hands-on care, and she disparaged those nurses who refuse to do basic hands-on tasks that are central to caregiving. She said PCTs need to maintain high self-esteem and pointed out that successful companies, like Microsoft, treat all their employees as if they can contribute important ideas. (Bill Gates was also used as a role model because he continued to work even after making so much money.)

Some trainers do recognize and even articulate the dilemmas of their role and of training within health care organizations. One consultant (the former social worker) who specialized in training nursing home workers remarked:

> There are certain facilities ... where I've already in my own mind established that management is part and parcel of the issue. They're going to offer conflict resolution, and I want to say ... "you just need to eradicate where the conflict comes from, not just conflict management." Why are we assuming that there has to be conflict?

Yet as people who want their work to mean something, the trainers with whom I had contact tried to persevere and figure out how to make a difference in the lives of patients and workers, even if they recognized the limits of what training itself could accomplish.

One way they did this was to whole-heartedly embrace the idea that radical changes were afoot in health care—namely, it was becoming more competitive and businesslike—and that they could, at the very least, provide health care workers with a "realistic" sense of the challenges they might face. At the same time staff were advised to take control of their attitudes and interactions, then, they were advised to accommodate these changes as inevitable. Sometimes trainers reacted to participants' complaints about understaffing or inadequate supplies not with sympathy, but a bit of old-fashioned tough love (and perhaps exasperation). At one point, the communication skills instructor responded to a participant who kept raising the problem of understaffing by mimicking what she had earlier demonstrated as an unprofessional way of talking and posturing, saying, "You got to learn to deal with it, girl, or you won't be able to work anywhere!"

The consultant who teaches at nursing homes said when issues of short-staffing or poor working conditions came up in her classes, she would explain to the class participants that it is simply the way the industry works. Workers can't really change that. "It takes the personalization out and allows us to see it from a broader perspective...hearing that from me as an outside instructor kind of helps them understand it, it neutralizes it." She went on:

> When we talk [in classes] about the institution...quite clearly we talk about the fact that the institution has its own goals and mission and it has to continue to thrive, and that's the primary goal. Make money and do resident care. That may seem like a conflict for the staff, or that it's somewhat distasteful to the staff, but we're all involved in that. If they don't make a profit, we don't have a job, so that's reality.

The instructors of the customer service retreat and in-services at the home health agency furthermore told workers that their employers' survival, and therefore their jobs, depended on their ability to sell their organization and provide high-quality customer service. At the home care in-service, an instructor reminded the aides that their agency's business came through a contract with the Visiting Nurse Service (VNS). If there were too many complaints about the agency, the VNS could simply cancel the contract and use another home care agency.

The former hospital training executive, turned private training consultant, explained why so many New York City hospitals, including her own, spent hundreds of thousands of dollars on customer service training:

> New York City hospitals, by the way, are notorious. They have totally bad customer service...I think that with the competition, there was a real feeling managed care was coming in, that one of the ways that you keep the people and you get more people to come in, is by word of mouth. I think everybody was saying that if one person has a good experience then they'll bring another person in, but if one person has a bad experience it will affect seven or eight people. So given what was happening with the competition coming, with managed care coming in, that one of the ways to ensure that you have a patient base is that people are treated nicely.

The idea that hospitals are driven by the need to make a profit and encourage more business may be consistent with the new ideology that health care is a commercial product rather than a public good, but it is a distorted presentation of what hospitals do. One nurse's published anecdote vividly captured how customer service seminars—implemented around the country as a component of restructuring—can play out in a health care setting:

> [I]n an effort to understand how the staffing cutbacks that compromised patient care contributed to our hospital's mission and enhanced our revenues, I attended a hospital-sponsored educational session on reorganization titled, ironically, "Delivering Exceptional Customer Care." I heard the business consultant, who was brought in by the hospital management for a multimillion-dollar initiative, tell a room full of nurses to avoid using the word "cancer." An oncology nurse asked, "What, then, do we say to a newly diagnosed patient?" "Try to say nothing," came this consultant's blunt and sincere reply. "The patient will associate the word with the hospital, and that's bad for repeat business."[5]

To this nurse, such an in-service was useless in the face of staffing cutbacks and the demands of patient care. It seemed completely irrational to spend millions of dollars on a customer service training program rather than hiring or recruiting nurses. More important, the consultant's lack of understanding of the nature of work in health care seemed potentially dangerous. She was apparently advocating that health care professionals avoid direct and honest conversations with patients about their conditions and treatment. To many who provide health care, this way of thinking would be comical if it did not also tend to dismiss and trivialize what they do.

It is no doubt true that hospitals develop reputations and it is in a hospital's interest to have a good one. But most people do not choose hospitals, or recommend them to one another, like they might restaurants or televisions. This is in part because they cannot: There is too much uncertainty to allow for an informed choice. In practice, most people go to the nearest hospital in an emergency or to the hospital that happens to be covered by their health insurance plan. Their choice may be limited by the admitting privileges of their physicians. For many, a lack of insurance coverage means they must go to any hospital that will accept them. People with money, good insurance coverage, and privileged access to information may be able to make decisions about their care that approach being fully informed, but that is a small group in this country. It is important that more patients have access to information on the quality of hospitals and doctors. But at a basic level, the "products" of health care are more complex and subject to a kind of uncertainty that makes them unlike standard commercial products.

The idea that hospitals view patients as regular customers or repeat business is of course also at odds with the idea that the aim of health care is to treat patients and minimize their business. Indeed, it is at odds with efforts to contain health care costs and services, about which the very same politicians and policy makers who advocate market-driven health care and a business mentality are fixated.

In such moments, trainers were trying to persuade workers to get used to, or accommodate, changes such as cuts in staffing or the resources they needed to do their jobs. While it is true that hospitals face considerable financial constraints, it is misleading to present these institutions as independent corporations which must make a profit to survive. Their survival depends to a significant degree on state and federal politics and on the policy makers who decide how health care is to be financed. But it also depends on the decisions of hospital administrators themselves. Furthermore, the argument that the survival of hospitals or nursing homes depends on the attitudes of individual health care workers depoliticizes the decisions of their employers as well as politicians and policy makers. These trainers' arguments removed the problems of short staffing and a lack of resources from the realm of collective debate and transformed a managerial claim—costs are too high—into a truism. At the retreat on customer service, the instructor explained very early in the day that staffing is not something "we" can control. It is an administrative, a "finance," problem, she said, and devoting energy to complaining about it was not conducive to team-work. In the new competitive environment, the hospital, she insisted, needed to show savings and cut back on patient stays, and staff could help by not wasting supplies.

The instructor similarly stressed that the hospital would soon be undergoing a survey and assessment by the Joint Commission on the Accreditation of Healthcare Organizations (JCAHO) and remarked that if any of the staff were angry enough to complain in front of the commission, they should quit. She quickly noticed this was not a well-received piece of advice, however, and tried to save the moment by saying, "After all, if you're angry, you hurt yourself—mentally and physically—as well as your colleagues." In the communication skills course, too, health care workers were asked to surrender their right to ask why, to call into question the way in which their work is organized, in order to save themselves the emotional and physical consequences of anger. At one point, the communication skills instructor advised that it is important not to aggravate people who are angry, especially when they are looking for an object upon which to take out their anger. She pointed out that one of the questions that can aggravate someone who is angry, which appears as a challenge to them, is "why?" In a couple of the course sessions, the instructor used the same example to illustrate her point. She asserted that when a staffing coordinator tells a PCT they have to "float" (move to another unit to cover an absence or staff shortage), they should not ask why because it will make the situation worse. In one session, a participant recounted that she had been asked to float to a floor where she didn't know how to do the job. The instructor reluctantly conceded that floating was not a good idea if staff didn't have the necessary skills. But in a later session, the instructor was prepared and preempted such a complaint by saying, "Floating is a fact of life," and the "sooner we get accustomed, the less we will get angry." Referring back to the physical effects of anger, the instructor noted once again that it is un-healthy to become angry.

The communication-skills instructor's emphasis on not aggravating people or making them more angry at times evaded an open discussion of why health care workers might often feel unsafe and vulnerable. She told staff never to say "no" to patients, using as an example the situation of a patient who brings a gun into the emergency room. She sensibly warned that telling the patient, "No, you can't bring a gun into the ER" might make him angry. The example, however, revealed as much about the unsafe situations in which health care workers can find themselves as it did about managing angry patients. One PCT, Georgia, described a situation in which a patient's husband threatened her. The instructor again warned Georgia not to confront such a person because they might take it as an attack and an opening for aggression. But the instructor did not discuss whether Georgia could call hospital security and expect them to arrive in a reasonable amount of time, a problem the participants had complained about. The instructor did not consider whether Georgia had a right to feel safe. Georgia said she felt so sick after the experience that she had a pain in her chest; she found comfort and security after the incident at her church. The instructor seemed not to want to take up this fundamental issue of security. Throughout the day, the instructor also evaded Georgia's comments about how she turned to her church to deal with anger and emotional issues. I was struck by just how necessary having a source of comfort and community, like a church, was for these care providers; certainly it seemed they could not expect to find such comfort at work.

In these courses, then, the hospital and its managers were not expected to produce the conditions necessary for good patient care and teamwork. The participants' complaints about being disrespected by their superiors were portrayed as, if not their own fault, then something that they could change—if, that is, they appropriately demonstrated responsibility and self-management. A lack of supplies and staffing were treated as inevitable. These courses also consistently emphasized persuading health care workers not only to compensate for inadequate resources and working conditions but also to take responsibility for managing the emotions of others and subordinating their own emotions to the larger cause of getting along. This seemed to be acutely problematic for the home care aides, who complained that they had neither enough education nor trustworthy, helpful supervision (not to mention pay commensurate with their responsibilities). The write-ups that the instructors read aloud in their in-services, and the aides' responses, raised a host of complicated situations that required skills and support far beyond those achievable in a self-help seminar or one-day refresher course. The aides described encounters with patients smoking marijuana (which might cause an aide to fail her next drug test if she was exposed to it), patients who are racist, and patients who hide their plan of care. They struggled with setting boundaries around their work, and described the difficulties that arise when a few aides do things beyond their job description, changing patients' expectations for all aides. Some were not sure whether they should or could go to church with their patients. Moreover, they were troubled that the touch-tone phone-in system for reporting completed tasks gave the aides no flexibility in documenting unusual situations.

The aides were cautioned by both agency instructors I observed to take the high road, to control their emotions and avoid angry confrontation with a supervisor because it would only reduce their legitimacy. Yet they often felt powerless to defend themselves and that there was little support for them in these situations. Health care workers must be able to manage the emotions of others—to calm and soothe patients, to work smoothly with people in a variety of occupations from stunningly diverse backgrounds. At moments, these courses seemed to add to the feelings of those on the frontlines that they are unfairly burdened—that they must take care of everyone else but no one will take care of them.

At bottom, these soft skills training courses taught that the responsibility for the effective completion of work is in the hands of those workers with the least autonomy, voice, and preparation. Workers were provided with a general set of aphorisms and principles for modulating communication and changing relationships on the shop floor, but the general framework in which they work was left unexamined. It was incumbent upon them as individuals to generate cooperation and improvements in patient care within the existing confines of their job descriptions or organizational structure. Attempts by those in charge to improve the jobs and working conditions of frontline staff were given up in favor of training them to have the right attitude.

Coincidentally but significantly, the instructors of both the communication skills and customer service courses used handouts with the same definition of attitude—though they edited the passage slightly differently and it was attributed by one instructor to an unknown author and by the other to Charles Swindoll, an evangelical preacher and author of numerous self-help books. According to the handouts, we "cannot change the inevitable," but our attitude is something we can control, something about which we can make a choice each day. Attitude "is more important than the past, than education, than money, than circumstances, than failures, than successes, than what other people think or say or do."

In such moments, the underlying logic of the training courses seemed to be to defuse discontent, to "cool out"[6] workers so that, in seeking explanations for workplace wrongs, they would turn their attention from the actions of their managers to themselves. Through restructuring and reengineering, managers and administrators were primarily attempting to cut costs and impose as much work as possible on lower-level workers. Soft skills training was seemingly intended to muffle the blow to morale such changes created. These courses were not meant to identify workers' complaints and remedy them, only head off and mitigate the conflict and discontent that cost-cutting and restructuring were creating. Moreover, the soft skills courses often reinforced the pro-market, managerial ideology behind such changes.

It should go without saying that the instructors and training industry figures I interviewed did not set out to create a cooling-out mechanism. Many involved in training and education genuinely hoped to create better conditions for health care workers, even if working with a limited amount of discretion and influence. Nonetheless, even though the position of the trainers I observed is fraught with difficulties and contradictions, it can never allow for critique of management, or the union, or health care as usual. Even the communication skills instructor, who so often recognized the difficult conditions under which health care workers attempted to create better patient care, never attributed these conditions to the policies promoted and implemented by managers, policy makers, and political figures such as Governor Pataki and 1199 President Rivera. She suggested individual solutions to problems that are far more complex and collective—solutions that at some points bordered on the absurd. Taking the power of positive thinking to its extreme, she once told her students, in relation to the shortage of basic supplies mentioned earlier, "If your positive attitude and professionalism increased, then maybe the hospital's market share and revenue would increase, and then the organization could afford supplies—it all comes down to you."

It would be a mistake, however, to think these courses were effective in this regard, that they convinced health care workers that the cause of inadequate supplies was their attitudes. Messages of self-help, a positive attitude, and individual responsibility are appealing, but only because these messages are widely disseminated in our culture and commonly internalized. When these messages were applied to course participants' work and working conditions, many health care workers were less than convinced.

Even though some similar messages emerged in the courses—about the inevitability of a market-driven health care system, the need to focus on the self, the equal importance of attitude and psychic imagery to that of material and structural conditions—the courses lacked impact in part simply because they could be haphazard. It seemed at times that the trainers I observed hadn't had the time or put in the effort to plan their way out of all of the cul-de-sacs of actual health care delivery into which their self-help guides could potentially lead them. Nor did they seem to anticipate all the possible effects of their exercises. When the retreat participants constructed a helicopter and played Pictionary, for instance, the overwhelming emotion in the room was that of stress and tension. None of the participants had played Pictionary before, and some were clearly intimidated by it. The course hardly seemed to be a "retreat" during the game. More important than the "unity" supposedly felt by members of the same team was the sense of competition with other teams. The exercises also created tension among team members, especially when some were perceived either to be too slow or showing off. I failed to see how such games introduced a spirit of cooperation—although the instructor was correct that they created a desire to win.

The courses also likely lacked impact for a more important reason: the nature of the work under consideration—providing care. Soft skills training is used in many other industries, but when it comes to caregiving work it seems inadequate, no matter how slickly presented. Studies of training courses in emotional management or customer service in the airline industry or at Disneyland have revealed highly organized and well-tuned training apparati.[7] Caring labor, however, unlike interpersonal service work more broadly,[8] may not be as amenable to standardization and control because the emotional, cognitive, and physical abilities required are of a different mixture; because the goals of caring labor are somewhat different; because there is a higher probability of the unexpected and unpredictable in health care work; and because patients are fundamentally more vulnerable than "clients," imposing different sorts of obligations on those who provide services to them. One union official I interviewed somewhat jarringly praised the management and customer service at Disneyland, though I am quite sure she had not thought through its applicability to health care. Veronica, a nursing assistant, talked about how she was taught in a customer service in-service that patients were "clientele" and the hospital was a "hotel." "I just go along with it," she said dryly. "I know it's a patient, because you go into a room and somebody asks you for a bed pan when you're bringing a meal."

While at times the participants "went along with it," at others they did not. Participants exposed the inapplicability of the courses to their specific situations by raising difficult questions, but also in other, more subtle ways. As mentioned, in the customer service retreat, in which the trainer emphasized that a hospital "is like any other corporation," participants wrote advertisements for their unit. The exercise did not necessarily have the intended effect, though it certainly tapped into the creativity of the hospital staff. The participants were asked to read their advertisements aloud, and one nursing assistant had to stop reading hers after the line "anyone is welcome—good credit, bad credit," because the laughter was so loud. The ad cleverly imitated common advertising directed at poor communities, where businesses offer loans to even those with bad credit, for outrageously high interest rates. Think for instance, about ads for renting furniture on credit, ads that are never seen in affluent neighborhoods. The participants' raucous laughter suggested that if they saw the hospital as a business, it was as one that serves and suckers the poor at the same time. It was also funny because the hospital could not pick and choose its "clientele"—the public hospital where these workers were employed could not deny someone care on the basis of their ability to pay. Staff have to care for all comers. The nursing assistant's ad called into question the premise of the exercise. And the exercise encouraged far more good will than Pictionary—participants even clapped for one another after each ad was read—but at the expense of the hospital and the instructor.

In a different, but no less political and significant, instance of participant resistance, the instructor of the customer service retreat asked participants to find out something new about the woman sitting next to her, a "dark secret," as she off-handedly put it. When the participants, largely nursing assistants (PCTs), went around the room to share what they had learned, one nursing assistant said about her neighbor, "I learned that her dark secret is she has eight children by eight different fathers." This was met by peals of laughter—"they'll be talking now!" said one woman. This moment produced some real solidarity in the room. The participants found this send-up of a racial stereotype hilarious. The only nonblack or Hispanic people in the room were myself and the instructor, and the joke was not meant for us. The bonding that this moment produced—bonding around the common experience of living with racism, being supervised and trained by people who do not experience race as a barrier—was different from the kind of bonding around loyalty to the hospital or the possibilities of customer service the trainer was aiming for.

Participants in the customer service retreat undermined the course in these indirect ways because the instructor was part of the hospital management and clearly established in the beginning of the day that she would not entertain complaints about short-staffing and other problems on the shop floor. The communication skills instructor, however, opened herself up to these issues, so that she in particular seemed to have trouble holding together the message of her course in the face of participants' questions. (Though perhaps that made the participants more receptive to her ideas. The participants in the customer service retreat seemed cool toward the instructor; in the communication skills training, many of the participants were obviously giving the instructor the benefit of a doubt.) The communications skills instructor would likely not have been pleased to learn that Gloria said she was empowered and inspired by the course to give her managers a piece of her mind. After attending communication skills classes for two days, Gloria was astonished and outraged that the following day she was pulled into a meeting for all unit clerks where management delineated new tasks and responsibilities they should perform. "It was an ambush," Gloria declared. From the communication skills classes she had taken "this feeling of security, about what our job description really was, what we're supposed to do, what we shouldn't tolerate." Yet the very next day she, along with several new and untrained clerks, was pressured to do tasks that she felt were part of a nursing assistant's job. Management asked the clerks to escort patients to their rooms, and Gloria argued, "That's not part of my job. What if the patient collapses? I have no medical training—that should be your nursing attendant or nurse." Gloria said she had been waiting to bring these issues up with management and the communication skills course had renewed her desire to do so. She could not restrain herself when the course was followed so quickly by what appeared to be fresh attempts to exploit her. News of Gloria's outburst even reached her mother, a nurse at another of the hospital's sites.

The participants found ways in the courses to raise the tangible issues about which they were most concerned and around which they might most readily mobilize, such as understaffing and the lack of seemingly mundane supplies like combs and toothpaste. There was also, always, the issue of livable wages. At the in-service at the home care agency, where aides' wages were capped at $7.50 an hour, one aide said proudly to the instructor, "to be a professional, you have to love your career," to which another responded sarcastically, "yes, because it sure ain't for the money."

These are collective issues that cannot be changed through individual attitude adjustment. Resolving such issues requires organizational and systemic changes—changes that could be guided by workers' concerns such as those identified in the training seminars. The federal waver monies allotted for "managed care readiness" or infrastructural and organizational reforms from which the need for much of the soft skills training ostensibly derived, however, were spent largely on building outpatient clinics and implementing new computerized information systems, especially for billing and accounting purposes. Indeed, when the CHCCDP funds for training were distributed, hospitals had difficulty determining how to spend them and do so quickly. Hospital and union staff, along with the trainers they hired, seemed to be caught off guard because the funds arrived suddenly and in unprecedented sums. Moreover, they were under pressure because the state would not release subsequent CHCCDP cycles of funding for infrastructure until the training funds had also been spent. 2003 reports filed by thirty voluntary hospitals show that those hospitals had by then spent on average only about one-third of the training grants allotted in the first three (of five) cycles of the grant program, suggesting the training grants were not driven by the urgent needs of hospitals or the health care workforce. There was little systematic planning for how to spend the training money, let alone planning for how to link training with creative organizational change. Soft skills training was, in my view, a readily available category for spending, since such courses were commonplace in the private sector. It also seemed to fit with the pro-market, pro-"customer" mindset behind restructuring.

In addition, some hospitals already had experience with customer service–type training because JCAHO rewarded it. The training consultant who taught at nursing homes had previously been a social worker at a highly regarded rehabilitation hospital. In 1998, she explained, the hospital implemented a training program as part of a total quality management (TQM) initiative leading up to JCAHO's survey. "And we passed with flying colors," she said. "They loved the project, they loved what we had done. And then when the survey was over it was a fight to keep it going, to keep the priority on that." The training consultant who had also been an executive at a large hospital that carried out customer service training said that even though "she never saw customer service training as a real need,"

> It's easier to train than to analyze the problem and say, hey, we need to change the structure.... The TQM was coming from the Joint Commission with an emphasis on customer service, but ... rather than deal with how you're really going to change customer service they went out and did a lot of customer service training ... So what they did, rather than really change the organization and structures and change the culture, they took the easiest way out. I think it was across the board in hospitals.

Later she quipped, "as they say in training, when you have a problem, you don't solve the problem: you train."

In 2002, when I noted, in interviews with several 1199 Training and Upgrading Fund officials who had coordinated the spending of CHCCDP grants, that often the infrastructure or institutional supports were not in place for workers to create the better workplaces soft skills trainers envisioned, one official said, "exactly. But that's where we come in and say this training is not meaningful." The official said they now intervened in the case of customer service training by "legislating" to hospitals that such training could be provided only if there was "buy in" from the top administrators, if everyone participated—including managers and doctors, and if there was some sort of "supported follow-up." Another training fund representative said they were going forward with customer service training only if it could be linked to "measured improvement" in both employee and patient satisfaction. There are some suggestions that by 2002 the proportion of grants spent on soft skills training was indeed diminishing. Training nurses became an obvious, necessary way to spend the money once the

nursing shortage became apparent in the late 1990s. By the 2002 reauthorization of HCRA, over $34.3 million of $56 million in grants made to the
New York City region under that program were spent on training new
nurses or on their "skill enhancement"[9] (although that might not preclude
soft skills).

This apparent recognition of the problems with soft skills training was
nevertheless unconvincing, in part because the actual programs I observed
placed so much emphasis on accepting the status quo. 1199 had by deed, if
not by word, endorsed the messages of these courses—that issues of short-
staffing or lack of resources are inevitable and beyond change and that
frontline health care workers alone must bear the burden of resolving conflict introduced by coworkers with far more power and discretion. Furthermore, by 2002, tens of thousands of workers had already been sent to
such training. 1199 officials undoubtedly knew before they commissioned
a study of it in 2003[10] that multiskilling and reengineering had devastating
effects on morale and that many hospitals had rolled back the reforms that
had supposedly necessitated communication and customer service skills
training. My perception was that they funded an evaluation of communication skills training in 2001, for which I was an investigator, because they
were concerned the training failed to address the real needs and concerns
of their members.

When I asked several representatives of the 1199 Training and Upgrading Fund whether the Fund's programs were evaluated, two of them referred me to a forthcoming Conference Board of Canada report, which was
to include the case of 1199's joint labor-management Funds. The report,
however, focused mostly on vague outcomes and cited only one evaluation
study: the study of communication skills training of which I was a part.
The Conference Board repeated our first conclusion that the communication skills program "contributed to workers' personal and professional
well-being. The newly learned communications skills improved the workers'
ability to cope with stressful situations in their jobs and also gave them
important skills with which to manage their professional relationships."[11]
But our second conclusion, reported in the executive summary with equal
standing, was ignored. We concluded that "communication skills training has a very limited effect on those factors that make health care work
conflict-prone, such as the hierarchical nature of health care occupations,
'jurisdictional negotiations' over job descriptions, staffing problems, or

racial and gender-based biases and inequalities." We argued that hospitals needed to train physicians and all managerial staff in communication skills if it was to have lasting effect. In addition, they needed to revise organizational structures in response to problems identified in communication skills training or follow-up and reduce reliance on floating and use of agency staff. We also suggested that hospitals manage patient care in interdisciplinary teams that include nursing assistants and develop regular mechanisms for staff feedback to management; minimize physical and spatial barriers to interdisciplinary communication; upgrade computer technology to facilitate information sharing; and design a more flexible system for constructing job descriptions.

Then, in 2003, the Training and Upgrading Fund reported that it had "secured state funding of almost $5 million to support customer service training."[12] Similarly, the 2003 reports New York City voluntary hospitals filed with the state on their use of CHCCDP funds showed that during the second and third cycles of the grant, most of which had yet to be spent, hospitals (public and private) planned to offer 53,095 "training encounters" in customer service training and 24,230 in cultural diversity/cultural competency.[13] Despite the union officials' seeming skepticism about soft skills training, one official at the Training and Upgrading Fund still talked about customer service training as a way of "reorganizing work," and the second remained optimistic about this kind of training. The hospital in which I observed the communication skills training in 2001 was continuing the training in 2003, both expanding the program and going back to do "follow-ups." Another training fund official who organized training grants for nursing homes spoke eloquently about the need to "restructure work to give people a voice," but then described training programs that involved only workers, not management, and put the impetus for providing better care with frontline staff. Even if this training has since been significantly reformed and repositioned, so that there is "buy-in" from the top or measured improvements or less pro-market ideology, soft skills training cannot accomplish what collective action might.

The idea that workers need to take greater control and responsibility for the conditions in which they find themselves cannot, however, be wholly dismissed. The need for change in health care settings is so urgent that administrators' and managers' failure to create it is no reason for frontline health care workers not to take some initiative. Furthermore, problems or conflicts health care workers encounter on the job cannot all be blamed on management or a lack of resources and staff; individuals can still make the decision to be more collegial, to cooperate more, and to make their workplace as positive and rewarding as possible. Undoubtedly there are individual workers with terrible and destructive attitudes, as in any other workplace. Still, one's attitude is decidedly not more important than the past, than education, than money, than circumstances, than failures, than successes, than what other people think or say or do—than the political and material circumstances that limit what kinds of change are and are not possible. And one's attitude is certainly not more important than these circumstances for those who face systematic and structural barriers to fair treatment at work and even economic self-sufficiency.

These courses unveiled the discontent that is always near the surface for these workers. Some of the training courses (inadvertently) provided a space and moment for collective engagement, which was clearly less likely to happen back on the unit floor, where increased workloads and pressing patient needs make it difficult to have sustained conversations or begin a process of collective reflection. Even if such moments of engagement were fleeting and quickly silenced by the drone of market metaphors, the "workforce" emerged in these moments not as a glob of skills and credentials to be molded as the labor market and managerial trends supposedly dictate, but as a collection of hard-working and good-humored women, whose tolerance for exploitation is not unlimited.[14]

The fact that workers were not actively rebelling against training programs such as soft skills or multiskilling cannot be read as an indication of a lack of critical awareness or an unwillingness to speak their minds.[15] We may not soon see soft skills training courses turned into grassroots campaigns against the organization of health care work and the U.S. health care system more broadly, but neither do I think we will soon see such courses turn out scores of allied health care workers convinced that their attitudes are destroying the health care system. These courses revealed the potential grounds for solidarity and collective action among these workers, an energy that might, under different conditions, form the basis for progressive change in the health care system and the organization of health care work. Soft skills training may be an attempt to harness that energy, depoliticize it, and turn it inward upon the self. It is, however, a crude attempt, in moments as likely to incite as to placate.

6

Training without End

Upgrading

In 1970, a prominent health care advocacy group commented, "the stagnant hierarchy, supported by elaborate credentialing requirements and arrogant professionalism, turns most hospital jobs into dead-end jobs: a porter or aide is stuck forever as a porter or aide."[1] Reports of how health care workforce training grants were spent in New York suggest that by the early 2000s, more efforts were directed toward individual upgrading and tuition assistance programs that supported workers' attempts to get out of dead-end jobs. This shift was driven by several factors. In light of the nursing shortage, nursing positions became an obvious means of mobility. Industry insiders also indicated that 1199 and the state had begun to question the long-term value of many soft skills training programs (though such training continued). Furthermore, because managed care failed to have radical effects on the health care industry, substantial changes at the organizational level requiring training were also less than anticipated. Finally, hospital and 1199 Training and Upgrading Fund personnel were under pressure to spend the training portion of the CHCCDP grants quickly (because future cycles of infrastructure grants would not be released until the training portion had been spent). Upgrading and tuition assistance programs were recognized as effective ways to spend down funds. Upgrading programs, in which individual workers are supported in external training or education programs, tend to involve more costs: tuition, paying a salary to the worker while they are released to attend school, and paying replacement salary costs to their employer.

In this chapter, we will encounter a number of examples of people who, thanks to training and education programs, have not been "stuck forever" as a porter or an aide. But we will also see the many hurdles that still exist to creating career ladders, including elaborate credentialing requirements and exclusive notions of professionalism, which training alone cannot overcome. The time and commitment required to make a career in health care is substantial, and the way that training and education plays out in the lives of health care workers requires costs and sacrifices inconsistent with the promise and potential of the most prosperous country in the world. Finally, implicit in the very nature of upgrading programs, as in the health care advocacy group's formulation, is the message that there is something wrong with being a porter or an aide forever. This message is demoralizing to health care workers and may have unintended negative consequences for labor unions such as 1199, for whom training and upgrading is now a signature piece of the benefit package they offer to members.

Individual upgrading programs represent the attempt to create career paths, to sustain the dream of upward mobility. As one training program administrator said, "For workers today, learning must be a lifetime pursuit." A highly touted feature of the so-called knowledge economy, lifelong learning conjures up the image of gradually ascending steps, rather than the circles, detours, and cul de sacs that often characterize it. Allied health care workers' experiences show what lifelong learning more likely entails for the majority of Americans in a service-dominated economy and the extent to which U.S. workers today must continually study, just to be.

Getting Ahead

While private corporations and public bureaucracies have traditionally created career ladders internal to the organization, in health care such ladders are virtually nonexistent. The historical dominance of the medical profession means the practices and responsibilities of allied health care providers, including nurses, were carved out of the physicians' role or obtained only on the condition—and sometimes fiction—of ultimate physician control. Occupations in health care are organized and regulated through state agencies or professional associations that function across organizations, rather than within them. In addition, professional associations, credentialing agencies, labor unions, and state regulations all contribute to the proliferation and ossification of specialized job titles in health care. Any career progression in health care requires going back to school for new certifications or licenses, and sometimes the "progression" that results is not very tangible. There is little articulation between various certificates and degrees in health care; one does not, for example, get credit toward medical school because of experience as a nurse. Nor does one get credit toward nursing school if one is an LPN or nursing assistant. The same holds true throughout the range and hierarchy of health care occupations. Creating career ladders for individual health care workers is therefore a considerable challenge.

Making a Career Ladder at Bayside Hospital

When Steve, the respiratory therapist studying to become a physician assistant (PA), walks into the community hospital on Long Island where he has worked since graduating from high school, he is greeted by staff and patients at every turn. "It's a small town," he said, "my whole life is at Bayside Hospital." He even met his wife there (with whom he has two young daughters), when she was doing her clinical rotation as part of her pharmacist training.

Steve started at Bayside[2] as a housekeeper, which was a union (1199) job, saying it was a way to get his foot in the door of the hospital and make money while he attended college. He obtained an associate's degree from Nassau Community College and in 1995 completed his bachelor's at St. John's University, majoring in biology. Steve always wanted to work in health care, though his specific aspirations changed along the way. He said, "PA school is something I've been wanting for a while, since I started in college," but when he was a kid "all I could ever think of was being a doctor." His grades at Nassau were not great, and though they improved at St. John's, he gave up the idea of medical school because of them. Entry into PA programs, however, is also competitive: Most require a bachelor's degree, substantial credits in the sciences, and several thousand hours of clinical experience. Steve therefore decided to become a respiratory therapist so he could acquire clinical experience while being paid for it. In 1996, he switched out of housekeeping to a part-time job in the central supply department while he pursued a second associate's degree in respiratory therapy, again from Nassau Community College. He was hired by Bayside Hospital as a respiratory therapist in 1997. In 2001, he began the 1199 Training and Upgrading Fund's PA program, a forgivable-loan arrangement that paid for him to attend a private, not-for-profit college on Long Island, and he continued to work part-time as a respiratory therapist at Bayside.

Steve identified himself as a caregiver. He did not want to go into the highest-paying PA specialty—surgery—because he wanted to interact with patients. He could not imagine doing anything outside of health care and explained this by saying, "my parents were older when they had me, like forty-two, so the majority of my time was spent with older people… I realized there's a need for older people to be taken care of." His father, a postal worker, volunteered at a local hospital on Sundays, giving patients the Eucharist, and took Steve along. Steve even remembered the smell of hospitals fondly. Steve's Catholicism inflected his talk about working in health care, describing the work as having a selfless and almost sacred dimension. "People working together in a collaborative fashion to save another life—to me that's incredible."

In the working-class area of Long Island where Steve grew up, health care rather than blue-collar industry is now more likely to provide the route into stable work. Though some men are going into predominantly female occupations like nursing, many are likely drawn to technical and paraprofessional positions that are not viewed, and therefore not penalized in terms of status and pay, as feminine. Steve spoke somewhat dismissively of the nursing profession. Even though he identified as a caregiver and had worked as a housekeeper, his attitude seemed to be informed by the notion that it was women's work. Daniel, also from Long Island, started his working life as a construction worker but after he was laid off went into the relatively new occupation of operating room technician (OR tech, sometimes called surgical technicians). He suggested the transition was less dramatic than it might seem, since he found that the operating room too was a decidedly masculine environment: "It's a rough, tough place...like being in the Army or the Navy."[3]

In addition to being a less "feminine" health care occupation, as a physician assistant Steve will have the status of a professional. His credential will signal that he has obtained substantial higher education and bring a degree of autonomy and responsibility. He won't enjoy the status of a physician, as Steve seemed acutely aware. Steve's experience represents one type of "upgrading" and upward mobility that can be facilitated by funded training opportunities—a best-case scenario given the nature of the health care occupational hierarchy and labor market. As a housekeeper just out of high school, he made less than $10.00 an hour. In 2001, the average starting salary of physician assistants was close to $60,000 a year.[4]

Steve's experience is typical, however, in terms of what needs to be done to make a career in a health care setting. Steve's path cannot accurately be called a "ladder" because each step forward required going back to school anew, so that Steve had spent almost fifteen years simultaneously working and going to school (not to mention getting married and starting a family). Steve said he has probably taken half a dozen courses in anatomy and physiology, though he said each program teaches it a "slightly different way." He moved from being a housekeeper, to a central supply clerk, to a respiratory therapist, and then to a physician assistant. By the time he finishes, he will have two associate's degrees, a bachelor's degree, and several credentials, not least his PA license. As the string of credentials after many health care professionals' names attests, this is not rare in health care.

It required tremendous initiative for Steve to put together a series of occupations that would work to his advantage. Driven to become a PA and with the skills and ability to make it through college, Steve seized a rare opportunity—a fully funded training program. There is no question that the opportunity to enroll in a full-time PA program, for which tuition was paid and provided salary replacement, allowed him to achieve his goals with less sacrifice and in less time. On the other hand, this training program did not create a career ladder that was previously unavailable. In addition the training Steve pursued was unrelated to sudden changes in the health care industry brought on by managed care and occupational restructuring. In fact, his training and education is exceptionally valuable because it transcended short-term fads and temporary reforms. He chose an occupation for which there is a growing demand across the United States and that has an established turf in the U.S. health care system.

Steve is an exemplar of success, but his experience draws attention to the amount of time and backtracking such success entails. Perhaps more important is the kind of lifestyle Steve was living: constant work and study with little "free" time. Steve's investment of time and energy may pay off once he is working as a PA. For him, like more and more working-class Americans, achieving a measure of security may involve spending many years beyond high school simultaneously working and studying to build a career ladder where others have been torn down. At the end of PA school, Steve will also sacrifice something very dear: As a condition of the forgivable loan program that financed his training, he will be required to work for several years in a hospital where PAs are 1199 members. Though his whole life is at Bayside, PAs there are not unionized.

Getting By in the World of Feminized Labor

Grace, the diet coordinator from Trinidad, was just about to graduate from a physical therapy assistant (PTA) program at New York University when I interviewed her. We met in a cramped office in the bowels of Grandview, a major academic medical center, next to the hospital kitchen. Grace was clearly pressed for time—the staff were preparing a luncheon for "secretary's day" at the hospital. Grace started at the hospital as a dietary aide in 1990 and had worked her way through the several jobs and promotions available in the kitchen. After twelve years, she was a dietary coordinator. Throughout her years at the hospital, Grace pursued other certificates or training programs and worked second jobs.

In 1993, the care nurses gave Grace's newborn son inspired her to complete the three-month certified nursing assistant (CNA) program. Grace said at one point she "always wanted to be a nurse." A state employment center paid for the CNA course—Grace qualified for the program's means-tested assistance even though she was working full-time. Grace then took a second job as a per diem nursing assistant on the night shift at a nursing home in Brooklyn, making about $15 an hour. At the same time, she became full-time at Grandview, working as an inventory clerk for the corporation newly subcontracted to run food services. Eventually, she said her "back went out" working at the nursing home: "This was like twenty patients to one person. I was too young for that." Feeling that she was young enough to still do other things, Grace quit the nursing home.

In the early 1990s, Grace also attended Technical Career Institutes (TCI)—a private, for-profit, two-year college offering occupational certificates and associate's degrees—to study computer technology. Grace said her decision to study computer technology was rooted in the same thing as her desire to be a nurse. "I love fixing things with my hands," she said. But after receiving financial aid and spending nearly two years of full-time study at TCI, Grace never obtained a degree or credential. The school abruptly shut down the computer technology program and "put me in electrical engineering. So I was in that program, then I decided I didn't like it any more so I got out of that."

By then, around 1995, Grace had been promoted to her current position of diet coordinator at Grandview, for which she was making $13.57 per hour in 2002. In 1996, she paid $500 to attend a 120-hour Dietary Manager certificate course at New York University (NYU). She said she might have been reimbursed by the 1199 Training and Upgrading Fund for that course if she had applied, "but I said not everything you do is for the money." At the same time, she also began working part-time for a home health care agency, caring for an elderly patient on nights and weekends until the patient's death in 1997. (Grace's mother was, by this time, also working as a home health attendant.) Along the way, to make extra money, Grace also worked as a bartender (off the books) and as a crew leader for the U.S. Census.

Hoping to combine her enjoyment of working with her hands, fixing things, and taking care of people, Grace looked into the PTA program at NYU (where she was also taking a sign-language class). When she took the entrance exam for the program in 1997, by chance she sat next to an 1199 member whom the Training and Upgrading Fund had sent to take the exam. Grace learned from her neighbor that the Fund offered financial assistance for the PTA program. After passing the exam, Grace signed up with the Fund, and was given paid release time from work while she attended school. Though there were a few hiccups along the way (she had to repeat a biology course), at the time of our interview Grace was one month from graduating, with an associate's degree, and had already been offered two jobs as a PTA—at a hospital and a nursing home. She said her starting wage as a PTA would be around $35–38,000 a year.[5] She hoped to eventually go back to NYU for a program in health and policy planning.

Being a second-generation immigrant, Grace finished high school in the United States and had the legal status, official diploma, and youthful lack of responsibility that made it possible for her to avoid working as a nanny or as a domestic in someone's home—work that many female immigrants from the English-speaking Caribbean do at some point. On the other hand, Grace did not avoid the realm of feminized service work altogether. Her first job in health care was essentially domestic work—preparing food for others—and her other jobs in health care did or will entail providing hands-on care. Though health care provides a crucial opportunity for women without a college education to make a decent wage, much of it is still feminized domestic and caring work, and as such it is underpaid and not recognized as a basis for promotion or responsibility.

Like Steve, Grace had been in near-constant contact with education and training programs since finishing high school, but she had by no means arrived in an occupational niche with built-in opportunities for upward mobility. As a PTA, there is no career ladder. One healthcare workforce analyst I interviewed singled out the gulf between the PTA and the physical therapist as an apt example of how poorly articulated the connections between occupations in health care are.

Grace has had more encounters than Steve with the insecurities of working and learning in the sub-baccalaureate labor market, such as for-profit educational institutions that suddenly shut down entire programs of study and nonunion service jobs that pay $3.35 an hour. Grace surmounted these obstacles by working two jobs or enrolling in a new educational program. She was always looking for a new opportunity, and she was never on public assistance. The main bread-winner for her family, she pays for her son to attend a private Catholic school, rather than the underfunded and struggling public school in her neighborhood. Still, fourteen years out of high school, Grace's only formal credential is an associate's degree. This degree is an important accomplishment, for it means she has also taken the basic college courses necessary if she later chooses or needs to go into a baccalaureate-degree program. Still, it is little to show for her years of effort. Her experience is by no means exceptional among the allied health care workers with whom I spoke.

Grace faced a number of barriers to mobility in a gender-segregated labor market, but they were mitigated to some extent by the presence and services of a strong union. Both Steve and Grace obtained entry-level jobs in hospitals and worked their way from support departments—where they did work not specific to health care—to jobs involving patient care and contact. This kind of pattern is not uncommon among New York City's allied health care workers because most of the jobs in these hospitals—from dishwashers to registered nurses—are unionized. Through union efforts and programs, 1199 members gain access to training opportunities and are, in many instances, given first consideration for job openings in the industry. Few other sectors of New York's economy offer such stability in the sub-baccalaureate labor market. Only unionized jobs in education and civil service offer comparable opportunities to the city's working class, and those sectors are under increasing financial duress in an era of cost-cutting and neoliberal government. Americans, however, continue to age and get sick, and health care steadily adds jobs.

"Anything I Can Learn"

Cesar, who came to the United States from the Dominican Republic as a teenager, lived with his wife and young son in a well-tended, prewar building just off the Grand Concourse.[6] The ornate, wrought-iron bars on the windows and intricate tile patterns in the hallway floors of his building reflected the neighborhood's more illustrious beginnings. His apartment, though not large, had high ceilings and was airy and bright, with large windows, a sunken living room, and shiny hardwood floors. Cesar's mother, who used to work in a garment factory but had retired, lived in the same building.

After high school, Cesar's first full-time job was as a security officer at Bronx Hospital. Cesar had no "real love" for security work, which was difficult and at times aggravating. Still, it was a secure 1199 job that paid the bills. There was also a lot of camaraderie in the department. Though the union was "always offering all types of programs," Cesar wasn't very interested in the health care field. In 1994, however, he signed up for a pharmacy technician program sponsored by the union and the hospital. He attended class five mornings a week for nine months. "I completed the program, but at that time the hospital was in the process of automating the pharmacy so they were actually getting rid of the personnel...and weren't willing to take anybody new to train." There was no job for him when he was done. He could have looked for a job at another hospital, but other hospitals were likewise transforming their pharmacy departments, and Cesar had seniority at Bronx Hospital. As we were talking, Cesar started to tell me the pharmacy tech training had been a waste of time, but he diplomatically stopped himself and said it had helped him later with the OR tech program.

In 2000, Cesar saw a bulletin board posting for an OR tech program for Bronx Hospital. After talking to a friend who worked in the operating room, he decided it was worth a try. He brushed up on his math skills to prepare for the entrance exam and was one of four hospital employees (out of at least a hundred who applied) to be accepted. Given paid release time from work, he attended the program at the Consortium for Worker Education Monday through Friday for nine months. After completing the program, Cesar worked in security for five more months while he waited for a position to open at Bronx Hospital. It finally did, and at the time of our interview he'd been an OR tech for about six months, making just over $18 an hour.

"I was never interested in the medical field before," Cesar said. He didn't know what he was getting into when he started the OR tech program: "When I first started I wasn't really sure that it was for me." The job is demanding—OR techs prepare the operating room, get instruments and equipment ready, and are at the surgeon's side throughout the procedure. The emotional demands—watching the surgeries and dealing with what several OR techs described as highly volatile surgeons—are just as great as the technical demands, but Cesar said he enjoyed working with the equipment and machines. He described how interesting it was to see an orthopedic knee surgery for the first time.

At the time of our interview, Cesar was finishing a ten-week film production class at a four-year City University of New York (CUNY) college in the Bronx, which would qualify him to produce a show for the CUNY cable television channel. He said he really likes school: "anything I can learn." He was interested in taking some of the computer courses (noncredit, certificate programs) at the recently opened CUNY on the Concourse. He also expressed interest in becoming a medical equipment salesperson, an occupation he discovered once he began working in the operating room.

As with Grace and Steve, school and education was a permanent presence in Cesar's life. For all three, school was either something about which they were constantly thinking and planning to do to keep moving forward, or they were actually enrolled in classes in one program or another. All three moved into and out of training and education programs for a variety of reasons—some of them personal but some of them created by a convoluted training and education industry. All three encountered obstacles that resulted from inadequate information about the status or requirements of the local labor market. Grace and Cesar, in particular, both devoted considerable amounts of time to a training or education program that they did not complete. The computer program Grace started at TCI was terminated before she could finish her degree. In Cesar's case, he never imagined that the union and hospital would pay for him to attend a training program for which there were no jobs. Not only did he not know the status of the labor market for pharmacy technicians, apparently neither did the union. Though the union presumably learned from that experience, it shows that it is not easy to predict employers' fluctuating demands. Similarly, Cesar's colleague in the security department, Linda, who also went through the OR tech program, had to wait even longer (eight months) to get a job as an OR tech at the hospital after she finished the program. During that time, she went back to being a security officer. Perhaps wary of giving the impression that they were somehow ungrateful, Grace, Cesar, and Linda did not express anger or resentment about these disruptions to their progress. Said Grace about not finishing at TCI: "It's just something I wanted to try, it's not what I wanted to do. It's not a big disappointment."

Unlike Grace, however, Cesar did not have any sort of college degree, even though postsecondary education and training had been a regular part of his life for about sixteen years. OR techs, while well-paid relative to their training, do not get college credits as part of the training program, and the job is not the first step in an internal career ladder. As Daniel, who had been an OR tech for some time and also taught in a hospital-based training program, explained, the OR tech position was created to take over some tasks formerly done by operating room nurses. It is an occupation carved out with cost factors in mind above all, not the possibilities for development and mobility for those who do the job. Indeed, it entails the downsizing of mid-level jobs above them. Cesar and Linda were also making less money as OR techs than they had as security officers, mostly because there was no longer the possibility of working overtime—which had been a crucial means of increasing their income when they were security officers. Like evenings and weekends spent in training programs, overtime is another way in which health care workers must sacrifice time to get by.[7]

The explanation for Grace and Cesar's failure to achieve more (if that's the perspective one chooses to take) is not poor individual choices or a lack of effort and motivation. Such patterns of engagement with education are an inevitable product of the way education and work are now organized. Moreover, it seems that experiences such as theirs are increasingly accepted as the norm for working-class Americans. Their experiences are indicative of a general shift in expectations and values in our culture. Education is reduced to credentials but also considered valuable regardless of the worth of those credentials. In the health care workforce training industry, there is a blurring of training and education, or an indifference to their distinction. Though the distinctions between these various types of training matter when asking certain types of questions, just as the potential earnings of a college graduate and a high school graduate differ very much, the reality for many workers entangled in the education and training industry is an active and near-perpetual deferment of traditional "outcomes." Examining the occupational and educational histories of allied health care workers, there are few orderly steps—where credentials lead to advancement and advancement to more credentials. Although Cesar and Grace have achieved a measure of mobility, what is remarkable is how modest their wages still are and how hard and long they had to study to obtain them.

"They Say This Is the Land of Opportunities"

"I'm not comfortable just working like that. I wanted to be a nurse," Wanda said about her most recent return to school at the age of forty-five. By "working like that" she meant working without also developing herself and her talents. When we spoke in 2002, Wanda, who became a nursing assistant shortly after she immigrated from Trinidad in 1987, was a licensed practical nurse (LPN) and hoped to become a registered nurse (RN). Like Cesar, Steve, and Grace, Wanda had been consistently involved in training and education programs for well over a decade, but her experience in particular shows how the "outcomes" commonly attributed to education and training—a new job, better pay, knowledge—do not always follow in an orderly manner.

Just after Wanda landed her first union (1199) job as a nursing assistant—a year after arriving from Trinidad in 1987—she spent six months in a union-sponsored training program for her GED. Then, in 1995, she completed her LPN certificate after attending a part-time, union-funded program for two years, each evening, after finishing her day shift at the Brooklyn hospital where she worked. Wanda intended to go on into an RN program, but was discouraged by the short-lived and ill-founded predictions of a registered nurse surplus in the mid-1990s. Describing her decision to stop after the LPN program, she said, "I shouldn't have done that because ... if I had continued I would have been finished by now [with the RN degree]." As late as 2002, some health care workers still seemed to have misperceptions of the state of the labor market; as Michelle, an ophthalmic technician and former unit clerk, commented, "there's no job security as nurse. You just don't know if you'll be able to get a job." On the other hand, and even though there is now a widespread nursing shortage, Michelle's perspective probably remains an accurate view of just how vulnerable nurses are to layoffs and managerial whims, made abundantly clear at the height of restructuring.

Several others I interviewed who had completed college courses found it difficult to take all the nursing prerequisites because the classes were full, offered at inconvenient times, or because of other bureaucratic problems with financial aid or tuition assistance. The confidence and near-apocalyptic pitch of predictions of the nursing surplus convinced universities to eliminate or contract their nurse training programs and they were unprepared for the nursing shortage that emerged only a few years later. Union-secured training funds helped them respond. As Wanda said:

> When I graduated [from the LPN program], they were not hiring RNs anymore. They were laying-off the RNs. So I said what's the point, you know? And I just kept on working as an LPN. And then the union also stopped giving the course, or paying for the course for RNs because it [the RN shortage] was not so extreme then. And until it was ... then we got some flyers saying that they had started paying for the RN course. So I said look, I'll take the opportunity.

After obtaining her LPN credential, Wanda continued to work as a nursing assistant for three years, a sustained period of underemployment (her skills were beyond those required by her job). Though she could have tried to get a job elsewhere as an LPN, she opted to wait for a job to open up at her hospital because she had seniority there and lived one block away, in a hospital-owned apartment. In the meantime, she took an introductory computer course at the union's training facility in Brooklyn and also completed a "nurse tech" course at a proprietary school, in which she was trained how to perform EKGs and hang intravenous (IV) bags. Although she had already learned these skills as part of her LPN training, she thought the nurse tech designation might be useful as long as she remained a nursing assistant. While waiting to get an LPN position, she moved through a number of units in the hospital as a nursing assistant.

After three years passed, Wanda was finally hired as an LPN in the emergency room. She was surprised, however, by her new wage: at $18 an hour, it was only two dollars more than what she earned on the evening shift as a nursing assistant—"which is no money," Wanda pointed out. In 2001, the median wage for registered nurses in New York City was, by contrast, $28.20 an hour.[8] Yet on a day-to-day basis, Wanda's responsibilities were much closer to those of an RN than a nursing assistant. Comparing her job to that of RNs, Wanda said, "We do everything. There are only certain things you don't do, like hang blood and blood product. But you do everything else: you have to give injections, you have to put in the IV, you have to put in the Hep-Lock [an IV access line]. We do everything as a nurse. So we need more money."

Many trainers and planners in the health workforce area present the LPN position as an important step up for nursing assistants. An official with DC37's training department said the LPN is "definitely a career ladder" for patient care associates (the public hospitals' multiskilled nursing assistant). Several nursing assistants I interviewed were thinking about becoming LPNs. Marie was hoping to get into the LPN program offered by CUNY on the Concourse. Even Linda, who had been a security officer and recently became an OR tech, still talked about going into nursing and mentioned that she went to CUNY on the Concourse to pick up information on the LPN program.

There are, however, a number of problems with this emphasis on the LPN credential. First, like OR tech programs, it is a non–credit bearing credential program. LPN programs require completing a nine-month, noncredit, certificate program—often extended into two years of part-time study—and passing a state exam. Students do not receive college credits for completing the LPN program, and the courses they complete do not count toward, or give them advanced standing in, an RN program. For example, when we spoke, Wanda was enrolled in the evenings and weekends in a union-run preparatory program for the CUNY entrance exam so she could get into CUNY and begin to take the nursing prerequisite courses. Though there are a few diploma programs for RNs still in existence, the vast majority of nursing programs require getting a college degree at the same time, either an associate's or bachelor's. Yet despite their lack of college training, LPNs do much of the same work as a college-educated staff nurse.

Marie had already proved her ability to do college-level work and had passed several college courses in the arts and social sciences. Although she had not yet passed the math section of the CUNY exam, this was due largely to a math phobia. If there were enough mentoring and tutoring available, Marie would probably be just as likely to succeed (or fail) in an RN program as an LPN. Linda, too, had already completed some college prerequisites for nursing and had an associate's degree. For her, pursuing a bachelor's degree in nursing would be a much more logical and promising option than an LPN program.

In addition, the widely used entrance exam for LPN programs is regarded by nursing program administrators to be more difficult than either the entrance exam for RN programs or CUNY four-year colleges. This creates a significant problem: People who take and fail the LPN entrance exam are likely to assume this means they have no chance of passing the RN or CUNY-entrance exam. In addition, LPN programs are intense. To prepare to do much of the same work as nurses, more information is in essence crammed into a shorter period of time. And LPN students are less likely to be in school full-time—they are typically working while going to school, which helps explain why the drop-out rates from LPN programs is higher. So, in exchange for passing a rigorous entrance exam, completing a difficult program of study, and dedicating one to two years of their lives, LPNs qualify for a job that pays substantially less than the RN and have a credential that is much less valuable and portable, but they essentially do the same work. In addition, LPNs will not qualify for most promotions within the nursing hierarchy and cannot move into nursing administration and management.

Though an LPN program may be a step up for some individuals in terms of pay and status, it doesn't actually build a ladder. This is especially true when viewed from the vantage point of the labor market as a whole. The LPN is a position developed and used, after all, like that of OR techs and PCTs, to substitute for more highly trained and highly paid workers. If the LPN profession is expanding, that is because the nursing profession is not, or not as much as it might be. The LPN position is a crucial part of hospitals' strategy to get by with the least-paid, least-trained staff possible.

"Miss Education"

Veronica started traveling to the United States from Trinidad in the 1970s to work as a nanny, but she "wanted something more." When we spoke, she was a nursing assistant at Parkview Hospital, a private facility in an affluent Manhattan neighborhood. Shortly after starting at the hospital and becoming an 1199 member in the early 1990s, Veronica enrolled in a GED preparatory class at the union's main training center on 42nd Street. Indeed, she had taken at least one class every semester since then. Before she passed it in 1996, she had taken the GED exam three times, then she stayed on with the same teacher in the 1199 reading and writing program to prepare for the CUNY entrance exam. She passed that the first time. "I said well, if I finished the CUNY exam I may as well try to get some courses in." At the time of our interview, she had completed four college courses. School had been an ongoing, concurrent activity to her work and home life for close to ten years.

Veronica said she wanted to get an associate's degree in nursing, but also said she was taking school one step at a time, not setting a goal too far ahead, while almost apologizing for what she thought must seem like a lack of ambition. "I know I should aim higher...but for me I always say if you go little by little—that's how I take it. I don't know if I'm holding myself back, but that's how I look at it." Veronica seemed above all to be enjoying learning, and was not focused on the credential she might obtain. She wanted to be a nurse so she could take vacations without working sixteen-hour days to save the money to do so. On the whole, however, Veronica seemed to think that being an "aide forever" might not be a bad thing. Her descriptions of her interactions with patients vividly portrayed that she is probably a conscientious and kind nursing assistant and that the work is rewarding to her. "Some tell you their stories," she said of the patients. "I mean you picture this person being head of household for so many years and ending up in the nursing home, and they tell you how many dinner parties they went to and how they felt, and you're there consoling them because you know your time is coming [too]. And you make them feel good."

Near the end of the interview, Veronica mentioned that she talks about the books she had read in her college and college-prep classes with patients at her hospital. Going over to a bookshelf in her living room, she pulled out a folder of hand-written notes from patients, some of which were lists of books they recommended. Among the suggestions were radical political books such as Howard Zinn's *People's History of the United States* and Noam Chomsky's *Understanding Power.Com*. Another list, written by a patient who had been a teacher, was three full pages and included novels on the experience of being an immigrant. Veronica had read some of these books and referred to the lists when she was choosing what to read next. She clearly used her education in interactions with her patients that were based on respect and sharing, in contrast to the disrespect she reported facing from her coworkers, especially nurses.

Yet as we know, Veronica started to say at one point that she wanted to become a nurse because then her work might "mean" something. A number of factors push allied health care workers into participating in education and training programs: the general cultural emphasis in the United States on making something of oneself, the availability of funded training opportunities, and the constant message, communicated in subtle and not-so-subtle ways, that their work and status are somehow inferior. No matter how successful the training and education industry is at providing the basis for individual mobility, in its current form it intensifies the sense of inferiority that so-called lower-level workers face and makes them feel that "I should aim higher." The education and training industry for allied health care workers prospers because workers feel that what they are doing is not important. Health care is a lucrative market for education and training providers because the hierarchical organization of the labor process and huge differences in power and autonomy among health care occupations make feelings of insecurity or inferiority particularly intense among those at the bottom of the hierarchy. Many allied health care workers experience irreconcilable emotions about their abilities and their work. On the one hand, they feel their work is trivial and that they should seek supposedly meaningful work. On the other hand, they know their work is meaningful but also inexplicably undervalued.

Veronica is among the few people I interviewed, all of whom have extensive, ongoing experiences with postsecondary education, who really expressed a love for her classes and studying in itself. Her teacher, whom I also interviewed, assigned students novels to read and stressed critical thinking in his classes. Veronica talked about reading those novels, and described becoming lost in them. But her enjoyment of learning is rewarded neither by the education and training system nor by her coworkers and employers. The training apparatus reinforces the message that she is in some way lacking and should be more ambitious. Moreover, at work, Veronica tells almost none of her coworkers about her studies for fear she will be considered insubordinate or seen as trying to move above her station. Similarly, there are no mechanisms in her workplace for acknowledging, let alone rewarding, the kinds of relationships and conversations she has with patients, which contribute immeasurably to the quality of care.

Veronica's experience raises troubling issues about how the training and education industry interfaces with inequalities of race in addition to those of class. When she discussed the disrespect she feels from nurses, Veronica hinted that it was in part because these nurses were white. Her exposure to racial and cultural discrimination, in addition to occupational and class discrimination, made her feel both that she should be doing more and that she could not discuss the "more" she was doing. The experience of being disrespected was common among nursing assistants I interviewed, and on several occasions they implied that specific instances of disrespect were also instances of racial discrimination. (If their interviewer—me—had not been white, perhaps they would have done more than imply.)

The experiences of Steve, Grace, Cesar, Wanda, and Veronica raise critical questions about the general emphasis on training and education as a remedy for inequality and economic restructuring. Upgrading is valuable for some individuals, but it nonetheless necessitates and normalizes a life of constant work and study. Such upgrading programs also subtly contribute to the idea that those who do not choose a life of constant work and study—in the sense of wage labor and formal training programs—are somehow inferior. They will remain stuck forever as a porter or an aide.

In addition, much of the training reinforced the image of the health care workforce as lacking, whether in skills or a good attitude. The constant emphasis on workers' lack of skills or their need to be multiskilled or upgraded exacerbates, rather than mitigates, workers' feelings that they are underemployed and undervalued. Multiskilling programs can increase the feeling among workers that their employer—and in this case their union—fails to understand the realities of health care work. Roiling just under the surface of the incessant assertion of their lack of skills is a basic dissatisfaction among allied health care workers with their working conditions. Workers know that training and education cannot solve the problems of their working conditions and nature of their work, although in some cases it may help them move out of their current jobs and into those that are better paid. Because of this, many workers see returning to school, quite pragmatically, as the only way to a better quality of life and more fulfilling work.

Of course, individual "upgrading" has long been one of the primary bases of social stability in the United States: the idea that if someone can make it, everyone can. The training and education industry helps some people to do this—though the criteria for "making it" are regularly deflated in light of the apparently unalterable realities of the labor market. 1199's Training and Upgrading Fund has been able to help a good many individuals move forward, but individual upgrading cannot be the basis of class mobility or the eradication of inequality.

Finally, in the lives of these health care workers, working and learning take so much time and energy that there is little left for labor and learning as ends in themselves, as play and as pleasure. Time is increasingly scarce—lifelong learning demands days that are crammed from dawn to dusk with work and school. When I asked health care workers what they did in their "free time," they would invariably laugh. Most claimed they could not remember, or never knew, what free time was. Stanley Aronowitz has argued that for many, work has been trivialized at the same time their leisure is colonized by the products and distractions of consumer culture.[9] For the workers I interviewed, their work is certainly trivialized, but their leisure has been eradicated by the demands of incessant study and work. Many allied health care workers exist on the margins of consumer culture in any case, barely able to afford the products it has to offer. Though wages ranging from $14 to $18 an hour, or roughly $29,000 to $37,000 a year before taxes (the wage range for most workers I interviewed), are better than those at Wal-Mart, in New York City they barely provide the conditions of self-subsistence.

7

From Skills to Meaning

Those with a stake in New York's health care workforce training industry mobilize several arguments in support of their programs. Most prominent is the ubiquitous argument that training and education programs are necessary to compensate for the gap between the skills of the workforce and the requirements of jobs. Common as well is the argument that the industry helps people gain access to working-class jobs and can even be the means of meaningful upward mobility. These rationales warrant further examination to come to a more nuanced, and accurate, explanation of this industry's endurance and ability to command substantial financial, even psychic and emotional, support.

There is little to examine, however, when it comes to the claim that the kinds of training that have been funded in New York City might improve the conditions of health care work or patient care. A glimpse into what multiskilling and soft skills training initiatives actually entailed is enough to show that they were far more likely to accommodate, rationalize, and even exacerbate the difficult working conditions frontline health care workers face. The sources of problems in health care work and pa-tient care are located much further upstream than the attitudes of indi-vidual workers, beyond the reach of short-term, narrow in-services and skills programs. Furthermore, no one in the city's health care sector, in-cluding 1199, has pressed for or developed systematic or ongoing evalua-tions of training programs that would assess their content and their impact on working conditions or the quality of care in health care facilities, even using measures as basic (and limited) as staff or patient satisfaction. A rep-resentative at the Consortium for Worker Education said they had trained 37,000 people in the public hospital system in communication skills, re-sulting in "tremendous changes in hospital environments." This was anec-dotal evidence and especially difficult to believe given what I had observed at one public hospital's customer service retreat and, as important, given that more than a quarter of the workforce in the public hospital system was being laid off at the same time. A nationwide study of the growing num-ber of labor-management training partnerships in health care confirmed that they remain unevaluated elsewhere too. "There are few initiatives to assess the impact of joint efforts on quality and performance," the report concluded.[1] I interpret the fact that those with a stake in the industry have not sought evaluations that might show the impact of their programs on working conditions and patient care as evidence they were never really the primary objects of such training.

Nonetheless, the training industry's self-justification must still rest on more than its supposed ability to provide skills, as we will see. The seeds of a more versatile and open-ended justification were evident when the training sessions I observed became an environment of mutual support, in striking contrast to the workplace. Trainers talked to me not only about skills, but about health care workers' need for meaning and respect, ac-knowledging a pervasive and deeply rooted problem. By tapping into this profound need, and attempting to meet it, training programs that fail to improve conditions in the workplace and rest on the tenuous notions of "skills" and a "skills gap" not only persist, but thrive.

Trainers and educators in many industries have always promised their courses will bridge the gap between the skills of workers and the de-mands of jobs. Recall the words of the administrator at the Consortium for Worker Education: "there's always going to be a need for training and upgrading and there will be other [training] monies available as time goes on because we understand that the economic development of the workforce depends on constantly being upgraded in order to have any kind of job security." In the 1990s in particular, both critics and advocates of restructuring and reengineering believed that the nature of work in health care facilities was soon to be radically transformed and the health care workforce was vastly underprepared for the demands of a market-driven health care sector.

Trainers and educators who justify skills training (whether for communication or performing EKGs) in this way use the same logic that has been ubiquitously used for decades to explain away the declining living standards and prospects of working Americans: It is workers themselves—not policy makers, economists, politicians, or employers—who are responsible for layoffs and declining real wages. Gordon Lafer has shown that since President Ronald Reagan signed the Job Training Partnership Act (JTPA) in 1982, job training funds have been a favorite tool of politicians—both Republican and Democrat—to create the impression, if not the reality, that steps are being made to right a sinking economy, to compensate for the disappearance of manufacturing jobs, to substitute for welfare in the age of a state withdrawal of services, and to help the poor without creating "dependency" on the state. The "skills gap" has even been offered as an explanation for expanding wage inequality in the United States since the 1970s and job training as its solution.[2]

In his classic 1970 account of the "great training robbery," Ivar Berg reported that he stopped interviewing human resources personnel in exasperation, preferring to look for concrete evidence of expanding skill needs prompted by occupational and technological change rather than taking their ritualistic claims that new skills were needed at face value. He found very little evidence. Berg showed there is no substantial disparity between the educational achievements of the U.S. workforce and the educational requirements of jobs. Certainly no such disparity could account for the tremendous growth of formal education.[3] Randall Collins also showed that inflation in employers' hiring requirements far outpaces any increases in the level of skills necessary to perform most jobs, creating what he termed a "credential society."[4]

More recently, in his 2006 book on the effects of layoffs and economic restructuring in the United States, Louis Uchitelle vividly portrayed the limits of job training when the economy simply does not provide enough well-paying, secure jobs. He described the fate of the several thousand airline mechanics laid off by United Airlines in 2002 and 2003 when the airline shut down its cutting-edge maintenance center in Indianapolis, to which the city and state contributed more than half of the $600 million total investment only ten years before. Out of the more than 800 laid-off mechanics sent to a federally funded job retraining program, only 185 were working a year after the center had closed and only 15 had regained or exceeded their United wage levels, which had ranged up to $31 an hour. Uchitelle pointed out that there are not enough high-wage jobs in the economy to soak up these displaced skilled workers. Most unfilled jobs in the U.S. economy have paid less than $10 or $11 an hour in recent years. As Uchitelle put it, "more than 45 percent of the nation's workers, whatever their skills, earned less than $13.25 an hour in 2004, or $27,600 a year for a full-time worker. That is roughly the income that a family of four must have in many parts of the country to maintain a standard of living minimally above poverty level. Surely lack of skill and education does not hold down the wages of nearly half the workforce. Something quite different seems to be true: The oversupply of skilled workers is driving people into jobs beneath their skills and driving down the pay of jobs equal to their skills."[5]

Yet supposed skill deficits was and is the most readily available and popularly accepted justification for the tremendous investment in training and retraining the health care workforce (and a way to avoid direct confrontation with the forces of economic restructuring and reengineering). The skills-gap argument was used both when it appeared health care workers were going to be laid off en masse and when the reality of widespread shortages was revealed. As we have seen, however, neither multiskilling programs nor communication skills training were required by a change in the nature of health care work or organizations. Only computer and coding trainings offered in workplaces when new technologies and systems were introduced seem to fit the traditional depiction of the need for skills training, and these short-term trainings taught a narrow range of skills. The expanding educational levels and credentials required to become a nursing assistant are not due to a change in the nature of the work. The increasing educational levels of nursing assistants, as well as the occupation's stagnating wages, are rather a result of greater competition for direct care jobs. People with higher educational levels are driven into direct care jobs, and employers can raise educational requirements without needing to raise wages. In addition, nursing assistant jobs are more likely to be in settings where the pay is less, such as home care and nursing homes.

Many in the health care workforce training industry nonetheless continue to insist that they are simply responding to employers' needs for more skilled workers. In so doing, they assume that workers' levels of education and training have a significant impact on the economic viability of businesses, in this case hospitals. As a recent review of the skills mismatch hypothesis concluded, "swings in macroeconomic forces had a far greater effect on the nation's fluctuating fortunes in the 1980s and 1990s than the modest trends in school quality or individual attainment." It is impossible to hold a skills mismatch or shortage accountable for economic performance when wide swings in productivity and employment levels occur while the extent of skills and education in the labor force change little. For example, the economic turnaround of the 1990s occurred without any sizeable change in the stock of skills among the U.S. workforce.[6] Employers, as Uchitelle also described, do not create and destroy high-quality or high-wage jobs based primarily on the skills or education of the labor force. They do so on the basis of the location of capital and the potential for profit.

Not unlike the United Airlines fiasco (though on a smaller scale), significant investments—in the form of CHCCDP grants for restructuring and training—were made in several New York City area hospitals that subsequently closed. St. Agnes hospital in Westchester county received over $1.6 million; Union Hospital of the Bronx received over $4.4 million; and Yonkers General Hospital received almost $6 million. These hospitals' fates did not ultimately depend on the skills of their workers or even the adequacy of their reengineering programs. The hospitals' positions were precarious because of the excess of hospital beds and the misalignment of the hospital sector with community needs, which has occurred under the watch of the private hospital sector, and poor financial decisions by their managers.

Many workforce experts tacitly recognize that high-skill jobs do not exist in abundance. They recognize that such jobs have to be created, and some believe that even if such jobs do not exist now, employers will create them once workers are more skilled. In New York City, labor officials argued that multiskilling programs in fact created new, higher quality jobs. When the Center for an Urban Future sought to identify successful workforce development programs in the city, it turned to joint labor-managements programs such as 1199's Training and Upgrading Fund.[7] Joint labor-management training programs are, however, exceptional because they are among the few "labor market intermediaries" with a remote chance at shaping the labor market.[8] In joint programs, unions may be in a better position to create better jobs or identify job shortages because employers are represented on their boards. Public job-training programs for unemployed or displaced workers (such as the Job Training Partnership Act or welfare-to-work programs), by contrast, have no defined ties to employers. Numerous studies have shown that such programs make no substantial difference in the living standards of the poor and poorly educated.[9]

Nonetheless, the case of the newly created patient care technician (PCT) job title proves how difficult it is even for joint labor-management programs to force employers to create better jobs. It is a stretch to claim that PCT positions are the high-skill, high-paying jobs employers have created or will create when workers become better trained and educated. There are some shortages of better jobs in health care into which individual workers with the right training and credentials can move, such as nursing. As we have seen, however, individual upgrading is a limited strategy that improves the quality of life for only a few. In any case, the availability of better jobs is always countered by employers' tendency to try to shift as much work as possible onto those workers who are the least formally trained and therefore least well paid. Even when quality and patient safety depends on using the most highly skilled caregivers, financial considerations may predominate.

Furthermore, as we have heard from workers concerned about "working out of description," in health care organizations, tasks are not always assigned to those who are better equipped to perform them. There is no simple relationship between training or skill levels and the actual work carried out. For example, Wanda, a licensed practical nurse (LPN), argued that her day-to-day work as an LPN was identical to that of a registered nurse (RN), making the lower pay of LPNs and the higher educational requirements for RNs seem irrational. Wanda may have underestimated the extent of education RNs receive, the number of tasks that they are trained to perform but do not necessarily carry out on a daily basis, and the added insight RNs might bring to even routine tasks. Nevertheless, as nurses have long recognized when they compare how their work is valued to that of physicians, who gets credit for—and assigned to do—particular tasks is often the result of what sociologists have called "turf battles" among competing occupational or professional groups, rather than a process of matching training and abilities to patient needs. On the health care playing field, more powerful occupational groups try to exclude some work from their territory because it *appears* to be less skilled or has less status, and therefore fails to advance the occupational group's standing as a profession.[10] The fact that many "less valuable" players often perform "valuable work" is often ignored or concealed by both powerless and powerful groups alike.[11]

In addition, there is evidence that employers, who claim the workforce is underskilled, are not effectively using the skills workers do have.[12] David Livingstone has argued there is an "underuse of knowledge and skills in current industrial market economies" on a "massive scale"; as a result, "we are already living in a 'knowledge society' in which the collective learning achievements of adults far outpace the requirements of the economy as paid work is currently organized."[13] He identifies several kinds of "underemployment" in contemporary market-driven society—all signs of the wasted ability of the workforce—including a talent-use gap, performance gap, and subjective underemployment. The talent-use gap refers to the difference in educational achievements between those of higher and lower social origins. Assuming that the distribution of talent is similar in groups from different origins, the higher level of educational achievement among those of higher social origin means that the school system is not developing the talents of a considerable number of people from lower social origins. The performance gap refers to the inability of workers to use their achieved level of skill and knowledge in their jobs. Subjective underemployment refers to people's sense of whether or not their knowledge and skills are being used in their jobs.[14] Returning to the experience of Marie, we can see aspects of each of these types of underemployment.

Marie's early experience in school represents the talent use gap. In junior high she was accepted to one of the city's elite public high schools, but did not have the resources or encouragement to attend that school; instead, she chose to go to another school with her cousin, where she was bullied and eventually dropped out. Her experience on the job suggests a performance gap. I observed Marie at work several times and found her to be a highly competent caregiver and PCT. She took satisfaction in caring for people yet also said that her job was boring and repetitive. Marie also feels that her skills and abilities are not fully used on the job—especially if caregiving is acknowledged as a skill. On paper Marie is underqualified and lacks the credentials she needs to move forward. In reality, she is underemployed.

Other people I interviewed were underemployed as well. Linda, the operating room technician (OR tech) and former security guard, has an associate's degree from a CUNY two-year college. This credential is not required for her current occupation and she completed it while trying to take the prerequisite courses for a nursing program. She was unable to complete all the prerequisites because many of the courses were full by the time she could register and/or were not available at times she could coordinate with her full-time job. When we spoke, she still hoped to finish the prerequisites and potentially enroll in a nursing program. Steve, a respiratory technician in school to become a physician assistant, has two associate's degrees and a bachelor's degree.

Similarly, some immigrants arrive in the United States with advanced health care training or credentials from their own countries, but because they are not recognized in the United States, find employment in occupations below their level of training. There are few mechanisms to ease their transition into U.S. health care settings or to obtain equivalent U.S. credentials. These workers do not suffer from a lack of abilities or skills.

Finally, and not insignificantly, when skills upgrading is touted as a way to end skill shortages, it disguises the fact that when most employers talk about "skills" they aren't referring to technical or cognitive skills but to workers' attitudes and behavior. In their surveys of employers, Philip Moss and Chris Tilly found that the majority mention some kind of soft skills as among their most important hiring criteria.[15] Michael Handel confirms, "cross-sectional studies often suggest employers are less concerned about cognitive skills deficits than what they consider poor work habits, motivation, demeanor, and attitudes." Such complaints are furthermore made chiefly about workers without a college education.[16]

The Conference Board of Canada's report on joint labor-management training programs, prepared for the Association of Joint Labor-Management Educational Programs, unsurprisingly included 1199's Training and Upgrading Fund as a case study. The report concluded that many of the "skill gains" the programs achieved were in areas such as improved communication, improved decision making, better personal management, increased self-confidence, and greater adaptability. The reported benefits of these programs to participants similarly included improved customer service, better personal management, better communication, better understanding of job tasks, improved attitude, and not least, a greater appreciation of learning—to which we will return.[17]

Terms like "better personal management," "greater adaptability," and "improved attitude," support Gordon Lafer's argument that communication skills or customer service training is often directed at ensuring workers' punctuality, discipline, and motivation. These, he argues, are not really skills at all, but "measures of commitment that one chooses to give or withhold based on the conditions of work offered."[18] Young, immigrant, and minority workers have long been exposed to implicit and explicit demands to conform to middle-class behavioral and emotional codes and have often chosen to ignore them. In the case of the health care workers with whom I have interacted, they are often very committed to patient care and need little external motivation to do their jobs. I would argue that self-discipline and commitment are not the products of skills seminars, they must be encouraged and supported by the culture, and material conditions, of the workplace. As we saw in the training in communication skills and customer service, if health care workers have bad attitudes it is likely due in large part to the fact that they are denied the tools, resources, and respect they need to do their work well. Finally, employer complaints about the poor attitudes of workers are hardly new or indicative of a growing gap in skill requirements.[19]

In summary, if there is a relationship between the skills of the workforce and the structure of employment or division of labor, at an aggregate level or within New York's health care sector, it is a loose one. The findings of national and macro-level studies show there is no necessary correspondence between the expansion of education and the demands of the economy. Nor is there a neat connection between the content of education and the skill demands of jobs. This does not mean that every specific instance of job training or education fails to correspond to the labor market or employer demands. Current upgrading programs in New York City prepare some workers for occupations for which there is an indubitable demand. Nonetheless, the belief among education and workforce policy makers that there is a stable set of business "needs" that it is their role to meet is a wishful view of how education and training relates to the labor market. This view of business needs presents employers' requirements as nonnegotiable and the ability and competencies of individual workers as perpetually inadequate. It fails to grasp how jobs change in response to factors unrelated to the kind of labor available, and it assumes that employers actually use the skills their employees already have.

In the case of the health workforce training industry in New York, the argument that training programs are merely a response to employer demands is further undermined by the almost total lack of interest in evaluating the programs, not only in terms of their impact on patient care but also in terms of their impact on the earnings and opportunities of health care workers. The limited state and hospital reports merely tallied up the number of people trained, and even those are not available for all programs, nor is there a central record of how the numerous funds for training health care workers have been spent.

Some trainers and educators with whom I spoke were aware that there are too few good jobs and that there is too much faith in the idea that if people are trained, such jobs will somehow appear—a leap of faith not supported by evidence of how economies work and employers behave. Faced with the criticism or realization that their programs do not really move workers into better or even better-paying jobs, trainers and consultants switched rhetorical gears. They emphasized the importance of any job at all to participants in their programs.

The dean of a proprietary, nonprofit training school for certified nursing assistants (CNAs) and medical assistants (one of those schools that places large ads in the New York City subway system, targeting new immigrant women) explained that their school "has its place":

> It does what it needs to do to offer people a chance to enter into the health care field, and I really do believe that we change people's lives, both on the receiving end by the skills they get...as well as in their own individual lives. They might be single parents and we're their last available chance at getting skills so they can work and raise their kids.

In truth, it is nearly impossible for a single parent working as a nursing assistant to work and raise their kids. Nationally in 2004, the mean annual wage of nursing assistants in nursing homes was $20,970 and for medical assistants in physicians' offices it was $25,600.

Those trainers and educators I interviewed who argued that what people need, above all, are jobs, seemed, in a way, proud of their awareness of the true state of the labor market and the barriers immigrant and nonwhite workers face. An administrator at a CUNY college in the Bronx said,

> We're in a borough that is made up mostly of middle- and lower-middle-class kids who are really anxious of figuring out a way of making more money and getting a better job.... So, we're essentially a liberal arts institution and always will be, but we also have a strong connection to the professions, what the students demand, what they want.

When institutions of higher education offer occupational training programs or short-term certificates, they insist they are not "vocationalizing" their programs by creating a second, inferior educational tier focused on narrow skills training, as some critics have contended.[20] They are, as the CUNY administrator explained, providing a gateway to more advanced liberal arts education and a college degree. Therefore, he said, "we are essentially a liberal arts institution and always will be" and students have *demanded* what is often quite narrow vocational and occupational training. Another administrator in the Bronx, at CUNY's new educational outpost, CUNY on the Concourse, confirmed this point: "[T]he fact of the matter is, especially here in Bronx, they want to go to work after they finish their training. They need to find a job and be able to hold onto that job."

It is indisputable that in the U.S. economy it is increasingly difficult to find well-paying work. Most people have to work and they welcome almost any sort of skills training as a chance for upward mobility. But we have seen how long and complicated the journey to a college degree can be as students move through programs like these. In addition, the emphasis on career training and vocational education as a reaction to what "they" want is simplistic. The assertion that "they" desire to work, "especially here in the Bronx," downplays, if inadvertently, a number of troubling issues. Nearly a third of Bronx residents lived below poverty in 1999, the fourth-highest poverty rate among populous counties in the nation in 2004. Over 35 percent of residents of the Bronx are black or African American, and over 48 percent are of Hispanic or Latino origin. The median household income is $27,611 a year, only 64 percent of the median income of $43,393 in New York as a whole.[21] If the desire to work is greater in the Bronx, it is because the inequalities faced by students in the Bronx are greater. The educators' circumspect references to "they" may be well-intended as a corrective to the conservative idea that "they" want to stay home and live off welfare. Such explanations nonetheless cut off any broader discussion of how inequalities of race, class, and gender inflect the educational system and labor market, converting such inequalities instead into facts of life. Certainly these programs cannot and do not intend to solve the problems of poverty and inequality, yet such rhetoric takes poverty and inequality for granted.

Some of these programs were not preparing students for specific jobs in any case. In its first semester of operations in the fall of 2002, CUNY on the Concourse offered a number of noncredit certificate programs, a GED program, a "bridge-to-college" program, and a select few programs for college credit. Its health-related noncredit certificate programs included pre-nursing for high school students, medical office operations, and translation studies in health care (for English/Spanish bilingual students). In addition, it offered a nine-credit managed care program, which included courses on the health care system and medical terminology and coding. It did offer a CNA program, which is a credential for a specific job, and the GED and bridge-to-college programs are essential steps for students seeking to improve their lives (but they are nonetheless an inadequate substitute for poor-quality high school education and unequal access to postsecondary education). On the whole, however, CUNY on the Concourse specializes in offering short-term credentials, many of which do not carry college credits and are not linked to specific jobs, such as the managed care certificate, or are for poorly paid jobs such as nursing assistants. The training industry for allied health care workers may be a bridge to university and better jobs for a few, but it is predominantly focused on narrow "skills" and short-term training. 1199 has cooperated in this. An official at one college said he spent months negotiating with 1199's Training and Upgrading Fund over his training proposals, trying to sell them several credit-bearing programs, but he succeeded only in selling a noncredit medical terminology course and an on-the-job program for a specific job title. For the latter, he said, "They couldn't sign fast enough."

Paul Willis, a sociologist of education and culture, wrote recently, "the highest ambition inculcated into the working-class student, indeed reflecting their own desperate needs, is for a job, often any job."[22] Health care trainers do indeed too readily blur the material necessity of getting a job with the desire to work or the inherent value of paid labor, even if they do not consciously or explicitly engage in a process of "inculcation." Some educators may use students' desperate need for work as an excuse to pay less attention to their hopes and dreams, reframing paid labor as their "highest ambition." This suggests these training programs attempt to lower expectations as much as they raise them. Nevertheless, working-class students may not be easily inculcated. They do not necessarily accept the way trainers equate their desire to realize their abilities with getting a paid job, particularly students and workers of color.[23] Though they want to work, I suspect few New York City health care workers equate paid labor and career ladders with social justice.

Another type of discourse therefore emerged in my interviews. Some trainers pointed to the rewards of various training programs that supplemented, or even substituted for, benefits like increased wages, a better job, or any job at all. They suggested that apart from skill building and ladder climbing, training programs are valuable because they enhance workers' sense of self-worth and self-esteem. They were less defensive about running programs that did not provide college credit and led only to entry-level work in health care. Though they might draw attention to the dire need for work, they also suggested that training programs, like the paid labor they ostensibly lead to, are inherently rewarding because they create a sense of self-worth and meaning. Despite (or perhaps because of) the limitations of the PCT program, the former hospital training executive director commented,

> One of the things which I think was a real boost to them [the nursing assistants] was that something like 98 percent passed the [PCT] course. And so, for their self-esteem—and these were people who never thought they could learn anything again, you know many of them were older.

She drew attention not to the skills the program helped nursing assistant students master, but to its role in enhancing their sense of self-esteem and self-confidence.

A large home health care agency has contracted with the city to hire and train welfare recipients for jobs as home health aides and attendants (after they have first been through a nine-week work preparation class run by the city). Wages for home care workers are even lower than for nursing assistants; in 2001, the median annual wage of home health aides was $17,000.[24] The agency's human resources director spoke with emotion about the program:

> It's a real self-empowering [program]; these are women that have been through a lot already and [we're] trying to get them back on their feet. Trying to get them to feel positive about themselves and their lives. I loved it...I still get letters from the first six months of classes that we hired here from these women because they're still with us. They're like the best employees we have.

His view that the training program, and the poorly paid work in which it terminated, helped women "feel positive about themselves and their lives" reinforces the American ethic that paid labor is the route to positive self-esteem and a socially valued life. Positive self-esteem also becomes an irrefutable defense of the training itself: Any training program that improves self-esteem is valuable on its own terms, regardless of its tangible or material outcomes.

The argument that these programs contribute to the workers' self-esteem and sense of worth is a window onto something profound—the need for meaning and respect—and not only among health care workers but also among those who train them. Many of the administrators and trainers involved in the industry also saw the programs they developed as indicators of their own self-worth, and they always described what they were doing as meaningful and important work, regardless of the kind of training or education they administered. Those trainers who started their own careers as health care workers, some even at the paraprofessional level, saw their own lives as models for the health care workers they met. An administrator at a training organization that primarily offers noncredit vocational programs and classes linked her previous work as a nurse to her later work as a teacher in vocational programs:

> I loved the direct education part, just as I used to like direct patient care, because I felt that I really impacted greatly on people's lives and was able to

have the gratification of seeing change in people...I still see people on the street that I remember from doing certain education programs, and they come up to me, "oh, how are you?"

A consultant who provides customized, on-the-job training on issues related to communication and working with geriatric patients (primarily to nursing assistants) described the impact of her seminars this way:

One [impact] is, they're very positive about the educational experience. Many of them come to the class saying this is just bunk and leave saying, wow, I really learned something, this has really helped, and everybody should take this course: management, my peers, everybody. My first couple of courses are—I've gotten cards from my participants, little gifts, flowers. I mean they've really been engaged by the process.

This trainer tried to reorient the worker-students' understanding of education, encouraging them to be "positive about the educational experience" and become "engaged" by the process of learning. She felt that her courses could dismantle a certain amount of skepticism and cynicism toward education. And she also found this process extremely rewarding, even if—as she surely knew as a former social worker who had herself burnt out—the long-term impact of her courses on nursing assistants' working conditions is limited.

The same administrator who reflected on her gratification of seeing a change in people, commented:

There has to be an administrative decision to constantly nurture the workforce. If I had my way, there would be all kinds of continuing opportunities for self-exploration and personal fulfillment. I think that those are linked to helping people to cope better with the kinds of jobs that they have in their lives, which are very rigorous and exhausting, emotionally and physically.

She described the kinds of courses that might provide such nurturance: in-services on topics such as nutrition, stress reduction, body mechanics, and health care workers' own physical problems.

The goal of nurturing the workforce is a laudable one. It acknowledges a real problem: the lack of caring and respect for those whose very jobs are to provide care and respect. Under such circumstances, allied health care workers create and covet ways to care for themselves, in the face of many obstacles. As we saw, soft skills training classes sometimes resembled group therapy sessions, in which participants could share their grievances and frustrations. During a lunch break at the communication skills training, one PCT told me that she had recently been transferred from a regular medical unit to a psychiatric unit. She had not, however, received any specific training or information on what turned out be a very different work environment. Visibly exhausted, she explained that she didn't know how to deal with patients who were often incoherent and combative. For her, the communication skills course was a break from her routine and a chance to decompress by reflecting on what she was experiencing. Although this woman did not learn the skills she needed to do her job at the seminar, just getting a break from such a taxing job was helpful. The training consultant who had been a social worker remarked that her classes succeeded in engaging the participants for two reasons: the participants were treated in a professional manner and "listened to"—an acknowledgment of the reality that the participants did not generally receive such courtesies back on the shop floor. That participants in these courses are so pleased to be both respected and heard attests again to how little they get this kind of attention in the workplace.

Because health care workers are asked to continually care for others when no one in their workplace cares for them, aspects of the training industry provide a short-term emotional antidote to growing inequality, inadequately rewarded work, and diminishing opportunities for upward mobility. Even if programs have no impact on the quality of health care jobs or upward mobility, they sometimes provide a place where people can express themselves and affirm one another.

Such training and education, regardless of its quality and outcomes, also becomes a place where workers turn to fulfill their desire to be challenged—to think about new things, encounter new people, learn new routines, and even reflect on themselves. Recall Wanda, who continued to work as a nursing assistant for three years after obtaining her LPN credential, tolerating a sustained period of underemployment. While waiting for an LPN position at her hospital, she moved through a number of units in the facility. When the hospital began downsizing, Wanda moved into an operating room job where she dealt with instruments rather than human beings. "As the instruments came out from the OR we had to wash them and we had to set them, set the trays. And then sometimes we had to sterilize them," she recounted. "So it was a different job altogether. I worked for three years in the OR." I asked her how she felt about this new job.

> I felt good about it. Because I think I needed a change. Because I welcomed the change, the work was different.... Learning different—learning, learning, learning. I learned how to set the trays for the different operations. I did that until I got the appointment to be an LPN.

Even when she was overcredentialed for her position, Wanda found aspects of her work engaging. She enjoyed the fact that she continually learned different things. Being an LPN in the emergency room, where she eventually landed, also challenged her. "I liked that change," she said, "because it was something new. Remember I was going as a nurse now."

Unfortunately, her stint in the ER was short because new hospital administrators decided they no longer needed LPNs there. So Wanda moved into pediatrics.

> The union took up the cause, because it was what we would call displacement, and then we had a meeting and they asked me where I wanted to work and I said I think I want to work in Peds, with the children. So that's where I went. It's nice working with the children.

On her long journey through different job categories, Wanda both sought out and was exposed to numerous training and education experiences. She received two months' training on the pediatrics floor, and when she worked on the general medical unit, all the unit's staff were sent to a mandatory communication class. When she was working in the OR, she voluntarily signed up for a computer class. "Learning, learning, learning," as she puts it, characterizes her occupational history.

Although she was subject to the whims of her employers and to the vicissitudes of the health care industry, Wanda was nonetheless pleased to learn. Wanda became animated when discussing her interactions with the mothers in the pediatrics unit in particular, and she lit up when describing working as a nursing assistant in the OR. Likewise Cesar, who had enrolled in postsecondary education programs on and off since finishing high school, several times without completing the credential he set out to obtain, nevertheless seemed to experience school as a kind of open-ended exploration; he said "I like school. I like learning, anything I can learn." Shirley told a similar story when she described with pleasure the many courses offered through her hospital's training department that she had volunteered to attend over the years:

> I'm always up to volunteer for classes...all these courses I'm taking now are voluntary [in coding and billing], but we used to have all kinds of little classes. They had a cooking class...And I was in a diversity class, everybody cooked something and brought it in and we saw the difference in food.

This emphasis on the pleasure of learning new things draws attention to the way in which training and education is valued apart from its effects in terms of career mobility or wages. When it comes to the types of rewards described above, distinctions among types of training programs are blurred; at this level, there are no differences between in-services on healthy eating, on-the-job training seminars, multiskilling programs, college prep courses, and university courses themselves.

Naturally, not all the health care workers I interviewed expressed such positive views of education and training. Some saw it as onerous—something in which they were more or less forced to participate in order to make a living. For some health care workers, there is nothing less pleasant than an in-service on customer service. Grace said she "hates the idea of school" but knew she had to further her education to become something other than a dietary worker. One trainer I interviewed explained that many health care workers, particularly in the heavily regulated nursing home sector, are bombarded with dull and stultifying in-services. Although some workers enjoy learning under almost any conditions, one should be careful not to assume their enjoyment is completely divorced from tangible results. Although Wanda was engaged by the various positions she'd held, she was still frustrated when she learned—after spending two years to become an LPN and waiting another three to get an LPN position—that her wages were closer to those of a nursing assistant than a registered nurse.

Indeed, the blurring of the material and immaterial that the focus on self-esteem and meaning enables is troubling. While trainers may be moved by a genuine desire to help the people they train, they are part of a larger culture, a set of values, beliefs, and expectations, in which promoting self-esteem and self-worth have become substitutes for responses to economic and material inequality. After she spoke of the PCT program as creating self-esteem, the hospital training executive added, "and it led to extra pay"—an acknowledgment, though almost an afterthought, that ultimately self-esteem cannot substitute for the devaluation of nursing assistants' work. Similarly, in-service courses on stress and nutrition will not change the physically and emotionally exhausting nature of jobs in health care.

The slippery logic that underlies this training industry, then, is that if training does not provide the skills necessary for good jobs (assuming there are such jobs), then it provides "skills" for any job, and any job is meaningful no matter the pay or prospects. If, however, health care workers feel, like Veronica, that their work is not meaningful, at least the training creates self-worth and confidence. This training industry is sustained by health care workers like Veronica who invest in training programs to find the meaning—the sense of worth and respect—that eludes them at work. The problem is that the training industry itself—by suggesting that workers are never quite good enough and always need to be enrolled in a training course or program to validate their self-worth—makes the search for meaning a futile one. By encouraging workers to enroll in course after course—without ever addressing the underlying problems that have made their work seem meaningless—it becomes harder for workers to identify what constitutes meaningful work and determine that they have finally reached the end point of their journey. Veronica, in her search for meaningful work, looks one step up the ladder, hoping the work of an LPN will be more meaningful than that of a nursing assistant—even though *she* knows what nursing assistants do is important. The education and training industry takes advantage of Veronica's desire for work that means something, but it does not provide such work. One can see how meaning might become perpetually deferred, but the engagement that the desire for meaning produces is continually reinforced.

In the end, the "need" that sustains this industry is the need for respect and for meaning, which is denied at work. While many workers certainly find comfort and a sense of worth at home and in their personal lives, in reality what one does for paid labor is, in America, a pivotal piece of one's identity, so that when your labor is devalued and trivialized the personal consequences are often severe. (In any case, the workers I interviewed were so busy working and going to school that they had little time at home.)

Trainers, too, saw in the training and education industry a means of verifying their own worth and value.

I interviewed the training administrator who spoke movingly about her desire to nurture health care workers, whose jobs are physically and emotionally rigorous and exhausting, on a gorgeous, sunny June day. Her office was in the corner of a spacious warehouse loft, with massive windows overlooking the lower Manhattan skyline where the World Trade Center had stood only a few months before. She had just moved into a newly created position to oversee workforce development projects implemented because of the economic downturn exacerbated (not caused) by the events of September 11, 2001. A dot-com firm gone bust had just vacated the loft, and some of the firm's boxes were still stacked on the floor, waiting to be moved. I pictured, for a moment, the space as it must have been only shortly before: teeming with what Robert Reich, a liberal economist and labor secretary in the Clinton administration, famously called "symbolic analysts."

These analysts—research scientists, design engineers, software engineers, civil engineers, biotechnology engineers, sound engineers, public relations executives, investment bankers, lawyers, real estate developers, and "even a few creative accountants"—were the "problem solvers" whose work Reich believed would sustain the U.S. economy and determine the fate of those consigned to ostensibly routine, repetitive personal service jobs. Reich described this polarization of the U.S. labor market in his 1991 book *The Work of Nations.* Although he proposed policies that would prevent layoffs and force employers to invest more in training their employees, he accepted the common myth that well-trained workers generate jobs for themselves. He similarly argued that workers with a college degree command higher wages than those without because they have the higher skills employers demand. Reich's faith that the emerging global economy would reward training and education made it easier for the Clinton administration to acquiesce to (and later, facilitate) large-scale corporate layoffs and shelve some of Reich's own more interventionist proposals for responding to economic restructuring.[25]

The vacated loft gave the lie to Reich's thesis. The "problem solvers" who had just left the building were now part of the problem: the group of U.S. workers who are overprepared and underemployed. More training cannot solve such a problem. The quality of jobs in the U.S. labor market is not closely related to, let alone determined by, the training and education levels of the workforce, as Reich believed. Moreover, the growing wage gap between university-educated and other workers is an outcome of the sharp decline in wages among the latter, not a product of the former's higher skills.[26]

This midtown loft, and the spatial transition from the world of new media to training for entry-level health care positions, expressed the fragility of the knowledge economy better than words.

8

A Common Cause

In the 1990s, 1199 and its leaders formed an alliance with hospital leaders to fight pro-market reforms and state budget cuts and preserve the jobs of its members. The state had been the unofficial third party to negotiations between 1199 and private hospitals since the passage of the Medicaid and Medicare programs in 1965, when federal and state governments became the single largest payers for health care services. Once the government became billable, health care costs skyrocketed, so that, by the late 1970s, state actors were focused above all on containing them. As government payers began to impose new payment restrictions on hospitals, wage increases obtained by 1199 slowed markedly.[1] Nonetheless, as late as 1989, Dennis Rivera confidently claimed to the media during his first contract negotiations as union president that it was "ridiculous" for hospitals to say they could not afford wage increases since "the state makes sure hospitals can survive."[2] While Rivera's immediate aim was to take a confrontational stance toward hospital leaders, his comment foreshadowed a significant and partially self-imposed narrowing of his strategic options: If the state did *not* make sure hospitals survived, Rivera's essential battle would have to be with the state, not hospital leaders.

Rivera was correct that public financing in New York State has sustained an unparalleled number and diversity of hospitals, blurring the lines between public and private. So too has the state issued periodic threats to drastically reduce funding or close hospitals outright, and it succeeded in doing so in the late 1970s. In the 1990s, those threats were renewed because the city and state both elected Republican, fiscally conservative leaders. Governor George Pataki and Mayor Rudolph Giuliani were eager to enact legislation and policies that would create greater competition among providers for payments, shift government-insured populations into private managed care plans, and cut public programs (especially Medicaid) across the board. Rivera joined with private hospital leaders to vigorously fight the program cuts and policy changes, many of which were intended to force hospitals to restructure their services. Together, they were able to wrest new kinds of subsidies and concessions from the state, especially money to train and, later, "retain" the workforce. Somewhat perversely, Rivera's efforts were made easier by these politicians' ideological antipathy to direct public ownership and control of health care services; if they were going to support the health care system, they were far more willing to support ostensibly private hospitals (where Rivera's members worked) than public ones.

By securing such funds from the state, 1199 and Rivera perhaps made it more difficult for hospitals leaders to justify and even implement some of the drastic restructuring measures they claimed were inevitable in the face of funding cuts. Voluntary hospital leaders also made a number of concessions to 1199 during collective bargaining, particularly in terms of job security, that were arguably the fruits of 1199's willingness to cooperate. However, the costs of 1199's strategy were rarely mentioned amid the glowing media reports of 1199's achievements in collective bargaining and the new era of labor-management "jointness." The union's united front with hospital leaders in the fight against cuts to public financing mutated into a united stance on the supposed underlying cause of the hospitals' woes: underskilled workers. This is a message that persisted after the health care worker surplus turned into a worker shortage at the end of the decade, when the union and employers continued to offer training and education programs rooted in the logic of an inadequate workforce.

Equally important, the jointness strategy absolved hospital leaders of responsibility for their precarious financial position—assuming it was as dire as they claimed—and for the problems faced by health care workers on the job. The union never challenged hospital leaders directly about the need for restructuring. In fact, it made aspects of restructuring such as multiskilling more feasible by directing new state funding to training and education programs that hospitals would have been unlikely to fund themselves. Union officials suggest that hospitals would have gone ahead with restructuring and laying off workers in any event; their efforts to secure state support, including for training, at least allowed them to have a say in the restructuring process and to use multiskilling to prevent layoffs. 1199's ability to establish a training and education industry for allied health care workers in New York City was certainly an accomplishment in the hostile political climate of the 1990s. As we have seen, however, much of the training and education grants, which were 1199's major coup in its fight against the state, were spent on programs that did not deliver many of the benefits they promised.

The focus on training as a panacea for instability in the hospital sector also made a number of other potential responses to the ideology of market reforms and restructuring less probable. To be sure, 1199 took advantage of the fact that in the era of neoliberal reform and economic restructuring, job training has been one of the few gifts politicians have been willing to bestow on workers in troubled or unstable industries, and the union tried to create new opportunities, new jobs, and career ladders. Still, 1199's embrace of training and education programs, instead of other potential responses to the dilemmas it faced, cannot be wholly attributed to making the best of a weak hand. In focusing on training health care workers, not shaping how health care is delivered or financed, 1199 has been consistent with its history. Unfortunately, given the nature of health care work and the state of the U.S. health care system today, that position seems increasingly short-sighted.

In addition, what began in theory as a safety net for vulnerable health care workers in specific occupations and institutions at risk eventually became pivotal to 1199's ability to show it could improve the lives of its members as a whole and expand its influence. In 2002, an official in 1199's joint labor-management training and education programs joked to me, "We went from being a bodega to being Wal-Mart overnight." Prior to early 1990s, the 1199/League joint Training and Upgrading Fund was financed primarily by employer contributions paid as a percentage of gross payroll. The Fund's primary service was arm's-length tuition reimbursement programs[3]—members who enrolled in career-related education courses at colleges such as the City University of New York could apply for reimbursement of their tuition for a limited number of courses. In any case, the Fund did not have enough money to allow all of its members to take courses and therefore did not systematically reach out to members, instead allowing interested workers to self-select. In the bleak 1980s, the Training and Upgrading Fund even atrophied as a result of reduced management payments.

The situation began to turn with increased state and employer contributions to the Fund under the 1989 contract. Soon after, new training programs were announced in the pages of *1199 News,* the union's newsletter, and the Training and Upgrading Fund began to emerge as a public-relations mechanism as well. The debut of the newsletter's new format in October 1990, printed on glossy paper with multiple colors and pictures, focused on the efforts of workers to move up in their careers. By the late 1990s, the Training and Upgrading Fund was bursting at the seams with more financing, staff, and an even greater role in the union's strategy. In 1998, after the announcement of the Health Care Worker Retraining Initiative (HWRI) and Community Health Care Conversion Demonstration Project (CHCCDP) programs, the Training and Upgrading Fund's income was predicted to "soar to some $45 million a year," of which only $9.5 million was from management contractual contributions.[4] In both 2002 and 2003, the Employment, Training and Job Security Program (ETJSP), the umbrella fund that contains Training and Upgrading, Job Security, as well as several other subfunds, reported grant incomes between $50 and $60 million.[5] A training and education superstore under de facto labor union control was the primary achievement of 1199's decision to form an alliance with hospital leaders in the 1990s. This achievement, however, entailed hidden costs for frontline health care providers and patients.

Within months of his election to the union presidency in April 1989, Dennis Rivera faced contract negotiations with fifty-three of the city's area hospitals and nursing homes, which negotiated collectively as part of the League of Voluntary Hospitals. At the same time, the union was in disarray and deeply scarred. Racial divides had arguably always been present, if submerged, in a labor union in which the leadership, though radical and sympathetic to the experience of the rank and file, was so culturally and ethnically distant from them. When Leon Davis, president since 1934, retired in 1982, race became a flashpoint in the decision about who would become his successor and in the assessment of his successor's job performance. It was a troubled period in the union's history: When 1199 finally elected leaders who came from the ranks—two black women who had been health care workers briefly served as presidents after Davis—bitter internal strife ensued. That strife in turn resulted in disastrous contract negotiations,[6] so that Rivera's efforts to heal the union and establish his presidency hinged upon successful contract negotiations in 1989.

Perhaps in rebuke for Rivera's publicly proclaimed confidence that the state would make sure hospitals survive, the governor (then a Democrat, Mario Cuomo) and health department officials insisted they would not get involved in the contract negotiations or underwrite any wage increases. The hospitals' negotiating representative claimed financial duress and told 1199 they could not expect to be saved by increased state funding.[7] Rivera chose to remind hospitals—and his rank and file—of the union's strength. He pursued a divide-and-conquer strategy, first negotiating a two-year contract with four hospitals owned by the Roman Catholic Archdiocese of New York for annual raises of 8.5 percent, a deal brokered by John Cardinal O'Connor, thereafter described as "the patron saint of health care workers" in the pages of *1199 News*. Rivera then applied steady pressure on League hospitals to match those contract terms by organizing well-attended demonstrations, mounting a public relations campaign, mobilizing political support in a mayoral election year, and conducting a series of walk-outs at individual hospitals. At first only a few of the most financially troubled hospitals gave in to the union's demands, but then Columbia Presbyterian, a major academic medical center, broke from the League to negotiate individually rather than face the costs of a strike. The League itself settled on a three-year contract in early October 1989 after the union membership voted to strike, providing workers with 7.5 percent raises in each of the first two years, 5 percent in the third year, and a one-time $500 bonus to be paid in 1991.[8]

During the next round of contract negotiations in 1992, by contrast, managed care and deregulation were on the horizon, and even though the union and hospitals had faced government-imposed cost restraints for years, new reforms were couched in the terminology and recommendations of the private, for-profit sector, heralding a new era of competition and market mechanisms. Health care "reformers" and private consultants focused critical attention on apparently anachronistic and expensive acute care hospitals (which employed most of 1199's members) and encouraged hospitals to adopt the same "restructuring" strategies that had already decimated much of the unionized U.S. workforce. As other labor unions have historically done when employers in their industry face or threaten contraction, 1199 turned from confrontation to cooperation with employers—the hospitals—to press for state interventions that would save jobs and, it was hoped, win a measure of control over changes in the industry.

In February, the union reached an early agreement with Beth Israel Medical Center in Manhattan that it hoped would set the terms for subsequent negotiations with the League. The remarkable deal provided full job security for the hospital's 4,000 employees for the duration of the forty-month contract and promised to match the wage increases negotiated with the League. In hindsight, however, the most significant contract element was the union's promise of partnership. In exchange for no layoffs, the union acquiesced to the idea that one of the main causes of instability in the hospital sector, and therefore the appropriate target of restructuring, was the paraprofessional health care workers the union represented—their skills, their flexibility, and their attitudes. Beth Israel's president at the time said the contract established a "Japanese workplace concept"[9]—presumably referring to notions of total quality management and reengineering which, in the hands of hospital administrators, became cost-cutting schemes focused above all on frontline health care workers.

In the contract negotiated with the League several months later, wage increases were less than stellar—3 percent for the first two years, 4 percent in the third, and a one-time $500 bonus—rates just above those of inflation in the same period. Moreover, League hospitals did not agree to a no-layoff guarantee. Instead, they promised to provide at least thirty days' notice of layoffs, give laid-off workers first rights to any comparable job opening at a League facility, supplement unemployment benefits until the worker was rehired, and make contributions to a newly created Job Security Fund—which would provide training and placement for laid-off workers.[10] Like the Beth Israel contract, the union and hospital agreed to develop a labor-management committee to increase employee "involvement" in the looming "transformations" of health care. Contract language confirmed a transition in labor-management relations: "This Contract represents a milestone in our relationship as Union and Management. In the interests of our patients, we have arrived at a mutually acceptable agreement in the spirit of compromise and conciliation. As people with a common cause, we seek to broaden this relationship."[11]

Between 1992 and 1994 private hospitals in New York City laid off almost 1,000 employees, including 380 members of 1199.[12] Many hospitals were beginning restructuring efforts, especially cross-training job titles.[13] Rivera suggested the hospitals' actions were undertaken largely in preparation for the anticipated effects of the Clinton administration's health reform plan,[14] which dominated the policy and legislative agenda in late 1993 and 1994, only to crumble by October of 1994. Rivera's major concern, naturally, was that Clinton's proposed reforms might lead to significant job losses in hospitals, and he pressed for inclusion of a "health care employment conversion plan," which would include a commitment of federal dollars for retraining and relocating displaced health care workers.[15] 1199 and hospital officials together organized and appeared at a number of rallies for universal health coverage in those months—that wouldn't hurt New York.

As we know, at the same time, Republicans devoted to cutting budgets and taxes defeated Democratic incumbents in both the city and state elections—incumbents the union had not only endorsed, but mobilized volunteers, phone banks, and mass mailings to support. Giuliani won the mayoral race in 1993, and Pataki the governor's in 1994. Giuliani proposed to cut the city's Health and Hospitals Corporation budget by a third (its chairman—a mayoral appointee—resigned that spring rather than support the proposed cuts), and both sought to substantially reduce the Medicaid program. In 1995, Pataki's budget proposed one of the largest cuts in state history, and Giuliani's city budget proposed the largest percentage reduction in spending since the Great Depression.[16] The cuts were drastic to all publicly funded programs and particularly deep for education and welfare. On one front, Rivera and hospital leaders together fought cuts to Medicaid, the biggest source of health care funding, and on another they fought—not entirely compatibly—to "manage the transition." Said Rivera, "We are going to have to work together to make sure that hospitals don't close. We hope there's a future for the American hospital. And we've got to manage the transition."[17]

To do so, Rivera turned decisively toward the possibilities of training and upgrading programs. In July 1994, the union announced it hoped to open contract negotiations with the League a year early, arguing that the pressures of restructuring, the uncertainties of national reform, and the threat of layoffs made a new contract with job security urgent. In *1199 News,* the term restructuring first appeared in the summer of 1993, in an article in which the union claimed defiantly, "we're not accepting lay-offs."[18] By the spring of 1994, however, another article in the newsletter referred to "softening restructuring's impact." As Executive Vice President Debby King (who would shortly thereafter become director of the training and job security Funds) said, "These changes are happening whether we like it or not."[19] In July, Rivera, joined by soon-to-be-defeated Governor Cuomo, President of the League of Voluntary Hospitals Bruce McIver, and others, led a procession of 910 Training and Upgrading Fund graduates down West 43rd Street, near Times Square, to a graduation ceremony. Rivera asked the crowd, "How many unions can say they've graduated nearly 1,000 members to higher skills in a single year?"[20]

The collective agreement reached with the League in September was noted above all for the job security clause for all workers with at least two years' seniority—about 32,000 of over 40,000 covered by the contract. Rivera credited the contract success to the union's willingness to cooperate with hospitals, which the union displayed during the Clinton reform debate. Although the union boasted the contract contained no give-backs, the union did consent to a one-year wage freeze in 1995, and wages in 1996 and 1997 would be raised by only 3 percent. Surpluses in the health and pension benefits funds also allowed the union to consent to reductions in management contributions.[21]

Along with job security, Rivera stressed that the contract gave workers a voice in how their jobs would be inevitably changed and their institutions run.[22] In particular, the contract created a new Planning and Placement Fund, which was to develop labor-management committees, provide employment services, and conduct research on health workforce issues. Together with the existing Job Security and Training and Upgrading Funds, it would be part of a new "superfund"—the Employment, Training and Job Security Program (ETJSP). The cover of the November issue of

1199 News featured a nursing attendant who had become an LPN. The accompanying five-page profile of the Training and Upgrading Fund urged members to "Go for it!"[23] Multiskilling and customer service training were also already on the Fund's agenda. Rivera said in the press, "We want to manage the transition so a clerk in a wing of a hospital that closes becomes the admitting person in a clinic, who can also take vital signs"; and the president of the United Hospital Fund said, "As the health care business goes more retail, the world of the future requires more decision-making ability and more interpersonal skills."[24]

Many groups and organizations went on the offensive against the proposed government cuts in the spring of 1995, including the state Democratic party, but "1199's multi-million-dollar advertising and grassroots mobilization against proposed budget cuts drove the Governor's poll numbers through the floor."[25] Pataki compromised on a number of cuts, in particular reducing to $700 million his proposed $1.2 billion cuts to Medicaid.[26] The chastened Pataki recognized the harm the union could to do him and his career, especially in heavily Democratic downstate areas.[27] As we know, when Pataki succeeded in deregulating state payment rates to hospitals in the Health Care Reform Act (HCRA) and obtained federal permission to make the enrollment of Medicaid recipients into managed care plans mandatory shortly thereafter, Rivera was able to win significant concessions on behalf of voluntary hospitals, including pools of state money to fund graduate medical education, "charity" care, and worker retraining. By 1995 therefore, Rivera had settled on an approach that circumscribed the union's possible approaches to serious problems in New York's health care system and in the organization of work on the shop floor. He would become the hospitals' most energetic advocate for state and federal support and funding.

Despite Rivera's cooperative spirit, the union's position in contract negotiations scheduled for 1998 was by no means secure. In June of 1996, during the first contract negotiations faced by the League of Voluntary Hospitals after the passage of HCRA, 6,000 hospital workers represented by Local 144 of the Service Employees International Union (SEIU) went on strike for sixty-three days against thirteen voluntary hospitals and nursing homes, rejecting management's demands to introduce a two-tier wage structure and reduce other benefits such as paid sick time. Local 144 workers had been without a contract for over six months and League president

McIver blamed cost-cutting pressures from HMOs and managed care for the need to reduce benefits and wages. Voluntary hospitals in the city announced they planned to layoff 500 workers in July, and several hospitals had fallen behind on their payments to union pension funds. Understood to be a test battle for negotiations with the much larger 1199 scheduled for 1998, Local 144 signed a contract in which it escaped a two-tier wage structure, but in which the only pay increases were one-time payments.[28]

In the summer of 1997, Rivera tried to open contract negotiations a year early, as he had done in 1994. The $1.25 billion in aid to hospitals (CHCCDP) had just been announced, and the union told its membership that 1199's role in securing the funds "made it certain that management entered into the negotiations knowing: (1) 1199 is a heavy hitter politically, and (2) 1199 can work with management to influence crucial decisions involving big bucks."[29] Hospital leaders, however, continued to argue that financial cuts were devastating—adding to the list of problems looming cuts contained in the 1997 federal Medicare reform legislation (the Balanced Budget Act).

Despite the new aid and union-supported efforts to mitigate pro-market, pro-managed care reforms, Rivera, along with his advisors, accepted the hospitals' depiction of their position and tried to convince union members to accept them as well. In May 1997, the ETJSP received a commissioned report on the likely impact of recent policy changes on the workforce. It predicted a loss of 15 percent of all hospital jobs, or 27,600 full-time positions, between 1997 and 2000, most in voluntary hospitals and including 11,000 1199 positions.[30] The 15 percent figure was widely disseminated, including in several *New York Times* articles and pieces in *1199 News* explaining why the union was attempting to open contract negotiations a year early.[31] The report also recommended that the Training and Upgrading Fund stop training RNs because of anticipated surpluses. The report played a role in how the CHCCDP training funds were eventually spent: Among other programs, the study recommended the union sponsor training in "customer relations and interpersonal skills" and create multiskilled patient care associates.[32] The union also produced a brochure for its members that explained why it was necessary to negotiate an early contract and repeated the litany of troubles hospital leaders themselves claimed: shorter hospital stays, managed care, cuts to Medicare and Medicaid. As the brochure stated: "Our worst fears have come to be reality with recent developments."[33] Rivera told members in *1199 News,* "Our employers are scared stiff about the future. Some CEOs have lost their jobs. Others probably will." He added that labor accounts for 75 percent of hospital costs, so it was no surprise managers' first impulse was to cut the workforce.[34]

The union's major demands were job security for all members working more than a year and part-timers and union recognition at hospital-operated satellite clinics and home care services. In return, Rivera proposed to use $100 million from the joint labor-management pension plan for $20,000 lump-sum payments to workers who would agree to retire early. He estimated 4,000 to 5,000 workers would take the offer, reducing the need for layoffs. Despite the union's willingness to go along with the hospitals' presentation of their position, management rejected the union's demands on September 4. Union negotiators reported that hospital managers said they would need to layoff 10,000 workers in the next three years. An angry Rivera wrote, "The bosses... do not deserve the cooperation they have received from us in recent years... New Yorkers can get ready to witness the biggest, toughest, most effective strike in the city's history."[35]

Before resuming the negotiations with the League, 1199 therefore finalized two mergers that had long been discussed but never brought to fruition because of political infighting in the labor movement: first, in January 1998, the 120,000-member 1199 merged with the national union SEIU. Rather than becoming another local of SEIU, the union took on peer status as "1199/SEIU," and Rivera became the head of SEIU (and all its locals) in New York State. This gave 1199 access to deeper pockets for organizing, political lobbying, and funding strikes if necessary. Second, later in the same month, 1199 became the largest union in New York City when it incorporated the 30,000-member SEIU Local 144, which had been recently placed under trusteeship by the national after its president was accused of financial misconduct.[36] By the time contract negotiations were reopened in March 1998, Rivera headed a much larger union with greater resources, and by June he was threatening a strike.

An agreement was reached on June 21, 1998, nine days before the strike deadline, and Rivera called off plans for 50,000 workers to go on strike.[37] Despite the union's new size and the positive gloss given to the contract in the media, terms of the contract show it was not an unmitigated victory.[38] In the forty-month contract, the union secured a 3 percent raise in the first year and final sixteen months of the contract, and a $1,800 lump-sum payment in the second year. By comparison, the consumer price index in the New York metropolitan area—a measure of increases to the cost of living—increased approximately 10 percent in the same period. The job security terms obtained in 1994 were extended to part-timers and made placement of laid-off workers into any League vacancies mandatory,[39] but the terms now applied only to workers hired before September 17, 1992— about three-quarters of the union's workers at the hospitals—rather than all workers with more than two years' seniority, as had been the case in the 1994 contract. 1199 again made it a priority to expand the safety net of training, but was able to do so largely because of the fortuitous boom on Wall Street. The union agreed to reduce hospitals' contributions to the flourishing labor-management pension fund and was allowed to divert $135 million from it to finance early retirements. In return, the contract specified that the hospitals and nursing homes covered in the contract would have to contribute $60 million a year to the retraining and job security fund (ETJSP). With the help of unemployment insurance and the job security fund, any workers laid off by the hospitals were to receive 80 percent pay for two years (extended from one), free training, and the first right to any job opening at the hospitals for which they were qualified.[40] The union was able to present the job security measures and increased funding for retraining laid-off workers as important achievements, but these did not require an increased financial commitment from the hospitals over the previous contract since they were offset by the pension fund. The union was also unable to extract a promise from the hospitals not to fight organizing efforts at the growing number of hospital out-patient clinics.

As it became clear the united front approach was not paying off in contract negotiations, Rivera's unquestioning support for hospitals was also being criticized by advocates for improving New York's health care system on the left and right, many of whom felt reductions in the acute care sector were essential to creating a more cost-effective, community-centered health care system. However, objections from the left were temporarily overshadowed in 1999, when Rivera achieved his biggest coup for the health care sector and his union's members while at the same time seeming to establish himself as a progressive force for meaningful reform of the health care system. For a brief moment, it seemed that in the process of furthering his union's interest, Rivera also furthered the interests of working-class, immigrant, and poor New Yorkers as a whole.

When negotiations over renewal of HCRA began in 1999, the union, in cooperation with the hospital trade association, the Greater New York Hospital Association (GNYHA), launched a massive lobbying and public relations campaign to press lawmakers to do more for the 3.2 million New Yorkers without health insurance. The lobbying campaign, which cost at least ten million dollars, was paid for through a subfund of the ETJSP (to which increased dollars were transferred as a result of the 1998 contract with the League of Voluntary Hospitals).[41] It resulted in a plan, as part of HCRA's renewal, for the state to spend over one billion dollars to extend health care insurance to about one million New Yorkers, primarily through an expansion of Medicaid called the Family Health Plus program. HCRA 2000 also maintained the pools for graduate medical education and charity care set up by HCRA 1996, and put another $150 million into the job retraining pool.[42] Other new provisions, such as demonstration programs to provide "enhanced" Medicaid rates to certified home health care agencies that provided health insurance to their workers, contributed to the sense that the bill was a substantial step forward in improving health care in New York. By extending insurance coverage, 1199 and the GNYHA were also hoping to make a dent in one source of hospitals' financial difficulties—"charity care." Still, it seemed 1199 was focused above all on doing something for the state's uninsured and needy populations, and only in the process accomplishing something for its members.

HCRA 2000 nonetheless established a trend that many would come to see as irresponsible: the reliance on short-term funding sources to create what would be long-term state commitments. Programs created under HCRA 2000 were to be funded in part by ongoing sources of funding, including already existing tax-levies on insurers and some health care services mandated by HCRA 1996, an increase in the cigarette tax, and a $300 million federal matching grant for the Medicaid program. In addition, however, the legislation counted on using the state's share of the settlement in the national lawsuit against tobacco companies (expected to total $25 billion over twenty-five years). The actual annual tobacco fund payments proved to be less than anticipated, however, in part because the amount was linked to the volume of cigarettes sold, which declined not least because of the increased taxes on cigarettes. In addition, a number of counties (including New York City) sold their rights to the payments to private investment firms in exchange for up-front payments that were less than the total expected over time.[43]

As was also noted at the time, 1199's awareness of problems in the health care system did not extend to voluntary hospitals. By the time another gubernatorial election year came around in 2002, and new contract negotiations with the League of Voluntary Hospitals, it seemed to many that Rivera would secure subsidies for the private, nonprofit hospitals at any cost and that 1199's institutional strength and self-interest took precedence over the well-being of working New Yorkers as a whole. The widespread acclaim derived from HCRA 2000 and the Family Health Plus program would be utterly silenced when HCRA was renewed again two years later.

Several of the union's contracts were due to expire late in 2001, including its 1998 contract with the League on October 31, just six weeks after the terrorist attacks on the World Trade Center. Contract negotiations were expected to be contentious, not least because the city had entered an economic slump exacerbated by the attacks. Rather than risk the public relations disaster of a strike in the midst of a political climate emphasizing loyalty and sacrifice above all, the League and 1199 extended the contract to March 31.[44] Kenneth Raske, president of the Greater New York Hospital Association, and Rivera used the time to pressure Pataki not to use Medicaid cuts as a solution the state's looming budget deficit. The contract extension also gave the state's political, labor, and health care leaders time to press the federal government for increased aid in the wake of September 11; Raske and Rivera now added the need for hospitals to prepare for bioterrorism to their requests for support.[45]

New federal aid for health care was not forthcoming from the Republican Congress and administration, however. So, in "one of the most brilliant and sordid chapters in the annals of health policy,"[46] Pataki and Rivera came to a secret deal, pushed through the state legislature on January 16, 2002,[47] that underwrote 1199's contract with the League and guaranteed—their denials notwithstanding—Rivera's endorsement of Pataki later that spring in his 2002 bid for reelection to a third term. The bill, known as the Health Care Workforce Recruitment and Retention Act, was the second expansion of HCRA and proposed to spend $2.7 billion (later increased to

$3.5 billion) on health care initiatives, including $1.8 billion to recruit and retain health care workers, primarily through salary increases. Wage increases were slated for hospitals, nursing homes, and personal care centers and community health centers statewide, but $750 million in wage subsidies was reportedly earmarked for 1199 members. The plan was predicated on a total of $4.5 billion in hoped-for new revenue from increases in federal contributions to the Medicaid program, another increase in the cigarette tax, and $1.1 billion in expected proceeds from the conversion of nonprofit insurer Empire Blue Cross and Blue Shield to for-profit status.[48] Anticipating the state financing, 1199 and the League announced an agreement on January 12, 2002, that would provide raises of slightly more than 13 percent over forty-two months to the 55,000 health care workers in the contract. The contract was similar to the 1998 contract in terms of job security guarantees, providing it to those hired before February 1996 (about three-quarters of those in the contract), and it raised employer contributions to the health care and child care Funds. 1199 members continued to have a health care plan to which they contributed neither premiums nor copayments, a rare achievement in contemporary labor relations.[49]

Though few commentators questioned that health care workers, especially nursing home workers, merited raises, criticism centered on the secret way in which the bill was negotiated and the wisdom of the way in which it was to be financed. Policy analysts correctly argued that the chances the feds would increase their share of New York State's Medicaid costs were virtually nil.[50] The most controversial aspect of the proposed funding was the use, again, of short-term proceeds, this time from the Empire Blue Cross conversion, to finance ongoing fiscal commitments and close the budget deficit. Empire Blue Cross, the nonprofit insurer of last resort in New York, had sought permission for years from the State Attorney General to convert to for-profit status, but it was granted in the 2002 health bill only on the condition that the state had the right to appropriate any profits from the sale of Blue Cross stocks. Several groups, including the state's Consumers' Union, brought a lawsuit shortly after the announcement contesting the state's right to appropriate the funds. In other states where Blues plans had been converted, profits had been used to set up permanent charitable foundations to expand access to health care. In New York by contrast, only 5 percent of the profits were allocated for a permanent charity fund, the rest were appropriated by the state and scheduled to be spent over the course of three years. There was a sense that, unlike in 1999, Rivera had sacrificed low-income and uninsured families in the deal.[51] In addition, the question of whether it was sound health care policy to convert the state's insurer of last resort to a for-profit company was abruptly silenced, even though 1199 had once been against the conversion on principle.[52]

The co-chair of New York's Working Families Party wrote in 2002 that while Rivera's endorsement of Pataki was a coup for his union's members, it was at the same time a "capitulation" to Pataki's larger "anti-worker corporate agenda." He noted that "Governor Pataki has faithfully carried out the wishes of employers and real estate interests, and during his tenure, New York's social wage—those parts of our standard of living that we win politically rather than as part of the paycheck—has withered."[53] While some in the labor movement were reluctant to criticize Rivera's endorsement of Pataki—recognizing the union's difficult strategic position and envying the deal he made for his workers—others felt that Rivera had sacrificed the very notion of a labor movement. "The last I remember we are not a special interest group," said Phil Wheeler, a New York official of the United Auto Workers.[54] A labor commentator pointed out that "deals that are good for the members of one union are not necessarily good for members of other unions, let alone working people in general. A governor [Pataki] who slashes welfare, cuts taxes, cuts and privatizes public services, locks people up, blocks efforts to redress the state's unequal education funding, campaigns for an antiunion president and can't even be bothered to raise the minimum wage *in an election year* is not likely to help the labor movement in the long run—and maybe not even in the next contract negotiations."[55]

The comment was prescient. Though the governor's press release for the bill declared the 2002 expansion of HCRA "fiscally sound,"[56] the actual magnitude of the state's budget shortfall—more than $11.5 billion—came to light only after Pataki's reelection to a third term later that year. Promised funding for health initiatives failed to materialize, and Pataki began to chip away at established extrabudget HCRA pools by shifting some programs included in the state budget into the HCRA pools and withdrawing "loans" from other HCRA pools. Only one month after his reelection he proposed using all of the tobacco settlement money, even the portion already going into health-related HCRA pools, toward guaranteeing the sale of tax-exempt bonds to close the state's growing budget deficit.[57] (That plan, along with the predicted sums from the settlement itself, withered).[58] The news also broke that several additional nonprofit insurers, including the Health Insurance Plan (HIP) of Greater New York, were considering converting to for-profit companies and that Pataki hoped to use those proceeds to close the budget gap.[59] Pataki also proposed, once again, cuts to Medicaid as well as substantial cuts in other areas such as education.[60]

Rivera must have felt swindled after Pataki's reelection. Reaction by the 1199 political machine was swift. On April 1, 2003, the union chartered 900 buses to carry between 25,000 and 35,000 people from around the state to the capitol to protest the budget. The buses clogged the New York State Thruway and the largest arena in Albany, rented by the union, could not hold all the protestors gathered to hear speeches by legislative and union leaders. Rivera and hospital leaders said the budget cuts would mean the firing of tens of thousands of workers. 1199 launched a television ad campaign against the budget, as did other major unions—though 1199's pragmatic approach was apparent: The ads did not mention Pataki by name. Rivera's public relations advisor told a *New York Times* reporter, "One thing he [Rivera] is not, is stupid."[61] In May, the state legislature, including the Republican-led senate and with the backing of most of the state's union leaders, passed a budget that, in defiance of Pataki's wishes, raised taxes and restored a number of cuts, including those to education and Medicaid. Pataki vetoed it and the legislature overrode a governor's veto of the budget for the first time in two decades.[62]

In the summer of 2004, 1199 reopened its contract with the League of Voluntary Hospitals a year early, a contract that by then covered over 71,500 workers. Several hospitals had announced they would close, and private hospitals had fallen significantly behind in their contributions to employee pension and benefit funds, including the 1199/League health plan. The union offered to give back 1 percent of the raise promised in the last year of the previous contract, in order to allow the hospitals to keep up with rising health care costs for their employees by diverting it into the Benefit Fund. The union also consented to a reduction in employers' pension contributions. In exchange, the union obtained a 12 percent raise over the following four years. The contract maintained job security language, this time applying a no-lay-off clause to workers hired before January 1, 2000.

Rivera indicated that the raises did not, unlike the previous contract, depend on any state financing.[63]

From early in Rivera's tenure, the union took a conciliatory tone toward hospital's presentation of their financial problems as well as their managerial decisions. The union's focus on the ameliorative possibilities of training and upgrading largely left intact the organization of the health care labor process—when it did not exacerbate the situation on the shop floor by shifting more work and responsibility onto workers themselves. The apparent reluctance to confront the problems of the workplace directly— and therefore the decisions of hospital managers and leaders—predates Rivera, however. 1199's original leaders were comforted by the criticism that they did not impact the organization of health care delivery: It had been a strategic condition of their organizing success. Leon Fink and Brian Greenberg write in their history of 1199, "from its very inception 1199 faced down industry charges that collective bargaining would seriously impair the functions of health care institutions, interposing a dangerous third party between patients and health professionals."[64] As early as 1199's 1970 contract negotiations, former union-staffer Elinor Langer lamented, "1199 has never questioned the hospitals' version of their economic situation."[65]

Over the course of the 1990s, the union was persuaded by the hospitals' argument that without state backing or guarantees, layoffs and restructuring were inevitable and substantial wage increases inconceivable. (Even if some union leaders were not persuaded, their tactics suggested otherwise.) Initially, there was a sense that the layoffs were unnecessary and unjust, not inevitable. A 1991 *1199 News* article on how to fight layoffs reported that when Maimonides Medical Center attempted to lay off workers in about a dozen full-time jobs, 1199ers there "met with the hospital president, demanded financial data and seniority lists, pointed out that cuts were aimed at the most vulnerable patient population...and began making plans for a demonstration outside the hospital."[66] Maimonides management withdrew the layoff request.

The brochure the union sent to its members in 1997, however, shows the union had decided not to question the hospitals' presentation of their financial position nor the implication that the wages of the workforce were the cause of declining operating margins. It was consistent with what had become 1199's long-term public relations campaign: to persuade not only the state but also union members that hospitals were in a bind not of their making. Workers probably needed persuading; after all, they were confronted on a daily basis with examples of irrational managerial decisions and costly misbegotten "reforms" like those described in chapter 1.

New York City hospitals have always had financially precarious balance sheets, some of which is due to the high proportion of New Yorkers without insurance; on that front, 1199 was able to make some progress through the Family Health Plus program in the late 1990s. But the burden of the uninsured was born disproportionately throughout the decade by the city's public hospital system, and (as I will argue in the next chapter) 1199's hesitancy to step between patients and hospital managers also extended to a reluctance to step between the patient-public and payers (insurers and government) more broadly. Pressure for more funding, which 1199 applied aggressively, is quite different than pressure to change how that funding is used and the health care system financed. In addition, the blame for this financial fragility could not simply be laid with public or private payers for health care services, as the case of Mount Sinai showed. Management itself bore much of it, and 1199 did not attempt to subject those managers to scrutiny. Such scrutiny would necessarily encompass not only the financial position of the hospitals, but managerial decisions about how to allocate their revenue. 1199, however, supported the presumption that hospital managers knew best—they knew best how to organize their finances and operations and to arrange work in their facilities.

At least by 1998, the union should have been suspicious of hospital leaders' unrelenting claims of fiscal unsustainability. In the lead-up to the 1998 contract talks, some voluntary hospitals, especially smaller nonteaching hospitals with a greater share of Medicaid patients, were unquestionably in a financially precarious position, but in 1997 and 1998 Pataki had not proposed to cut Medicaid—as he did in 1995 when his first reelection campaign neared—and total operating margins at voluntary hospitals actually increased on average in 1997. Payments according to managed care arrangements (as opposed to fee-for-service), which were repeatedly invoked by hospital officials as a cause of their problems, accounted for only about one-fifth of discharged patients at large hospitals and academic medical centers, and the most financially distressed voluntary hospitals were those that relied disproportionately on payments from Medicaid under traditional, fee-for-service arrangements.[67] It is true that operating margins at most voluntary hospitals were falling in 1998, when contract negotiations took place, and the recently passed federal Balanced Budget Act included provisions for substantial Medicare cuts. Still, there were grounds for arguing that their position was not nearly as precarious as they had been claiming for years. The United Hospital Fund's updates on city voluntary hospitals spuriously tied the operating losses to increases in the hospital workforce (the first increases since 1995),[68] but as is customary in New York health care politics, the lack of detailed information on how hospitals spent their revenues made it impossible to identify other probable causes of losses, especially managerial decisions. Moreover, acute care hospitals had, with Rivera's help, managed to consolidate their power and position in the market in a number of ways, especially through mergers and by becoming health insurers themselves. Finally, before the 1998 contract negotiations, the national and regional economies began to emerge from their slump.

An unusually lengthy 1997 article in *1199 News* on health policy, co-authored by health policy specialist Howard Berliner, contained some atypically critical observations. The article stated that restructuring and reengineering "generally boils down to making fewer workers do more work," and trying to make "workers more flexible" and have "them perform more tasks." The article also pointed out that managers needed to look beyond 1199ers for the sources of their cost problems—"to extravagant compensation of doctors and some other professionals, top heavy administration, and duplication of equipment and services." Still, the union had already embraced multiskilling as a solution to layoffs, not their cause, and the article also claimed workers "will have to be more flexible and adaptable, since it will be more difficult to precisely prescribe a particular job routine," and "will have to be taught to do multiple jobs." It also contained the first, and one of the few, mentions of communication skills training in the newsletter, under the unsurprising subheading "tomorrow's health care skills." In addition, the article noted that for some hospitals, "sometimes...across the board staff reductions are a real financial requirement."[69] The article reflected the tensions in the union's position. Its critical observations were perhaps intended to demonstrate to union members that at least the union was aware of the difficulties they faced on the job, but they were also tempered by accommodation and did not inform the union's external strategy.

Even accepting that some voluntary hospitals were operating under tight financial conditions, there are reasons to think that 1199 could or should have called into question the necessity of restructuring and market-based solutions. Most important should have been the reports and experiences of workers themselves. The dangers and limitations of restructuring could have been predicted from the angry letters that nurses around the country wrote to their professional journals (until they burnt out and quit); but 1199's own members recognized as well the problems with hospital management and were willing to tell almost anyone who spent some time with them, as I did.

Furthermore, by 1998, evidence was in to suggest that cost-cutting and restructuring carried out under the catch-all rubric of "managed care" did not in fact contain costs. Public opinion showed that the climate for managed care had become considerably more hostile than in the past, with over half of Americans expressing support for increased government regulation of managed care.[70] In addition, annual cost increases of health benefits for employees jumped in 1997 after having been fairly stable for several years. (By 2002, when health care premiums increased on average by 14.7 percent, and some markets reported increases as high as 20 percent, the heyday of managed care was a distant memory.)[71]

Although multiskilling programs funded by HCRA were already underway in 1997 and 1998, millions of dollars of training funds were yet to be received and spent. In 1999, after a two-year delay, the first cycle of federal waiver transition aid (CHCCDP), $250 million, of which at least 25 percent was to be for training programs, was disbursed to hospitals. This wave of funding for training, coming on top of the HCRA state grants, began to attract the attention of critics who argued the money was no longer necessary. They noted that not all of the state funds for training had even been spent, let alone this new stream of federal funds. (Rivera had reportedly allowed $148 million in the HCRA workforce retraining pool to be diverted to the pool for hospitals' charity care.)[72] 1199ers countered that the state funds, which were spent both for retraining those laid off and for on-the-job training such as the patient care technician upgrading program, had averted layoffs and the new federal funds were now needed to fill shortages. 1199 estimated that 4,000 of its members had so far received training under the HWRI grants and 35,000 people a year would benefit from the federal waiver funds.[73]

1199 was able to justify the continuation of training grants in part because hospital administrators continued to threaten layoffs and claim they were under financial duress, which was perhaps one reason the union did not more aggressively challenge those claims. After Pataki won reelection in 1998—a campaign in which 1199 remained ostensibly neutral even though Rivera publicly appeared at the governor's side[74]—he tried again to drastically cut Medicaid. The 1199-hospital coalition launched a TV ad campaign against Pataki's proposed cuts not unlike that of 1995. The campaign asserted that the cuts would result in hospital closures and layoffs. Rivera told the media in June that New York City's private hospitals had already allowed 2,571 employees to take early retirement and 600 additional workers had lost their jobs because of Medicaid cuts since April.[75] But the broader trends suggested the period of intense threats of layoffs was coming to a close. Rivera and other political power brokers in New York State continued to seek and receive increased funding for the health care sector, including the training of health care workers, but the rationale behind such training shifted from that of potential layoffs to that of potential shortages. In June of 2000, reporter Jennifer Steinhauer wrote a story buried in the metropolitan section of the *New York Times* titled "Workers Cut as Hospitals Tighten Belts." On Christmas Day of the same year, she wrote a front-page article with the headline "Worker Shortage in Health Fields Worst in Decades."[76] In the governor's January 2001 press release announcing $28.1 million in grants for worker retraining aid funded by HCRA's 2000 renewal, the term layoff does not appear, as it did in his 1997 press releases for prior versions of the same funding. Instead, the funding is referred to as a "worker recruitment and retention" effort. (However, a second press release from the same month announcing the disbursement of cycles two and three of the federal waiver aid still maintained the original rationale attached to this funding—that it was required for the adjustment to managed care.)[77]

During the 1990s, the union also let management off the hook by refraining from making a direct connection between managerial actions and the quality of patient care. It is true that throughout the decade, articles in *1199 News* described, or more often noted, that patient care was threatened by continual cost-cutting and an overstretched workforce. Most consistently, however, problems with patient care were linked to the state budget and the layoffs cuts to Medicaid would entail. Rather than focusing on

the longer-term management of the hospital industry, 1199's political energies were siphoned into the almost-annual fight against cuts proposed in
the state budget. Thus, a connection was established between patient care
and the state that bypassed managerial and organizational decisions. "Restructuring," as an organizational-level change entailing job redesign and
layoffs was treated as inevitable in the face of budget cuts. While this fight
waged on with the state, most New York City hospitals—especially the
academic medical centers—persevered and some even prospered (despite
their meager operating margins on paper).[78]

With 1199's help, hospital leaders were able to exempt themselves from
responsibility for patient care. In their attack on Pataki's 1999 proposed
budget, the hospital association and union launched a radio ad that said,
"Governor Pataki's $1 billion in health care cuts will force some hospitals
to close. They will mean fewer nurses, less care in nursing homes, and
they'll devastate the high quality of care we expect when we get sick."[79]
Such ads enabled hospitals to mask, with union support, that they wanted
to cut some staff as a cost-saving measure. Their aims were not identical
to the union, except in these annual budget fights. The hospitals wanted,
above all, to be able to cut staff to save costs *and* retain federal and state
funding.

1199 took the position that the only way to prevent staffing cuts was to
secure enough federal and state funding for hospitals that it could persuade
them not to do so. An alternative strategy might have been for the union
to implicate management in staffing cuts and restructuring and the dangers they created for patient care. That approach, however, would have
endangered the union's partnership with hospital leaders and the united
front they presented to those legislators and policy makers that controlled
health care financing. The union might have argued—to the public, its
members, and the state—that the hospitals were not as financially weak as
they claimed and that the financial difficulties they did face were not due to
problems with its frontline workforce (whether its wages, the organization
of work, or its attitudes). This would suggest that wage reductions, layoffs,
and restructuring were not inevitable—even in the event of budget cuts.
Making such an argument, however, would have required becoming the
"dangerous third party" that 1199 had long promised not to be. It would
have required taking a more activist role in how hospitals were run and
how they spent payments for care. 1199 instead opted to go along with

changes in the workplace that put pressure on workers individually—even facilitating them through on-the-job training—but to offer compensatory benefits outside the workplace (such as upgrading programs) while working with management to maintain employment.

Some amount of change of New York City's health care sector is long overdue—for the benefit of patients and to reduce costs, such as the lack of health care services within many poor urban neighborhoods and the overemphasis on acute care at the cost of primary care. But 1199, by allying with hospital leaders, became an obstacle to some of those changes and allowed hospitals to link justifiable calls for change with a host of unnecessary "reforms" aimed at 1199 members. 1199's members became, in a sense, the hostages in the union and hospitals' fight with the state. While 1199's position was surely a difficult one, its public relations campaign repeatedly linked its members' fates not to the decisions of hospital management but to the decisions of the state. Paradoxically, the union's strategy during this period reinforced the public perception that workers' wages were the causes of health care cost increases, by continually linking its contract demands to the demands for greater public funding of private hospitals. It seemed that 1199 could not obtain a contract without state concessions to hospitals, culminating in direct underwriting of the contract in 2002. The interests of 1199 members were in that way pitted against the interests of those who consume health care and pay taxes. Rivera was correct to observe that ultimately it is the state that ensures hospitals, even private ones, can survive. In refusing to confront hospital managers and by securing subsidies for private hospitals through shady and secretive deals, however, 1199 seemed to be an accomplice in what many saw as irresponsible if not corrupt uses of taxpayer dollars. Paradoxically, this reinforced a widely held notion that health care would be better operated under private, market principles than public auspices, an ideology 1199 ostensibly rejects.

Despite all the union's efforts on the hospitals' behalf, the wage increases 1199 obtained under Rivera barely kept pace with increases in the cost of living. From 1989 to 2005, the cumulative value of raises negotiated by 1199 in League contracts was 62.5 percent (excluding one-time bonus payments that were not built into base wages) and the consumer price index in the New York metropolitan area increased by 62.9 percent. In other words, a health care worker making $343.59 a week in the summer of 1989 (the weekly minimum rate for the lowest-paid workers) could expect to make

$558.26 a week in the summer of 2005 because of raises, while the same amount of consumer goods increased to $559.58. By contrast, the consumer price index in urban areas for hospital services alone increased by 174 percent in the same period.[80]

The charge that 1199 was unwilling to interfere in hospital affairs, in particular in terms of how care was organized and delivered, may seem exaggerated. After all, the 1994 contract laid the basis for joint labor-management committees at facilities where its members worked, a move not unique to 1199. Health sector labor-management projects were established around the country in the 1990s explicitly to "promote employee involvement in the implementation of organizational changes prompted by increasing competitive pressures and decreasing reimbursements."[81] These included an alliance in California between the giant health plan Kaiser Permanente and twenty-five locals of the American Federation of Labor and Congress of Industrial Organizations (AFL-CIO). In the few New York City hospitals receptive to labor management projects, 1199 officials claimed that labor management relations improved, formal grievances declined as workers and management learned to work through their problems independently, and the union was able to play a direct part in negotiating how restructuring and reengineering was carried out in several hospital units, in particular avoiding layoffs. The small registered nurse division of 1199, which established a staff-patient ratio project in its 1999 collective agreement, was able to negotiate staffing ratios for some facilities using a "methodology" of "interest-based problem-solving" rather than "traditional methods of adversarial negotiation processes."[82] Rather than become a dangerous third party, the union aligned itself with a branch of new unionism that promises to "add value" to enterprise.[83]

Yet, the long-term wisdom of such labor-management partnerships for the labor movement are unclear, and the short-term effects of their programs largely unknown. Partnership rather than confrontation may not always be desirable. A representative of the militant California Nurses Association, which advocates legislated minimum nurse staffing ratios, characterized the Kaiser Permanente Labor-Management Partnership as one "in which the company accepts unions and the unions actively market Kaiser, while agreeing to a gag clause on Kaiser's decisions that harm patients, from hospital closures to worker deskilling to notorious HMO gatekeeping practices."[84] There are hints that 1199ers are skeptical of their union's relationship with management. One 1199 executive vice president commented, "More worker education about the external reality (industry forces affecting the employer) is needed to overcome the lack of buy-in among rank-and-filers" to the concept of partnership.[85] We have seen that many trainers and educators tried to convey just these "realities" in courses implemented around the city. As TechLeaders Consulting promises on its website, their training shows workers "the big picture and how their jobs may be affected when cash flow turns negative" and will increase employee morale.[86]

In a 1999 analysis of the allied, "hidden" health care workforce in California, the authors praised the creation of joint labor-management partnerships in health care and sanguinely concluded, "job preservation in this dynamic environment may not be possible. Therefore, it will be the responsibility of the unions to collaboratively work with industry to reposition the workforce, particularly at the lowest skills levels, and to retrain workers for the new jobs of the twenty-first century."[87] Such an approach has also been called "high-road partnerships," in which firms and unions cooperate to create high-paying, high-skilled jobs under the assumption that higher productivity and quality will compensate for higher labor costs. Firms on the "low road," by contrast, pay the lowest wages possible to the lowest skilled workers possible and hope that the higher profit margin will compensate for higher rates of turnover and problems with quality.[88] For instance, the AFL-CIO formed the Working for America Institute in 1998, which is "dedicated to building a high value-added, socially inclusive, high-road economy."[89]

Many high-road partnerships are focused on trying to save and create good jobs, which has long been the missing element of U.S. workforce policy. The major result of 1199's involvement in restructuring in the 1990s, however, was the creation of the patient care technician (PCT) position, which was achieved only on the condition that certain more highly skilled or specialized and highly paid positions (RNs, phlebotomists, EKG technicians) were downsized. The troubling aspect of the message that those with the "lowest skill levels" must be "repositioned" is that the core of what many of these workers do is provide care, which is a job that is neither low-skilled nor likely to be outmoded by the advances of the twenty-first century. Certainly some jobs will change, and people should be trained to adjust to those changes; registrars need to learn to use computers and lab techs new automated technology. But nursing assistants, now PCTs, were trained in exactly those skills that are most likely to be automated and rendered obsolete by wondrous new technologies, such as "smart" bandages that can take a patient's temperature and blood sugar or remote devices that can measure and report blood pressure. Maybe such devices will one day be able to draw and analyze blood samples (perhaps with patient or family assistance). Far less likely are machines that will comfort patients and clean their butts. Such jobs may be downloaded unto unpaid caregivers or outsourced to countries and places with cheaper labor, but there would seem to be some limits on this as well (unless we can envision a dystopia of America's elderly being shipped to nursing homes in less de-veloped nations or "right to work" states). But regardless of the location or century, caring labor remains the basis of what many health care workers do. This is still a task that is systematically undervalued and obscured by talk of "jobs of the twenty-first century" and the creation of training pro-grams that continually exhort workers to prepare for them.

As we know, much of the training funds in New York were also spent on individual upgrading; in which the responsibility for overcoming the limits of the labor market is assigned to individual workers. (As the direc-tor of a joint labor-management training program in the airline industry reported to the *New York Times,* he tells his workers, "You're in control of your career path."[90]) Much of the rest was spent on soft skills training un-related to job creation. The Conference Board of Canada report confirms that joint labor-management training programs in sectors such as trans-portation and hospitality have also emphasized customer service, com-munication, and soft skills training, which ultimately makes individual workers responsible for accommodating and improving the conditions of the jobs in which they find themselves. While 1199 did not invent such training, or the idea that training should be the primary response to eco-nomic restructuring, virtually all of the state- or federally funded training programs at voluntary hospitals in New York City had to be approved by the 1199 joint labor-management training fund. Sometimes the approval was only tacit. In many instances, however, the fund took on a planning and coordinating role: recommending vendors/trainers, communicating between various hospital human resources directors about what their col-leagues were doing, and filing reports on how funds were spent with the public granting agencies.

In 1971, former 1199 staffer Elinor Langer argued in the *New York Review of Books* that the union's best opportunity to effect a radical agenda was in the "fundamental texture of the industrial system itself," so it should more carefully address the economics of hospitals and take a "fundamental look at the whole notion of skills and training in this society, since in the hospitals it is the rigid classification of skills and jobs which plays a key role in keeping the workers down." She speculated on what might happen "if skills could be demystified and training programs initiated which were realistic (instead of, as at present, immensely costly because they help to reinforce the divisions in the system they are trying to reform)." Thus Langer was disappointed when a 1970 contract proposal that would have considerably expanded the recently created Training and Upgrading Fund, revealingly titled "Establishment of Career Ladders Within Each Hospital," was shelved.[91]

The Training and Upgrading Fund is now a behemoth—"Wal-Mart," as one official joked—compared to what it was in 1968. Despite its new resources, the training fund has not been used to pursue the path suggested by Langer; the counselors and assessment test administrators who stand as sentries to training programs and occupations do not suggest that skills have been demystified. Rather, in the process of securing hundreds of millions of dollars in state and federal funding for training, the union and health care workforce planners employed a discourse of worker inadequacies, not competence and ability. Wal-Mart is devoted to maximizing size and growth. The company's mission does not include providing the best possible working conditions, wages, and benefits. This makes it an apt metaphor for 1199's turn toward offering training that either is outside the workplace—and therefore disconnected from conditions on the hospital floor—or that facilitates deteriorating conditions on the shop floor and then appeals to workers to accommodate them. The metaphor tells the whole story: defined as an enterprise to enhance the bottom line above all, the training and education industry, like Wal-Mart, bends both trainers (producers) and health care workers (consumers) to an impoverished vision of what it means to get by in America.

9

Education as a Benefit

Labor unions have long struck questionable bargains to survive to fight another day, but 1199's training and education programs are the basis of a strategy that will have lasting consequences and shape future choices about how to respond to the inequities and insecurities that face growing numbers of Americans. Education that is a benefit of employment is a potential obstacle to a public education system that is universal, accessible, and of high quality. At least that is a plausible lesson to draw from the historical record on health insurance in the United States. In the years following World War II, health care was established as a benefit of employment, often collectively bargained, rather than a right, creating a private insurance system that has become an insurmountable obstacle to universal health security. The United States is the only industrialized nation that does not provide universal health insurance to its citizens, and unions played a pivotal role in shaping this reality. Collectively bargained health benefits have reinforced a health care system in which access is stratified, insurers (now largely for-profit companies) "cherry-pick" and cover the healthiest populations while government payers cover the most costly and vulnerable groups, and providers of services (including physicians, hospitals, but also pharmaceutical companies) focus on developing products and services for which there is a viable market—for which they will be paid. The question is whether trends in education might point toward a parallel future.

The analogy between health care and education developed below may at first seem dubious: education through high school is ostensibly a well-established universal right and education at the postsecondary level is readily available through public and community colleges. 1199's joint labor-management training programs therefore might be seen as opening access to a level of training and education beyond that which is a basic right, supplementing the security that is provided publicly. Many of the programs to which 1199 members now have access through their employment attempt, however, to make up for the inequities in access to basic kinds of education. Bridge-to-college programs, for instance, provide core competencies in reading and math that should be the responsibility of high schools or, in the case of newcomers, accessible to immigrants no matter their employer. Programs to support union members in college courses—whether toward a general degree or a specific occupational credential—are necessary because college is not readily accessible, even to those who are unquestionably qualified. Students face growing costs, high rates of indebtedness, and other obstacles created by the continual underfunding of public institutions like City University of New York (CUNY). Despite the abstract agreement that education is a universal right, education in the United States is in reality a service made available on discriminatory terms.

On-the-job training, such as in-services or job-specific training, has been, traditionally and logically, the responsibility of employers (though such training has long been subsidized by the state in various ways, and, as in New York, employers seem to increasingly expect public educational institutions to provide such training). This chapter, however, focuses on the significance of union-organized programs such as individual upgrading, college preparation, and tuition assistance—programs that compensate for deficiencies in what has been the traditional role of public education. Like private health care benefits, such programs receive large amounts of public financing and subsidies, which are channeled through private, even profit-driven organizations charged with the task of designing and administering benefits.

Much can be learned about the possible consequences of these programs—for working Americans and the unions who represent them—from the historical case of health care benefits.

In the short term, the training and education industry for allied health care workers in New York City offers access to education to a group of working Americans who have historically been discriminated against in education as in the labor market. Union programs offer tuition assistance, and in some cases even salary replacement, in an era when more and more Americans go into significant debt to acquire even entry-level skills and credentials. In the long term, however, the risk is that the employment-based training and education industry will become an obstacle to an adequate universal, public education system. It is an industry in which public resources support narrowly conceived programs open only to people lucky enough to have the right job with the right employer or union. Those not among the lucky few do not have the same access to training and education that is promoted as the key to social mobility.

Moreover, this private training system potentially forecloses alternative responses to the growing inequality in the labor market and in educational outcomes and achievement, especially on the part of Labor. As long as union members receive educational benefits, unions may feel less inclined to use their political force to press for a more radical response to economic restructuring than training and upgrading. This worry may seem overly pessimistic, even misplaced given labor's decline, but the legacy of labor's role in shaping the current health care system warrants such concern. And in New York City, at least, labor unions, especially 1199, still play a significant role in shaping the lives and prospects of the working class as a whole. Today's training programs are at odds with 1199's other efforts to create classwide solidarities and represent the voices of the marginalized in the U.S. economy. History matters, in the sense that we must attend not only to the specific institutions, policies, and power relations that are the conditions for social change in the present but also to a whole series of past decisions and policies that have shaped the possibilities available today.[1] Thus, we must consider health workforce training and education programs in a comparative historical context. 1199 is certainly *willing* to fight for broader social rights, including universal education and health security, but at the same time its institutional interests and strategies make some kinds of fights and policy changes practically less likely.

Private Benefits and Security

Collectively bargained welfare and benefit funds became a major aspect of the social safety net in the United States in the wake of World War II. Although many labor leaders at the time recognized that employment-based benefit funds were inadequate remedies to the failures of the state to provide basic economic and social security, they energetically advocated for their expansion in the collective bargaining process. Some historians view welfare and benefit funds as a payoff business leaders and conservative politicians made to labor leaders in exchange for heavy restrictions on unions' scope of action. Other historians view them as a significant labor achievement in an increasingly hostile political climate. In either case, the decades of labor-management accommodation and "business unionism" that followed the war were viable only while the economy produced new and better jobs, an era whose end was marked by the "energy crisis" and stagflation of the early 1970s that precipitated labor's stunning decline. The debate over labor's role in securing welfare and benefit funds applies as well to the circumstances that 1199 faced in the 1990s. One lesson from the postwar struggle over health security is that labor leaders have always downplayed how their choices at one moment might foreclose possibilities in the future.

The 1935 National Labor Relations Act (also known as the Wagner Act) strengthened workers' rights to form unions and reinvigorated the U.S. labor movement, but World War II provided the political cloak for employers and conservatives to dismantle many of labor's advances. Most important for my purposes, wartime policies enforced the notion that the legitimate way for unions to handle disputes was through bargaining and contracts, rather than action and activism on the shop floor or in political arenas.[2] Many labor leaders were co-opted through the war-planning process: They were invited to sit on wartime boards that would govern labor relations, such as the National War Labor Board (NWLB), and became part of a tripartite structure governing the economy, with employers and the state.[3]

At one level, it would seem these arrangements allowed labor leaders to ensure that workers' interests were considered during exceptional wartime conditions. Even though the NWLB imposed strict limits on wages and profits during the war, it also ruled that contributions to employee benefit plans would not be counted as wages, making fringe benefits (non-wage benefits) an obvious substitute for wage increases and a possible stake in collective bargaining. Labor leaders might not have been enthusiastic about bargaining for fringe benefits, but many employers had unilaterally offered benefit plans during the war in part because of a 1943 IRS tax-ruling allowing businesses to deduct contributions to health and welfare funds (essentially hiding profits that would otherwise have been subject to the wartime excess profits tax by transferring them to benefit plans).[4] There was therefore a risk unions would have no control over the structure and aims of benefit plans.

Jennifer Klein has argued, however, that the NWLB's aim in encouraging negotiation over fringe benefits was to ensure stability in labor-management relations during wartime by institutionalizing contracts and collective bargaining, not to expand employees' rights or entitlements.[5] Indeed, stability was by no means guaranteed. Even though most unions in the American Federation of Labor (AFL) and leaders of the Congress of Industrial Organizations (CIO) had made no-strike pledges for the war's duration,[6] which most union members probably supported, the combination of wage limits, deteriorating working conditions, and soaring corporate profits generated considerable unrest among the rank and file, who instigated an uncounted number of wildcat (unauthorized) strikes during this period. While labor leaders began to see themselves as partners and equals to their corporate counterparts, the latter took advantage of the climate of patriotism and duty by speeding up production and ignoring safety regulations: More than ten times the number of Americans were injured on the job than those injured fighting in the war.[7] Employment-based, collectively bargained health benefits grew explosively during the war and became a key means of enforcing a labor-management accord in the face of the ongoing struggle and resistance of the rank and file.

When profit and wage restrictions were lifted after the war, employers fought vigorously against every type of union demand. Unions at the time represented an unprecedented number and density of U.S. workers—roughly one-third—and 1945 and 1946 were the "most strike-filled years in American history."[8] Unions attempted to capitalize on their wartime status and expand the scope of collective bargaining. In 1946, John L. Lewis led his United Mine Workers (UMW) on strike against the horrific conditions in the mines and the inadequacy of health and safety provisions in the industry. The strike was capable of slowing post-war economic growth, so when the mine owners refused to settle, the Truman administration seized control of the mines and signed a contract giving the mine workers an employer-financed health and welfare fund under union control.[9] Inspired in part by the mine workers, other unions began to seek not only fringe benefits as part of the collective bargaining process but also benefit funds they controlled. In turn, many companies accelerated their unilateral purchase of health benefit plans from commercial insurers to ward off the twin threats of universal benefits imposed by a "socialist" state and labor union control.[10] Unions also tried to expand their role in industrial planning. For instance, as the war came to an end, Walter Reuther, president of the United Auto Workers (UAW), demanded that General Motors provide a 30 percent wage increase without increasing its prices, which "[put] the corporation's price policies on the bargaining table" and sought to undermine the supposed contradiction between workers' and consumers' interests.[11]

Even though Reuther and the CIO won 18.5 percent wage increases in the round of strikes and bargaining that ended in the winter of 1946, those wage increases evaporated when the government lifted price controls the same summer and industry leaders turned wage increases into price increases, forcing unions back to the bargaining table. Nelson Lichtenstein has pointed out "the frequent strikes and annual pay boosts of this era, which industry used to raise prices, were at least partially responsible for creating the conservative, antilabor political climate that gave Republicans their large victory in the 1946 elections."[12] When Republicans gained control of both houses of Congress that year, one of their first actions was to cripple the labor movement through the Taft-Hartley Act, legislation of which the most notorious feature required union leaders to pledge that they were not communists and drove a devastating wedge between leaders and members of some unions and among unions themselves.

The Act, however, went far beyond red-baiting. Among other provisions, it banned secondary boycotts, prohibited closed shops, imposed severe penalties for labor leaders whose members engaged in wildcat strikes, eliminated informal methods the National Labor Relations Board (NLRB) previously used to determine if a majority of workers favored a union, made it possible for a union to be decertified, and allowed individual states to pass laws further restricting union security. Describing the bureaucratized and formalized labor relations system created by Taft-Hartley, Rick Fantasia and Kim Voss write, "all the effervescence of the collective dynamic, with its capacity to generate wonderment, creativity, and group solidarity among participants (and therefore the source of its strength), would now give way to regulation, individualization, and atomization that are the inevitable products of judicial proceedings, electoral procedures, and the systematic delegation of authority to those of higher rank."[13] Or as Lichtenstein puts it, if Taft-Hartley "did not destroy the union movement, it did impose upon it a legal/administrative straitjacket that encouraged contractual parochialism and penalized any serious attempt to project a classwide political-economic strategy."[14]

Part of that classwide political-economic strategy would have been the creation of universal health security. When the NLRB ruled in 1948 that employers were obligated to negotiate fringe benefits under the terms of the Taft-Hartley Act, a ruling upheld in 1949 in federal court, labor leaders understood that this ruling was intended to buy their acquiescence to the Act's other provisions. The government encouraged labor to seek fringe benefits while government and the courts blocked unions in their efforts to unionize supervisory personnel, bargain on an industrywide basis, and (most notably) influence decisions on production and prices by forcing corporations to open their books or negotiate job content. Labor leaders were excluded from government policy making in which they had participated during the war, and new campaign laws made it difficult for labor to organize voters and back candidates that might undo antiunion legislation.[15]

Given these huge losses, it was difficult for labor to resist the opportunity to take credit for securing fringe benefits. Moreover, even this would require a fight: The requirement that employers negotiate benefits did not mean they had to provide, or make unions partners in planning and administering, them. The 1948 NLRB ruling merely made unions' efforts to secure these benefits credible. In this environment, labor unions aggressively pursued private benefits. The largest push was during bargaining in 1949, when major union leaders such as Philip Murray, president of the CIO, and Walter Reuther declared that social insurance, not wage increases, would be the center of their collective bargaining strategy. By the end of 1954, twelve million workers and seventeen million dependents were enrolled in collectively bargained health plans, representing three-quarters of union members.[16] Yet unions' embrace of employment-based, collectively negotiated benefits made the fight for universal health care immeasurably more difficult. Welfare and benefit funds became the core clients of a private insurance industry and diluted the political will among labor leaders and Americans with secure employment to fight for a universal health care system.[17]

Despite their push for private benefits, no labor unions were able to negotiate for benefit plans over which they had as much control as the mine workers. Under Taft-Hartley, if employers were to contribute to benefit funds in which unions played a role, they had to be under joint control and placed in a trust—the same structure that governs 1199's benefit plans today. Taft-Hartley plans, moreover, represented a minority of the benefit plans negotiated. Employers retained effective administrative and financial control of most of the health benefit plans (as well as pension plans) negotiated in the 1940s and 50s—unions merely had a say in what benefits would be included. The vast majority of benefit plans were furthermore implemented on a firm-by-firm basis. Unions could not standardize benefits across their membership, and many employers contracted the management of benefits to firms in the burgeoning commercial insurance industry and refused to share the financial details of the plans with unions.[18] Unions themselves favored contracting health benefits to Blue Cross and Blue Shield plans,[19] which were nonprofit and pooled risk over entire communities (not just low-risk population groups). They too, however, became a major force in opposition to universal health care. In addition, benefit plans varied greatly in terms of the services they provided, and employers did not necessarily pay the majority of health care costs.[20] In a 2003 article depicting organized labor's "century-long struggle to achieve universal coverage," Andrew Stern, SEIU's president, accurately noted that the failure of labor unions' postwar campaigns for a national health plan was due in part to the opposition of the commercial insurance industry, "which had become firmly entrenched thanks to labor's success in winning benefits at the bargaining table."[21]

Stern's comment shows that despite the limits of many collectively bargained benefit plans and their role in reducing the possibilities for a universal health plan, union leaders continue to understand the course of events as an achievement. It is true that securing pension and health benefits was a remarkable feat. Things could have been worse. In reaction to the mine workers' victory, the original draft of the Taft-Hartley Act sought to bar union involvement in health and welfare funds entirely. Only after pressure from Democrats was the Act amended so that it barred employer contributions to funds under unilateral control of unions.[22] At least benefits secured through the collective bargaining process gave unions an opportunity to ensure that those benefits were more than corporate public relations stunts and met workers' needs. Evidence shows that private wage supplements were indeed highest in union-dense industries. In the absence of union pressure, which forced employers either to bargain for such benefits or provide them to ward off organizing campaigns, employers would likely have done little to compensate for the absence of public services.[23] Such benefits—not only for health, but also for pensions and paid vacations—might never have become part of the social wage at all were it not for unions' resolve. And while the economy produced well-paying full-time jobs and union membership grew, union leaders might have justifiably felt that employment-based health and pension benefits were tantamount to a social right.

"Realistic" labor leaders, too, argued that the chances of achieving universal health security, even with their might behind it, were not good. There is indeed no guarantee that had labor fought more vigorously for universal health security, as opposed to employment-based benefits, it would have been victorious. Those opposed to a government-sponsored health plan or government-mandated insurance had long nurtured reactionary and highly effective arguments against a role for government. Labor-supported legislation for a national health plan—which the American Medical Association and conservatives relentlessly branded as "socialized medicine"—was repeatedly introduced and defeated as early as the mid-1930s. Such rhetoric only intensified after the war.[24]

Some labor leaders, however, continued to support a national health system after the war. They believed that their role was to fight for the security of working Americans as a whole and not just their members. The more conservative group of craft unions, the American Federation of Labor, was least inclined to give up the fight for universal health security, largely because its members were employed by small and widely dispersed employers with whom it was more difficult to negotiate uniform benefits.[25] Reuther indicated he thought the escalating costs of privately negotiated benefits would inevitably lead employers to the conclusion that universal, state-sponsored benefits were more efficient and less onerous.

Nonetheless, Michael Brown has argued the idea that private insurance would force employers to join the fight for universal health insurance can be viewed in retrospect as nothing more than labor's rationalization of its collective bargaining strategy.[26] Even as early as the late 1940s, "most industrial unionists gave national health insurance only lip service."[27] Many observers at the time, including some within the labor movement, foresaw that the growth of private insurance would diminish, rather than escalate, the pressure to create a universal, state-sponsored health system.[28]

Labor leaders' support for collectively bargained benefits cannot be explained entirely by the fact that their strategic choices were limited. According to Brown, many labor elites welcomed the chance to negotiate for private benefits because of the advantages and prestige that would accrue to them as individuals. Brown has argued that in labor leaders' debates about the consequences of collective bargaining for social rights, the slim political chances of achieving universal health insurance "was always less relevant to unions than the question of their status and power with respect to that of managers."[29]

What seems more sure is that in the postwar era, nonwage benefits achieved through collective bargaining became "central to the viability of unions as institutions," and trade unions "came to view collectively bargained health benefits as the best weapon for recruiting and retaining members."[30] This was especially important in the wake of the Taft-Hartley provision banning closed shops (in which union membership had been required as a condition of employment). Benefit funds effectively created closed shops because employees who did not join the union would not have access to collectively bargained benefits.[31] They also played a strong symbolic role. Benefit funds were one way unions could maintain an image of strength, the sense that they could achieve concrete gains for workers in the face of devastating blows to their real power. The jointly administered Taft-Hartley plans, in particular, became important sources of institutional cohesiveness and symbolic identity for many unions, which in most cases handled the daily management of the funds.[32]

Brown has argued many unions became "welfare fiefs" more concerned with the operation of their internal bureaucracy than with organizing or struggling to improve social conditions. Indications that becoming benefits administrators and service providers had a conservative effect on labor unions appeared rather quickly in the debate over expanding health care benefits. When Harry Truman pressed for national health insurance after his reelection in 1948, John L. Lewis refused to support it in part because the mine workers' benefits were so much better.[33] By the late 1950s, unions were focused on managing and refining the private benefits they had secured for their members rather than on the extension of such benefits to all Americans or, in the case of health care, handing over such benefits to an expanded, universal public plan.[34]

Examining how labor unions today have responded to the failures of the health care system, Marie Gottschalk has argued that Taft-Hartley funds continue to operate as an "institutional straitjacket" that prevents many labor unions from taking the lead or even supporting more comprehensive health care reform efforts, especially those modeled after the Canadian system, in which the government is the single payer for most services. She argues that, at least in the case of health care, the interests of unions, as institutionalized payers for health care, now resemble those of large employers and insurers.[35]

The case of 1199, which operates one of the largest joint labor-management benefit funds in the country, lends some—though not unequivocal—support for Gottschalk's argument. In 1990, the union headed a coalition that called for universal health insurance, and Rivera cited the "tremendous problems in our [health] Benefit Fund" as contributing to the need for a public plan.[36] Similarly, according to a major 1992 profile published in the *New York Times Sunday Magazine,* Rivera's "larger agenda" was a "system of government-paid national health care patterned on the Canadian model."[37] But as the Clintons prepared their health care reform proposal in the same period, commentators noted that Rivera did not endorse a single-payer, Canadian-style health care reform, despite a number of voices in his union supporting it.[38] He preferred to wait until the Clinton proposal was released and then push it in a "progressive" direction.[39] In 1993, Rivera told *New York Newsday* that Hillary Rodham Clinton "makes you feel we're really in this together, that it's a very inclusive thing."[40] But in 1997, after the Clinton reform plan had failed, Rivera said, "[T]he effort was done in a very sloppy way. There were 500 secretive meetings led by the First Lady, who had great intentions and a great desire to achieve the goal, but, who, unfortunately, alienated the people who had to pass it—the lawmakers."[41] Rivera's disenchantment with the process was understandable, but blaming the plan's failure on the Clintons' lack of vision and organizational skill was overly simple.

Rivera did not himself push forcefully for something more radical, and his support for universal health insurance was not unqualified. Rivera was concerned that the Clinton plan did not include measures to protect and retrain the health care workforce, especially in hospitals. By 1994, the recovering health Benefit Fund also played a role in the union's strategic calculations. Rivera expressed concern that the Clinton plan could reduce the union's control over the benefits provided to its members.[42] As important, while 1199 members whose employers did not contribute to the Benefit Fund (such as home care workers) would have gained from any type of national plan, the core of the union membership was receiving benefits superior to those in most workplaces and those likely to be offered under a public plan—like the mine workers fifty years earlier. Rivera noted that through the creation of preferred provider organizations (PPOs) at specific hospitals—contracts for privileged access to union members in exchange for expanded benefits—the Benefit Fund was "moving toward a situation where 1199ers pay no out-of-pocket expenses for health care. But we could face dramatic out-of-pocket expenses for health care under the Clinton plan as it is now constituted."[43] By late 1993, nine hospitals had created such PPOs with the Benefit Fund, and by 1997 Rivera described the union's intention to "build our own health care delivery system" by allowing other unions to join the Fund.[44] The same year, the Benefit Fund severed its contract with Blue Cross and began to administer and manage its benefits in-house.

When the Clinton plan collapsed, it was barely mentioned in *1199 News,* even though it had been the newsletter's major topic for almost a year and the rationale behind the early contract negotiations in 1994. Rivera said later, "we did not get universal health care coverage from the failed health care reform of 1994, we got HMOs—insurance companies that basically have taken over the health care industry and are siphoning our dollars from the health care industry for their Wall Street bankers and investment folks...We need to put health care reform back on the forefront of the national agenda."[45] Never mind that insurance companies had been in charge of the health industry for decades, that HMOs were once models of community-controlled and determined health care, or that 1199 itself would soon support the conversion of Blue Cross Blue Shield to a for-profit insurance company. SEIU President Stern wrote, "labor did everything possible to hold off the inevitable demise of the Clinton plan," but also noted that Taft-Hartley benefit funds, in addition to large employers, were in part responsible for its failure as they "scrambled to maintain their independence" as insurers and payers.[46]

The importance of the Benefit Fund to the union was due to its symbolic and institutional power, in addition to the material support it provided union members. The Fund created its first PPO during the union's pivotal 1992 negotiations with Beth Israel Medical Center—negotiations that produced the union's first contract with a job security clause. By allowing a group of Beth Israel doctors to form a PPO under the union's health plan, the hospital secured a guaranteed patient base (especially since the workers who sought care from the PPO would have expanded benefits and no out-of-pocket expenses).[47] Similarly, in 1997 Rivera thought management might be more inclined to negotiate a contract early because of the "potential benefits to 1199 hospitals as the 1199 Benefit Fund prepares to expand into a not-for-profit HMO" and invite other unions to join the Fund.[48] The plan, which covered 400,000 thousand people by 2007, offers preferred provider contracts only to hospitals where 1199 workers are represented. In addition, "the [Benefit] Fund's growth helps as an organizing incentive," Rivera pointed out.[49] Similarly, in 1998, 1199 announced that the health plan would only cover pharmaceuticals purchased at unionized retailers, in return for which the giant drugstore chain Rite Aid agreed not to fight 1199's organizing drives in its stores.[50] Finally, the health benefits became pivotal to the image of what the union could do for its members, especially in an era when the union was unable to win wage increases beyond increasing rates of the cost of living.

On the other hand, the Benefit Fund has been in periodic fiscal trouble; health care costs have grown across the board, and hospitals have at times fallen behind in their payments to the Fund. For several years, 1199 was able to subsidize the health fund using excesses from the pension fund. In a different market environment, however, the pension fund is a less reliable safety net. Rising health care costs might be controlled more effectively under a universal, government plan and wage increases easier to obtain if health care benefits were not a major factor in the bargaining process.[51]

Today, the union has again endorsed the notion of single-payer universal health insurance.[52] Its commitment to a tax supported, non–employment-based universal health system, however, is belied by its immediate strategy on health care reform. In addition to the possible institutional constraints posed by its Benefit Fund, the union's common cause with private, voluntary hospitals has arguably moderated its stance on health care reform and financing. 1199's strategy of obtaining public funds for private hospitals has expanded the public role in private industry, but through the backdoor, with little accountability and via one-time cash infusions and funds earmarked for specific ends, which cannot provide the continuity or security of benefits that entitlements under a public welfare state would. In addition, though hospitals in a single-payer system like Canada's are private in principle, they have less fiscal autonomy than their private counterparts in the United States. The creation of a single-payer health care system would render obsolete most forms of private insurance, including the union's health plan, but it would also make private hospitals much less independent, and the union has consistently argued throughout its history that private hospitals deliver much better care than public ones.[53]

The Family Health Plus program, one of Rivera's biggest accomplishments in the arena of health policy, exemplifies the limits of an incremental approach to health care reform. While the Family Health Plus program did expand health insurance, it nonetheless covers only one hole in a patchy, poorly designed health care system. It was a progressive program in so far as it expanded a public insurance program, Medicaid, rather than employment-based insurance. But the Family Health Plus program paid for participants to enroll in managed care plans, thus bolstering the private insurance industry rather than consolidating the administration of and payment for benefits under public auspices.[54] Enrollment in the program was furthermore slowed by difficulties in contracting with managed care plans and by the same complex eligibility rules and application processes that plagued the broader Medicaid managed care program, as they would any "public" health insurance plan conceived as a privately administered means-tested assistance program, rather than a universal right.[55]

With nearly forty-seven million Americans uninsured in 2008, the employment-based system has proved itself to be utterly inadequate. Labor leaders continue to optimistically believe, however, that the rising costs of health care will force employers to embrace public health insurance. SEIU hopes that laws like the one passed in Maryland in 2005—which mandated that companies with more than ten thousand workers (in effect, Wal-Mart) spend at least 8 percent of their payroll on health care—will force employers to realize the cost advantages of a universal, public system not linked to employment. SEIU President Stern recognizes that should "fair share" laws like Maryland's succeed, they could hinder the creation of a national plan by further entrenching an employment-based system of benefits, but he has continued to endorse employer-mandate plans (sometimes called "pay or play" schemes). Wal-Mart's CEO, Lee Scott, has dutifully criticized the lack of a comprehensive health care system in the wake of union-led attacks on the company's abysmal health benefits.[56] Yet even though business leaders have vocally protested rising health care costs, few have become allies in the campaign for universal health insurance. Between 2001 and 2005, when insurance premiums for employer-sponsored plans grew by no less than 9 percent each year, employers showed that they would sooner cut benefits than join the campaign for "socialized" medicine.[57] Maryland's law was in any case struck down by the courts on the basis of federal legislation that exempts self-insured health plans from state regulations.[58] Americans have proved themselves to be highly tolerant of inequality and suffering in their midst,[59] but the increasing number of middle-class Americans who have found themselves un- or underinsured may prove to be more reliable allies in the fight for universal health insurance.

Health care, which is considered by some a basic human right, is now in the United States a service for which access and quality are based on one's success in the labor market and ability to pay. This is true for aspects of the education system as well. The phenomenon of joint labor-management training funds has not yet reached nearly the scale of collectively bargained private health plans. Nonetheless, they raise some of the same dilemmas. 1199 relied on the expansion of its job-training fund to maintain a semblance of security for its workers in a threatening climate. Yet the story of 1199's contract negotiations and political machinations indicates that the training funds may settle into a role other than the protection of health care workers from layoffs and uncertainty.

Like its health Benefit Fund, the Funds for training and job security have become pivotal to the union's image, a symbolic substitute for lackluster wage increases (especially in depicting the results of collective bargaining). They too have become an important organizing tool. In 1998, Rivera told the media that 1199's Training and Upgrading Fund would be a major feature of an image-building and organizing campaign.[60] The job training funds have become a benefit that no other competing union, or employer for that matter, can offer. 1199's initial attempts to direct all federal waiver aid (CHCCDP) to voluntary, downstate hospitals was undoubtedly so it could be used as a carrot for workers and managers in hospitals not yet organized by the union. Reports of site visits conducted by the New York State Department of Health to track the use of the training portion of the federal waiver funds—though skeletal—indicate that in at least one hospital where a sizeable proportion of the workers were not unionized, 1199 argued training funds could be used only for union members.[61]

In 2005, 1199 boosted its efforts to expand beyond New York by finalizing a merger with SEIU 2020, whose members work at Boston Medical Center and some nursing homes and small hospitals in Massachusetts. The first, and "most visible effect" of 1199's move was that it persuaded Boston Medical Center to contribute $300,000 a year to the union's training fund, which would be used to pay hospital workers to take up to twenty-four college credits a year.[62] Boston's mayor indicated he would be supportive if 1199 attempted to organize other hospitals in the city, citing the SEIU training programs as a sign of the constructive labor-management relationship the union fostered.[63] A cook at one Boston-area hospital, who was helping to bring the hospital workers into the 1199 Training and Upgrading Fund, nicely summed up the various ways the training programs were framed as valuable: "If a hospital needs certain things, their workers will be prepared. They won't need to go outside to find somebody else. That's something we've been pushing for. Plus, it gives people an A-plus feeling for the union. If they're feeling like they're in a dead end, they see the union can help them. The union can build their self-esteem."[64]

1199 now counts on the political and institutional benefits of extensive training and education programs—benefits independent of the programs' outcomes for workers. It is not alone in opening education and training as the latest frontier of the private welfare state; DC37, New York City's largest municipal union whose members include public hospital workers, "is a leader in the transformation of many unions into a private welfare state."[65] It has adopted a similar emphasis on services for its members and job training and upgrading in particular. Though the DC37 Training Fund has far less autonomy and money than its 1199 counterpart, the College of New Rochelle runs a branch for union members at DC37 headquarters in lower Manhattan. There is today even an association of joint labor-management education programs, which fosters efforts to expand these programs around the country.[66]

Education, like health care, has become a fractured system, in which it is difficult to ensure uniform standards of quality and accessibility. Just as people receive widely varying levels of care and types of health insurance based on their social or economic position, so too do they have access to very different educational experiences. Seen as part of a broader political process, blurring various types of education and training by saying that they all provide an opportunity for self-expression or self-esteem disguises real differences in quality. Of course, as one trainer remarked, it is important to help health care workers whom the education system has failed to feel "positive about the educational experience." After all, as one teacher in a GED-prep program (Veronica's teacher) observed of his students:

> They have an idea about education because they see it—they see it in their workplaces. But the vast majority of people who are highly educated in their workplaces are busy exploiting them. So they don't particularly like the people with educations, and they have a knee-jerk feeling that people with educations have no common sense. And in a lot of ways I think they're right.

This teacher, however, was thinking about how to get his students involved in reading books and engaging in creative thought for which there seems to be an ever-shrinking amount of time. The trainer who spoke of the positive "educational experience," by contrast, was referring to on-the-job training seminars. Among some people in the training and education industry there is a tacit acceptance of, or at least resignation to, the idea that it is acceptable and possible for education and learning to occur in short snippets, in almost randomly disbursed moments of attention and insight, in cross-training programs, soft skills seminars, and short-term certificate or skills programs.

In the training and education industry for allied health care workers, education has become a marketplace "where knowledge (or skills) brokers barter for the sale of their cost effective, efficient, truncated pedagogical packages" and "the notion of curriculum has been displaced by content-poor, outcomes-oriented 'packages.'" Moreover, "educators are [being] replaced by trainers and assessors, most with minimalist pedagogical education."[67] Though accreditation standards require that universities and colleges hire faculty with formal credentials, new patterns of organizing academic labor—such as the reliance on part-time and adjunct faculty—undermine the consistency of teachers and curriculum. Consider the variety of the teachers that I interviewed. Daniel, an instructor at a hospital-based OR tech program, was hired because of his previous experience as an OR tech and because he had a bachelor's degree. Similarly, the director of health sciences at Monroe College was hired because he had experience as a health information technologist and a bachelor's degree, which was necessary for accreditation purposes. For many education or training jobs, prior health care experience and a degree are the formal hiring requirements. Several other trainers and administrators I interviewed started their careers as nurses or social workers. Health care experience is useful to teaching in the health care field, but these trainers do not necessarily end up teaching in areas in which they have formal experience or knowledge. Neither does health care experience nor a degree equate with pedagogical ability. Health care facility–based human resources personnel could, in particular, be called on to teach almost anything that was deemed necessary, from technical skills to communication skills. Again, this does not mean the quality of those classes is necessarily poor, but there is un-regulated variety in terms of the background of trainers and educators in many organizations.

Most of the sub-baccalaureate certificate programs (e.g., for OR techs, certified nursing assistants, or home health care aides) considered in this study relied on nurses or foreign-trained nurses and doctors who did not or could not (because of licensing issues) practice in the United States. While I only have information on their salaries and wages from interview respondents, and some programs paid their instructors relatively well, it is difficult to make a living on what is usually part-time work. In this situation, an instructor who wants higher wages is not in a strong bargaining position. One teacher at the Consortium for Worker Education explained that the Consortium's continual efforts to replace full-time teachers with part-timers was "one of the first indications that the goal of this organization really isn't to educate people."

One administrator and former nurse pointed out the grants and contracts on which many training programs and organizations rely typically do not allow for spending on teacher preparation and education (i.e., faculty development). Moreover, education and training on a contract basis—particularly if it is training that takes workers away from their current jobs—is forced to conform to a schedule that many would argue is not conducive to learning. Sometimes students have classroom instruction for seven or eight hours a day, five days a week. This produces exhausted instructors and students and little time for the independent digestion and exploration of curriculum.

The Conference Board of Canada report on several joint labor-management training programs, including 1199's Training and Upgrading Fund, indicated that one of the major outcomes of training included in the report was a "greater appreciation of learning." Notice that the outcome is not learning, as might be measured by tests or essays, but rather an "appreciation" of learning. The Report is symptomatic of the general culture around education and training that has taken shape. In this culture, eliciting engagement has equal standing to learning. Indeed, other outcomes praised in the report, such as "increased self-confidence" and "better personal management," confirm the extent to which many education and training programs are now removed from learning, regardless of whether it is vocational skills training or an education in the liberal arts. One can see, too, how this rhetoric masks the gradual entrenchment of a two-tiered educational system, in which allied health care workers in the lower tier must spend years building bridges between vocational and on-the-job training programs that only rarely form a road out of the day-to-day struggle to get by.

Although CUNY is a world-class university system with a history as the gateway to opportunity for New York City's immigrants, working-class, and minority students, its latest outpost—CUNY on the Concourse—represents an accommodation of this two-tier system. CUNY on the Concourse is admirable in so far as it provides access to the degree-granting CUNY colleges for students who otherwise would not have attended them. When many of its programs steer students into a dead-end and perpetual cycle of training and low-wage work, however, it deserves to be disparaged. An official at CUNY on the Concourse described its role this way:

> In adult education you have to realize…it's like shopping. People, they're just walking off the street, they're doing window shopping, they look at what you're offering, they come upstairs, and then they ask questions. That's the way that it works, especially when you offer courses to the community.

In this model of education, the "community" becomes analogous to individual consumers and education a product that can be displayed in shop windows. It is a model in which the consumer has minimal input into the design and production of the product except in so far as they periodically participate in marketing surveys and focus groups. While in the waiting room of CUNY on the Concourse, I watched a young man from "off the street," who wanted to register for a noncredit computer course, struggle with the receptionist who said he could not pay for half of the course on his credit card and the other half on his debit card; only reluctantly, he swallowed his pride and admitted that he didn't have enough money in his checking account to pay for the entire course. For these types of noncredit programs, students cannot qualify for financial aid or scholarships. Do we really want to liken education to shopping? Do we want to liken health care to shopping? Do we want people who are struggling to get an education and improve their lives to feel shame?

1199's Bread and Roses Cultural Project is an informative counterpoint to the programs offered by CUNY on the Concourse and the Taft-Hartley Training and Upgrading Fund. In the early 1950s, 1199 initiated a series of cultural and educational programs under the stewardship of Moe Foner, well before it organized its first hospital in 1957. In his 2002 memoir, Foner, who was in charge of 1199's communications and was its public relations guru for thirty years, described how theatrical and staged performances were central to the union's organizing campaign at the hospitals. In one case, the union staged a "mock funeral" for the meager, two-cents-an-hour wage increase offered by a Brooklyn hospital. Said Foner, "The workers loved this kind of thing."[68]

In 1978, Foner founded the 1199 Bread and Roses Cultural Project with a planning grant from the National Endowment for the Arts. The name came from the motto of the 1912 Lawrence, Massachusetts, textile workers strike: We Want Bread and Roses Too. "It captured what I envisioned for 1199ers: economic gains to meet their material needs and cultural programs to enrich their lives," Foner recalled.[69] Among other things, the Project organized concerts, musical revues, street fairs, exhibitions, theater programs, concerts at worksites, and conferences and lectures. Professional artists were involved in many of these events, but they were also often written or performed by union members and workers. For Foner, the Bread and Roses Project was simultaneously a public relations vehicle for 1199, a space for union members to express themselves, a source of entertainment, and a way to "advance union principles such as solidarity, opposition to racism, and support for women's rights."[70] Foner perceived it as a source of cultural capital and enrichment for 1199ers.

The Bread and Roses Cultural Project reflects an impulse to move away from established institutions and create independent sources of knowledge and culture, whereas the Training and Upgrading Fund further embeds workers' aspirations in those existing institutions and structures. The readings that Ossie Davis and Ruby Dee performed of Langston Hughes poems on workers' lunch breaks, recorded in a 1980 television documentary on the Project, are funny and subversive. The Project aimed for the kind of consciousness raising consistent with its political era. Similarly, 1199 and other unions maintain political education departments (not Taft-Hartley Funds) to train organizers and members on issues ranging from collective bargaining to raising class consciousness.[71] In the last decade, however, the human and financial resources poured into training and upgrading far exceed those poured into projects like Bread and Roses or union education.

Even projects like Bread and Roses suggest problems in the way that the union conceives of its members. Or at least, such projects show the extent to which trade unions like 1199 are fundamentally bureaucratic, top-down organizations, with a tendency to impose on their members what they think is best for them. In the case of 1199, black and Hispanic workers were essentially organized from the outside by a group of white radicals. In 1974, Al Nash, who wrote his doctoral dissertation on labor-management relations at Montefiore hospital, concluded that the 1199 leadership desired and cultivated intensive membership involvement in activities like "dances, boat rides, sports, civil rights celebrations, rallies, peace demonstrations, political rallies, and utilization of union services," while it blocked member participation in decision-making activities.[72] Foner's phrase—"the workers loved this kind of thing"—contains a paternalistic kernel that inflected, though did not dominate, the cultural projects. The union leadership and the rank and file were, particularly in the union's early years, divided by vast differences of class, race, gender, education, and culture. Though the Bread and Roses Project expressed a "conscious opposition culture," it was not organized by the workers themselves.[73]

While Nash found 1199's headquarters "modern but modest" and its officials "easily accessible to the members,"[74] today the lobby of the Training and Upgrading Fund is separated from the huge floor where staff work by doors that open only with key-card access. Junior training fund staff work in identical cubicles—a sine qua non of bureaucracy—while executives, naturally, occupy the windowed offices around the perimeter of the building. One union insider described the offices angrily, asserting the space symbolized how the union had traded "struggle for service." This charge is not new,[75] but it continues to be relevant.

There is no question that as part of its public commitment to social justice, 1199 in principle supports a stronger, better public education system as it in principle supports a better public health system. The limits of private benefits for the health and welfare of working Americans *as a whole,* however, are clear. In a period of diminishing union membership, the private benefits negotiated by employers and unions cover an ever-fewer number of working Americans. The private welfare state does not compensate for the inadequacies of the public welfare state, as it appeared it might in the wake of the New Deal, and seems even to block the latter's expansion or enable its retrenchment. And even if union membership were to increase, the changed nature of the labor market—with its higher reliance on contract employees, part-timers, and agency staff—indicates that an employment-based system of health benefits will be inadequate.

Based on my description of some of the programs, it might seem that these training grants were a waste of public dollars, part of a package of subsidies that were ultimately a disincentive for health care organizations to become self-reliant market competitors.[76] The fact that labor unions and hospital leaders could successfully argue for the necessity of training grants was certainly confirmation of just how dependent the private health care system is on the state. I share the perspective, however, that a private health care system, driven by the logic of the market and profits, can never provide a public good. The training grants made to private, voluntary health care providers (mostly hospitals) are another in a long line of public subsidies required to make a private health care system responsive to public needs. The largest federal training grants were, it was claimed, intended to facilitate the creation of a more community-based health care system because the private health care system had failed to create it independently. In practice, the reform policies of the period were fundamentally flawed—such a community-oriented heath care system could not be created on the basis of cost-cutting and competition for revenue. Nonetheless, the subsidies—including those for training—were an acknowledgment that the private system could not produce a rational system of care on its own, especially for the most vulnerable, and that competition and markets were not a solution.

Though I have serious qualms with how some of the training funds have been spent (and I do not know how *all* of them have been spent), I have no qualms about public subsidies for health care and the need to continually train health care workers. A private system of financing and delivering health care has repeatedly failed to meet the needs of patients and workers, and without public financing and regulations it would be a more inequitable system than it already is. When public funds are construed as subsidies, however, it maintains the fiction that the private health care system is essentially functioning well, only on occasion requiring a boost from government. It makes increasingly less sense for the extensive public funds that support not only New York's, but also the U.S., health care system to be detoured through private insurers and providers whose decisions about how to spend that money are not necessarily driven by the needs of frontline caregivers or the patients and communities they serve. Many of the training grants I have described are another such detour of public funds—funds that should be used for better education for all, rather than for programs that serve only a narrow segment of the population, one lucky enough to be represented by 1199.

In the early twentieth century, there was considerable disagreement in the U.S. labor movement about the wisdom of government-sponsored, compulsory health insurance. AFL President Samuel Gompers saw both government and employer involvement in union benefit plans as paternalistic.[77] The Great Depression, however, revealed the vulnerability of capitalist firms while it also destroyed many of the associations for health, disability, and pension benefits that unions had established independent of employers. In the New Deal political climate that followed, unions along with many other community and activist groups began to experiment with new ways of providing economic and health security. Communities and unions in many places developed "prepayment plans," which were organized around the communitywide collective pooling of resources (both rich and poor, sick and healthy, union and nonunion) and often hired physicians or paid hospitals and clinics on a salaried or flat-rate basis. These groups might be considered nascent HMOs, whose principles were originally inclusive and expansive. Today, they have become organizations focused on cost-cutting alone and driven by managerial concerns rather than community needs.[78]

At the same time, labor unions expressed interest in a state role to either support such community plans or provide insurance directly. Although a few unions had begun to negotiate with employers for private, "fringe" benefits in addition to wages during the 1930s, and some employers had also begun to develop their own internal benefit plans (in large part to deter unionization), efforts to expand social security were by and large not part of a process of collective bargaining.[79] William Green, president of the AFL from 1924 to 1952, felt employment-based benefits were inadequate and wanted compulsory, government-administered health insurance even while his unions created benefit funds.[80] The radical, industrial unions of the CIO, which John Lewis played a key role in organizing in 1935, initially rejected the formation of union benefit plans altogether, believing the extra dues and contributions required to run them would make organizing new workers more difficult.[81] The New Deal was a period, therefore, in which labor leaders more readily perceived economic and health security as a natural extension of the relationship between citizens and the state than between employees and employers. Labor unions were among those, along with activists from every section of the working class, arguing that universal health and disability benefits were the right of all Americans.[82]

Dennis Rivera has said, "the labor movement is the greatest self-help organization that exists in our country. We are doing for ourselves. Republicans who believe in quote-unquote self-help thinking should support the labor movement, because the labor movement basically tries to advances its members."[83] Yet the services 1199 provides to its members as part of its joint labor-management plans are a far cry from both the mutual aid and self-help societies of the early years of the twentieth century and the universal benefits envisioned under the New Deal. 1199's benefit funds are predicated on employer and state support—through employers' payments to the funds, indirect public subsidies of employers that offset their benefit fund contributions, and public grants such as those that support much of the union's workforce training programs—but they also remain exclusive, private benefits. They have been an obstacle to universal health security and may now hamper efforts to sustain education security for all Americans. And, of course, there is the troublesome nature of the message of the training and education programs I have studied: that workers are primarily to blame for problems hospitals face. Much of the training was consistent with a managerial perspective and in some instances exacerbated problems on the shop floor.

Just as important, welfare and benefit funds did not prevent the decline of the labor movement nor are they an adequate basis for its revival. Lewis's benefit fund did not stem the decline of the mining industry as a whole and the erosion of his membership. Even at the height of its power immediately following World War II, the UMW agreed to what employers said they must to do survive, such as mechanize production, even if it meant the loss of union members and workers.[84] Welfare and benefit funds have in many cases allowed unions to temper the effects of layoffs and workforce contraction because they provided some security to those who are laid off. When most U.S. unions pursued the same policy in the face of economic threats to their industries, however, the result was not just the demise of individual unions along with their industries but the erosion of union-density and the U.S. labor movement as a whole.

Rivera too has sought to use training and upgrading funds both to protect members and—if Rivera's explanations for the need for communication skills and multiskilling is to be believed—to protect the industry itself. 1199's fate may not be the same as the United Mine Workers', but not because of the skills and credentials its training and education programs supposedly provide to workers, or even its other benefit programs. The health care sector is expanding, and hospital employment within that sector is declining, so that 1199's future hinges on organizing the unorganized in home care agencies and nursing homes, in which job growth is especially rapid and working conditions especially shameful. There, the substantial benefits that 1199 can offer its members, including those of training and education, are an important, but still paradoxical, organizing tool. The contradiction between private benefits and universal security remains, whether for health or education. As early as 1966, just after the passage of Medicare and Medicaid and just before the economic contraction that marked the end of the postwar age of prosperity, Raymond Munts, a pro-union analyst, observed the United Mine Workers' decision to curtail their pension and health benefits and asked whether "we are witnessing the beginning of a proof that 'private social security' is really a contradiction in terms, that a program cannot be both private and secure?"[85] His question resounds today.

Conclusion

A Dose of Idealism

Many frontline health care workers need and want more education. As Marisol, a home health aide, said to the instructor of an in-service I attended, "We don't have enough education. We have all the responsibility, but we don't know. Then what we do doesn't count." Marisol wanted education both because it might allow her to do her job better and because it might make what she does count. Of course, her job should count, regardless of the credentials behind her name. Health care providers like Marisol, regardless of whether they work in patients' homes, nursing homes, or hospitals, already have a tremendous amount of responsibility and make important decisions every day, but they do not receive the support and preparation necessary to do their work as well as they could. It is quite possible to be simultaneously underemployed and need more education for one's current job: Both are evidence of a lack of investment in these workers.

Education and training programs could be an essential part of a greater investment in health care workers, and consistent with efforts to enhance their ability to deliver better care and improve their jobs—even their lives. Organizations like the Paraprofessional Healthcare Institute (PHI) and its closely affiliated home care worker cooperative in New York City, for instance, have developed alternative training models for direct caregivers. PHI allows greater time for training—home care workers in agencies adopting PHI's model complete three to five weeks of full-time training before beginning their jobs, which meets or exceeds the requirements for home care workers and Certified Nursing Assistants in most states (and PCTs in New York City hospitals, whose scope of practice includes more clinical and technical skills).[1] Equally important, the organization provides intensive follow-up and support, including peer mentoring and three to six months of additional on-the-job-training and supervision, and has mechanisms for trainers to develop their own skills and receive and respond to regular feedback from trainees.[2] The training also includes modules on relational skills, such as team building, communication, resolving conflict, and problem-solving. The latter are no doubt crucial to high-quality care and to building the relationships and work environments that will support those who provide it. But as we have seen, the circumstances under which such training was carried out in many hospitals, the way it was structured, and indeed the messages some trainers conveyed, suggests that "soft skills" played a very different role in the dynamics of work and labor relations in New York City hospitals than it does for organizations like PHI.

Training might also play a role in progressive efforts to improve the health care system, rather than being used in the defense of detrimental and impractical ideologies of self-help, restructuring, and market miracles. Aspects of the training industry that emerged in New York City in the mid-1990s—both its role in a larger political struggle and the content of specific programs—not only failed to change the conditions of health care work, they undermined a more progressive agenda. The most crucial plank of such an agenda would attempt to redress the devaluation of caring labor and what is conceptualized as unskilled labor. This devaluation occurs at the level of individuals—in terms of the way people who provide that labor are treated every day—but also at a broader level, in terms of cultural values, economics, and the structure of the labor market. When trainers and educators justify their "skills" programs by noting that they improve the self-esteem and self-worth of allied health care workers, it is because they recognize that many health care workers suffer—financially and psychically—from the trivialization of their work.

Despite the hopes and efforts of many trainers, however, the training and education industry in many respects reinforces what those health care workers who are lowest in the hierarchy of health care jobs are made to feel regularly at work—that they are never good enough. The multiskilling program conveyed to nursing assistants that the only way to obtain a raise and improve their status was to learn new, technical skills such as EKGs and drawing blood. The widespread discourse about health care jobs of the twenty-first century and health care workers' lack of preparation for them quite pointedly ignores the jobs of the present that require, and are done by, committed, skilled, and knowledgeable workers. While soft skills courses stressed the need for these workers to adjust their expectations about what they can and cannot change, they seemed simultaneously to blame problems both large and small on the workers themselves, implying that if they just fixed themselves, as individuals, the health care system might also be saved.

The training and education industry in some respects also fuels the rather common view that health care workers do not "care" enough, that "customer service" in New York City hospitals is poor because of workers' attitudes. Unionization is often blamed for this. Unions, apparently, have committed the sin of making health care jobs the most secure possible in the sub-baccalaureate labor market of the service economy. Thus, according to this view, many health care workers are no longer "called" to or motivated by the altruism that is supposedly at the heart of health care work.

It is true that many workers—especially women, people of color, and immigrants—work in health care because, as a unionized sector of the economy, it offers relatively decent jobs (see chapter 1). Yet, if a major problem with health care in the United States is the motives of those who enter care work, it can hardly be blamed on unionization. In fact, if unionization makes health care jobs better, in terms of wages and benefits, one could just as easily assume this would make workers more committed to them. It is rare for anyone to ask whether nursing assistants in New York City hospitals might have worse attitudes without unionization. Moreover, because of unionization, New York City does not have the same problems with quality care created by the constant turnover of nursing staff that exist elsewhere. Finally, to claim in the context of New York City that unionization makes workers more adversarial and less altruistic seems ironic given that 1199 has become less confrontational and drawn much closer to management in its views of health care and how it should be organized.

Finally, the focus on individual motives is a distraction from more urgent and perhaps more effective initiatives to improve health care. Whether they are motivated largely by the security health care work offers or the intrinsic rewards of caring for others, frontline health care workers are bound to lose.[3] Both can be used to justify paying them less and dismissing their work. On the one hand, there is concern that if they have not freely chosen to do such work because of its intrinsic rewards, caregiving will suffer—a concern found on both the left and right. It is a fear rooted in what Viviana Zelizer calls the "hostile-worlds" view, in which commodified relations are seen as incompatible with intimate, caring ones. "Explicitly or implicitly," Zelizer writes, "most analysts of intimate social relations join ordinary people in assuming that the entry of instrumental means such as monetization and cost accounting into the worlds of caring, friendship, sexuality, parent-child relations, and personal information depletes them of their richness."[4] This common assumption drives, for instance, efforts to make health care more "meaningful." Reports such as the American Hospital Association's "In Our Hands," imply what is missing from health care today is the kind of selfless commitment a mother presumably has toward her children.[5]

However, the problem is not so much that health care workers don't take meaning from their jobs, but that the meaning they take may be the awareness that what they do is not considered very important—as evidenced by their employers' reluctance to support and invest in them and their work. The people I observed and interviewed do find their work rewarding and are committed to their patients, even if they feel disrespected and undervalued. Many of the health care workers I have interviewed attested to their enjoyment in taking care of people, their sense of a calling to this kind of work, and its rewards, even if they never entirely planned or chose to go into caregiving work. It is, I contend, perfectly possible for people to find their work rewarding and do it well even though they did not "choose" it and may desire a "better" job. Yet, the idea that these workers are somehow less committed to their jobs, and are merely mercenaries out to make the highest buck, can be used as an excuse to clamp down on their wages and refuse to improve their working conditions. This is, I think, part of the circular, self-defeating dynamic some hospitals have created with their employees, most recently through the vehicle of soft skills training, by telling them, in essence, we won't reward or support you until you improve your attitude. This in turn creates greater resentment and discontent.

On the other hand, there are also risks in overemphasizing how much health care workers really do care. Health care workers may indeed feel called to their work and may be motivated by strong personal feelings of compassion for, and attachment to, their patients. This emphasis is, I think, an important corrective to the notion that those who are paid to care are necessarily less compassionate or caring and is part of a broader strategy to account for the true value—both social and economic—of caring labor and make a case for improving the wages and working conditions of those who do it. I once, however, attended a conference for nursing attendants where one of the keynote speakers praised at great length a nursing attendant from Africa who gave exemplary care because she was raised in a tradition of caring and community values absent in the United States. Though the story was intended to valorize the contribution of immigrants to the health care system, it relegated them to caregiving jobs that are underpaid and disrespected by suggesting this is a kind of work such immigrants are naturally raised to do. (And the speaker's exaggerated characterization of an amoral U.S. culture—and implied, if inadvert, slight of native-born nursing assistants—made her description of African village life equally suspect.)

While caring is a real and important part of ensuring that ours is a healthy society, that patients get well, that children grow up feeling secure, there is also a troubling tendency to romanticize caring or to reduce it to some simple, natural phenomenon.[6] This emphasis too can play into the assumption that paid caregiving is a "natural" process driven by emotions, therefore requiring little training and warranting minimal pay. There is indeed a branch of economic theory that maintains that workers who provide care can be paid less because of the work's inherent rewards.[7] This dismissal of the skills and abilities it takes to provide high-quality care also extends to those allied health care workers who are not directly involved in hands-on care. They too are financially and culturally stigmatized by working in health care.[8] And even though hospital housekeepers and unit clerks, for instance, aren't in jobs that explicitly call for hands-on care, they do often talk to and touch patients. And they are involved in another kind of caregiving, cleaning up the messes patients and even "professionals" leave in their wake.

I do not think it is necessary to portray health care workers, whether they provide hands-on care or indirect care, firstly as altruistic and compassionate (which, of course, they can be) to make a credible case for improving their work and lives.[9] I also do not think, ultimately, that the solution to the devaluation of health care workers' labor and injustice of their wages can rest on econometric estimates of the true contribution of their work to the economy. The latter are important, but today there is only a weak link between the "value" of people's work and their wages or remuneration, as we can see by the exorbitant pay and benefit packages of corporate CEOs. Health care workers deserve better pay and respect as a matter of ethics and principle. Such an idea requires that health care workers and their unions bring a measure of idealism with them to the bargaining table, in an attempt to dismantle the myth that pay in our society is somehow a direct reflection of the "skills" workers bring to the job, which in turn are recognized only if the workers also have formal credentials. 1199, on the contrary, has in recent years reinforced that myth.

Training that values caregiving and recognizes it as a process rooted in cognitive understanding and practice, rather than personal feelings and motives, might have a very different character. It might emphasize improving care rather than "new," technical skills. It might make caregiving a more visible, a less "natural process," which is therefore more likely to be rewarded with adequate pay and respect. Rather than dismissing caregiving during training, training could be one aspect of a larger investment in these workers, not with the aim of giving them more "skills" or moving them into "better" jobs, but in terms of making the jobs they have better and improving their ability to do them.

Above all, if we aim to improve health care services and patient care in addition to the pay and well-being of health care workers, it is as important— and perhaps more fruitful—to focus our attention on the organization of health care work rather than the motives of individual health care workers. Care (and its quality) is a relational and situational process, affected—but not determined—by individual motives and intentions. The "organizational aspects of caring"—such as whether care providers have a sense of control of their work, feel empowered, have the opportunity to use their abilities, and gain feedback on the value of their roles—are just as important. These aspects impact care providers' level of stress and ability to cope with it and are shaped by organizational and administrative practices. Studies have shown organizational factors such as adequate staffing, decentralized decision making, and self-scheduling flexibility to be associated with higher job satisfaction and lower turnover among nurses.[10] Currently, we expect health care workers to provide good health care under difficult circumstances. Such circumstances do not bring out the best in health care workers; they do their best work in spite of them.

Absent among the reforms to which U.S. health care is continually subject have been the kinds of support and change that might give workers greater autonomy and decision-making power over issues related to their working conditions and patient care, when appropriate; take advantage of the creativity and commitment already present in the workforce; and minimize the strict divisions of status and power in health care settings that leave many of those workers on the front lines feeling undervalued and disrespected. Frontline health care workers and their attitudes and wages are not to blame for the dysfunctional ways of many health care organizations and the health care system as a whole. Rather, we might look to the policy makers, politicians, hospital leaders, lobbyists, and even union leaders who have made America's health care system the most expensive and inequitable in the industrialized world.

The training programs I encountered do not help workers to understand the systemic roots of their problems. The solidarities and collective awareness they may inadvertently stimulate do not become political or critical conversations about injustice and inequality in the health care system. There are no bosses visible or present, and physicians were not similarly trained. 1199 has argued that more training is needed to convince health care workers of the dire situation facing health care organizations and hospitals in particular, but it has not argued for training in a critical politics and economics of health care, and certainly not on how its own so-called pragmatic decisions have at times undermined the cause of a better health care system. Nor has it argued for "training" on how the dire situation in which health care organizations supposedly find themselves might be changed or fixed.

Quite the opposite is true. Most of the training programs I observed reinforced the notion that markets can fix health care. In the context of

New York, this perspective has been especially appealing because the state and its bureaucracy have given little reason to feel confident it can manage and direct a health care system that provides high-quality care in the most appropriate settings for a fair price. Health care in the United States has become a growth industry, driven by profit-making institutions and providers of services and products. Politicians have therefore been willing to tolerate waste and inefficiencies, and thus far their careers have not suffered because they fail to fix the system. When they do make gestures toward comprehensive health care reform that are not distorted by a blind faith in the market, their efforts are thwarted by the sheer number and power of payers and providers, all of whom have taken advantage of the chaos to create their own lucrative market niches. Those patients who fall through the cracks—the sickest, the most vulnerable, the costliest—are left to rely on insufficiently funded government programs or make do with little or nothing.

I have spent the last few years teaching at a university in Canada. I am convinced the best remedy would be a single-payer health care system, in which the government pays for the majority of necessary services out of tax revenue and coordinates and negotiates with those groups with an interest in health care about how that revenue will be allotted. Central to such a system are measures for public accountability and transparency, so that $1.3 billion is not spent without some sort of mechanism for ensuring that it is done so wisely. The U.S. government, after all, is already knee-deep in health care. Its repeated attempts to extricate itself have only further mired it in the mud. Through direct funding, indirect subsidies, and regulations, federal and state agencies play a major role in shaping the health care system, but in a way that is not coordinated and subject to unusual sway from special interest groups. Moreover, government financing is filtered through a number of organizations and institutions whose missions revolve around private gain, not public good. There are many excellent institutions, well-trained health care providers, life-saving medical technologies and procedures, and even moments of caring, in the U.S. health care system, but these are increasingly jeopardized by backward ways of financing and organizing it.

Despite the lessons from health care, we have also recently seen efforts by the state to divest itself of direct responsibility for education, to leave it to the entrepreneurs and assume that what is good for them is good for everyone. Not only has education become, for many, reduced to depoliticized, vocationalized, and privatized seminars, but it has become routinized. It is held up as a sign that our society is providing paths to upward mobility, that politicians and employers care about the fates of U.S. workers who have to get by in an economy defined by deteriorating jobs, and that individuals are worth something. The actual nature of education (and training) programs, the presence or absence of opportunities for an improved quality of life, and the psychic security of working Americans seem to have little relationship to these symbolic functions.

Milagros, an immigrant from the Dominican Republic, who had worked for years in a light industrial factory in New Jersey making around $6.00 an hour but was employed as a school bus driver and training to become a nuclear medicine technician when we spoke, put it this way:

> When you go to school and you try to get a degree for yourself, people look at you a different way…when you say "I work and I go to school" they look at you with—I feel, with some kind of respect, or different than everybody. It doesn't matter what you study, it's the fact that you go to school. It means that you're looking for something in life, that you don't just want to be chilling and doing nothing.

Milagros suggests that merely enrolling in school or education programs is, symbolically, a vehicle for obtaining more status and respect. Her perspective, however, would not be possible in a society in which access to education was truly universal. Her observation is possible only because education is, like health care, a commodity made scarce and distributed unequally, so that to gain access to education is a means of differentiating between those who are worthy and those less so. Moreover, Milagros's comment exposes an important feature of participation in education for poor and minority community members in particular. For them, it is a socially accepted response to the many permutations of the judgment that they are responsible for the conditions in which they find themselves. For members of marginalized groups, education is a way to signal that they are in fact hard-working people who deserve respect and fair treatment. In a society defined by a growing disparity between those who have and those who don't, and in an economy defined by the relentless creation of low-wage service jobs, education and training—of any sort—is one of the only ways

of claiming worth and respect. Such respect can be claimed only by participating in *organized,* formally sanctioned education and training programs.
This is because learning itself does not earn respect if it is unaccompanied
by certificates and credentials. Moreover, as Milagros points out, "it doesn't
matter what you study," the content of education is beside the point.

The idea that education is primarily a sign that "you are looking for
something in life," is a warning that the content of education matters very
much. The prospect of large numbers of Americans continuously cycled
through low-wage jobs and short-term training programs, sustained by
the notion that at least they are "looking for something in life," means that
we should be critical indeed of the quality of education and the promises
of those who provide it. So, too, we must be critical of economic and social
policies that create an endless supply of low-wage jobs and ad-hoc training
programs.

Finally, Milagros's feeling that "chilling and doing nothing" is to be
avoided at all costs presents a fitting way to close. Milagros implicitly cat-
egorizes her time into three areas: that spent working, that spent training for (in official programs) paid labor—both considered inherently
worthwhile—and that spent "doing nothing." What she does not, even
cannot, consider—perhaps for her own well-being—is that for many
Americans, time is *wasted* training for or even doing paid labor when the
abilities and talents of many workers are already and seemingly perpetually underused and many such training programs do not lead to decent
jobs. Milagros also excludes the possibility that she might spend time outside of both work and formal training being creative and productive, that
she and other Americans do not necessarily use their "free" time to "do
nothing." Even more unimaginable is that she might deserve time to chill.
Milagros's division of her time is consistent with what critic Ellen Willis
has described as a culture in which austerity is "not just an economic but
a moral imperative," so that free time becomes a kind of sin, especially
for people like those I have interviewed—people who are always already
suspected of being lazy and unmotivated.[11]

The taken-for-granted valorization of paid labor and continual need
for economic and emotional thrift is not innate to American culture, but
a product of concerted institutional and political efforts, among which we
might now count the training and education industry for allied health
care workers. The soft skills training courses involved convincing health

care workers that the money to alleviate basic problems with health care work and patient care simply was not there. Multiskilling initiatives, communication skills training, and individual upgrading alike proposed self-discipline as the "realistic" alternative to the misallocation of wealth and resources that is rampant in the health care industry. Such programs told workers they are never good enough and reduced the problems of health care to their lack of skills and poor attitudes. If this is the result of pragmatic responses to economic restructuring and the dismantling of universal health and social security, how much better might we do with a dose of idealism?

Appendix: A Note on Methods

As I described in the introduction, the interviews and observations in this book are drawn from three research projects carried out between 1999 and 2003. Here I will provide more detail on those I interviewed and observed, the purpose of the interviews, how participants were recruited to participate in the research, and how I analyzed the evidence from observations and interviews.

The subacute care study and communication skills evaluation were funded by grants from the 1199 joint labor-management Training and Upgrading Fund, made to the Center for the Study of Culture, Technology and Work at the City University of New York (CUNY) Graduate Center, directed by Stanley Aronowitz. I was hired by the Center, as a graduate student, to conduct observations and interviews, analyze the results, and write reports for the funder. For the subacute care study, I conducted observations at three subacute care units from September 1999 to February 2000, for ten to twelve hours each week. For the evaluation of a communication skills training program, I was joined by two other graduate students,

Heather Gautney and Dominic Wetzel, and we observed seven eight-hour sessions of the training program, conducted semi-structured follow-up interviews with twenty-one staff members (of whom I personally interviewed six), and conducted follow-up observations of staff and their interactions on six of the hospital's units. The focus of our interviews and observations were nursing assistants (patient care technicians [PCTs] at that hospital) and unit clerks. In addition, I attended several meetings of the hospital education committee and interviewed two consultants hired by the hospital to run training, including the communication skills instructor. In this book, I have relied on my own fieldnotes (from observations of the training sessions and hospital units) and the interviews I conducted. However, I am indebted to Heather and Dominic for ideas and insights generated in their own fieldnotes and interviews and in our process of analyzing the data together and preparing an article for publication.[1] The article we cowrote is a partial basis for chapter 5. I have added information from my later research to the chapter and substantially revised it, however. Neither Heather nor Dominic are responsible for any changes in my perspective or flaws in the chapter. And, of course, I am indebted to Stanley Aronowitz for his intellectual guidance and support.

For my dissertation research, carried out between 2002 and 2003, I conducted in-depth interviews with seventeen allied health care workers about their educational, occupational, and personal histories, as well as with twenty-one people involved in the planning and implementation of the health care workforce training industry. I also observed several sessions of two additional training seminars: a customer service training program at a public hospital and an in-service on communication at one of the city's largest home health care agencies. I also examined additional evidence in the process of writing this book, including articles involving 1199 published in New York City's major newspapers from 1989 to 2005 (*New York Times, New York Post, Daily News*) and a content analysis of the union's newspaper, *1199 News,* from 1989 to 2000 (now known as *Our Life and Times*). I also studied reports and articles published by research centers, trade associations, and advocacy groups with interests in New York's health care sector and health workforce training. These are cited throughout the book.

The interviews I conducted for the dissertation served two purposes: first, to document the occupational and educational histories of workers and trainers. As part of this, I also asked trainers and administrators about how the education and training industry for health care workers operates and its history. The second aim was to explore how workers and trainers understood and felt about their experiences in the industry. This interview approach enabled me to both explore what the industry was, what it did, and how it worked and discuss with participants how they felt it should be. I constructed my interview guides to avoid leading questions as much as possible and to ensure consistency across the interviews, but the interviews were carried out as conversations. They lasted from one to two hours, and though I did not pay the respondents for participating, I usually tried to buy or bring them coffee or lunch (they invariably refused—one fellow even bought me coffee). Interviews, like any conversation, are never a mere reporting of what happened, but simultaneously a search by the participants in the conversation (including the interviewer) for how to interpret and understand what happened. This makes the observations of health care settings and training seminars I conducted particularly valuable because the interviews and observations together enabled me to recognize likely differences between what health care workers do and how they describe and explain what they do.

For the interviews with health care workers in particular, I purposefully sought out allied health care workers who were engaged in training, education, or "upgrading" programs of some sort. I was especially interested in talking to workers who were moving into "tech" or paraprofessional occupations that constitute a growing, and understudied, portion of the health care workforce. I recruited the health care worker respondents in several ways. I sent out a letter and postage-paid response card to a random sample of participants in the 1199 Training and Upgrading Fund's "professional training programs." I also recruited respondents through training programs at hospitals, referrals by other health care workers, and through my contacts at several hospitals who distributed flyers on my research, including at the hospital where we conducted the communication skills study.

It is possible that enrollment in a training program with the aim of getting a better job is an indicator of dissatisfaction, so one bias in this research could be that I was less likely to interview health care workers who were satisfied with their work. But my ethnographic observations, during which I interacted with dozens of health care workers in numerous settings, leads me to believe health care workers who are "satisfied" are few and far between, and satisfaction is not a clear indicator of whether they would seek out training and upgrading opportunities. "Satisfaction" and "dissatisfaction" are in any case overly simplistic conceptualizations of these workers' experience. Many of the people I observed and interviewed liked and were committed to their work; at the same time they felt frustrated by a lack of respect for, and attention to, their needs on the job. I make no claims to having interviewed and observed a representative "sample" of allied health care workers in New York City, but I did attempt to capture the experience of workers in a variety of occupations and from varying backgrounds.

Table 1 includes some basic demographics of the twenty-three people I interviewed as part of my dissertation research and the communication skills training evaluation.

TABLE 1. Demographics of Health Care Workers Interviewed (*N* = 23)

Age	Age range	21–55
	Average	37
Gender	Women	18
	Men	5
Race	Hispanic	6
	White	4
	Mixed	2
	Black	11
Highest level of formal schooling	High school diploma	8
	Some college/postsecondary credential	6
	Associate's degree	5
	Bachelor's degree	4
Children	Yes	19
	No	4
Marital status	Never married	8
	Married or partnered	9
	Divorced or separated	5
	Widowed	1
Place of birth	United States	9
	Dominican Republic	4
	Trinidad	3
	Romania	1
	Canada	1
	Jamaica	2
	Ghana	1
	St. Vincent's	1
	Barbados	1

Table 2 shows the health care occupations respondents held at the time we spoke and that they reported holding previously. Most of the interview respondents worked in hospitals when we spoke, unless they were in training for their first health care job. Of course, many of the respondents had also worked in occupations not in the health care sector, especially in retail and domestic work. I also suspect that some respondents forgot some of their previous jobs, simply because the nature of the sub-baccalaureate labor market means people often take on short-term or part-time work with which they don't strongly identify. The column total for the occupations respondents held at the time of our interview is greater than 23 because it includes occupations for which respondents were in training and because some respondents held more than one job at the time of the interview.

I recruited the trainers and administrators to interview for my dissertation research through existing contacts and referrals to one another—this is a true network of people, some of whom have known each other for a long time and many of whom have held positions at several organizations central to the training and education industry. While I by no means interviewed everyone in this network, I tried to interview people in a variety of positions and organizations. I also interviewed some people off-the-record and informally, especially during the exploratory phases of the research.

TABLE 2. Occupations Held by Health Care Workers Interviewed (N = 23)

	Occupation in at Time of Interview	Total Ever in Occupation
Dietary/Kitchen Aide	1	3
EMT/Paramedic	1	1
Home Health Aide	—	3
Housekeeper	—	1
Licensed Practical or Registered Nurse	1	2
Nuclear Medicine Technologist	3	3
Nursing Assistant/Patient Care Tech	4	7
Ophthalmology Technician	2	2
Physical Therapy Assistant	2	2
Physicians' Assistant	1	1
Registrar/Clerk	7	8
Respiratory Technician	1	2
Security Officer	—	2
Surgical Technologist	2	3
Trainer for allied health care occupation	2	2

Table 3 identifies the type of organization with which people I formally interviewed were affiliated, and the types of organizations at which they previously worked. It is also notable that at least seven of the trainers and administrators started their careers as health care providers, and they were able to reflect on their own experiences building a career in the health care sector and their personal experiences with various kinds of training and education.

In accordance with the human subjects' approval to carry out this research, I have protected the confidentiality of those health care workers interviewed and observed for this study. Their identities are disguised in two ways—I refer to each worker by a first-name pseudonym (for those I observed, I sometimes use a last-name pseudonym, which is consistent with how workers in many health care facilities address one another and how I addressed them during fieldwork). In addition, in chapter 6, where I describe specific workers' occupations and educational backgrounds, I have also used a pseudonym for the hospital or health care facility at which they worked. In the rest of the book, however, I use the actual names of hospitals and health care organizations. Throughout the book I use the actual names of schools and educational entities because I believe so many students pass through these schools that the identity of workers I interviewed will not be compromised and because naming these institutions is important for understanding the scope of the health care workforce training industry.

The trainers and educators who participated in this research were not offered the opportunity for their identities to remain confidential. They were, however, informed of the purposes and nature of the study. This decision was made because they are in quasi-public and official positions,

TABLE 3. Organizational Affiliation of Trainers, Educators, and Workforce Planners (N = 21)

	Affiliation at Time of Interview	Total Ever with Affiliation
College or university	5	5
Community or nonacademic training organization	3	4
Hospital or health care organization	5	6
Independent training consultant	1	4
Labor union	5	5
Policy and workforce planning organization	2	2

and they were asked to speak "on the record" about their organization's activities. Moreover, most of the organizations receive public funding and are therefore in principle obligated to report on the nature of their activities in a way that is accessible to the public. Nonetheless, I have chosen not to identify the trainers and administrators interviewed by name, and I have in some cases slightly altered their job titles to obscure their identity, though I do at times refer to the organizations for which they work. This is for several reasons. First, the respondents at times made personal remarks or discussed their personal feelings, and I think it is respectful to provide them a measure of privacy in thanks for their participation and openness. Second, I would argue—in sociological fashion—this industry as a whole exhibits tendencies and has effects that are more and other than the aggregation of individual decisions. Therefore, though I rely on in-depth interviews, this is not a story about the merits of the decisions and perspectives of particular trainers and workforce planners—it is the story of an industry and its embeddedness within larger political and cultural forces. If the reader takes from this book the feeling that something should be done about how health care policy in New York is conducted, then it will be obvious who is to blame and to whom one should talk. I have not, for instance, disguised the names of those officials whose roles in establishing health policy and this training industry are well-known and well-documented in public documents and the press, such as George Pataki, Dennis Rivera, or Kenneth Raske. The book is also full of references to people and organizations involved in the debate over health care and health workforce policy, which can be a source for the reader. Nonetheless, having said all that, some industry insiders might be able to identify themselves and their colleagues in this study. I hope they find here a fair reflection of the nature of the industry in which they work.

In regard to my analysis of the evidence, in preparation for writing this book, I imported all of my fieldnotes and interviews, from all the studies, into a qualitative data analysis software program. I read through the fieldnotes and interviews initially looking for common themes and issues ("codes"). Then, using the software program, I assigned codes to pieces and sections of the data. I was then able to create reports on each theme, which collated relevant sections from the fieldnotes and interviews. I also regularly reread entire interviews during the analysis and writing phases, in order to better place particular quotes in the context of the entire set of interviews or within the particular history of the person being quoted. I have reconsidered and revised the codes at regular intervals in the years since I collected the data and published this book, especially as my own understanding of the issues at stake has changed and evolved. While I make no claim to objectivity, I have attempted not to mold the data to any particular story, but to present the contradictions and inconsistencies among the stories people tell, the experiences they have, and the settings and interactions I observed.

As I mentioned, there are some gaps in this research given the methods I employed. It is a compilation of evidence that I collected as my own understanding of the industry evolved, and in some ways the structure of the book—moving from ethnographic observations of particular facilities to a sociopolitical analysis of health care and labor politics—reflects the development of my own thought. The evidence presented is valuable, I think, because as a result of my various research projects I have been able to present multiple perspectives on the health care workforce training industry, its emergence, and its effects. I would also contend that it is entirely legitimate, and in fact urgent, to draw conclusions and make speculations even in the absence of so-called representative data. Those with the power to fund, design, and implement training programs for New York City's health care workers do not make their decisions about whether to go forward on the basis of such evidence. Why should we, as researchers or concerned readers, wait for such evidence to assess the penetration of education and training programs into ever greater areas of our lives?

NOTES

Health Care and Getting By in America

1. Health Resources and Services Administration (HRSA), *State Health Workforce Profiles 2000: New York* (U.S. Department of Health and Human Services, HRSA, 2004), iv; Center for Health Workforce Studies (CHWS), *The Health Care Workforce in New York City, 2002* (Albany: Center for Health Workforce Studies, School of Public Health, University at Albany, 2002), v.

2. Fiscal Policy Institute, *Health Care Industry Trends and Issues* (Albany, NY: Fiscal Policy Institute, 2002), 3.

3. See Joshua Benjamin Freeman, *Working-Class New York: Life and Labor since World War II* (New York: New Press: Distributed by W.W. Norton, 2000).

4. Alan G. Hevesi, *Current Trends in the New York City Economy* (Albany: New York State, Office of the State Comptroller, 2004).

5. David Leonhardt, "Growing Health Care Economy Gives Northeast a Needed Boost," *New York Times,* December 30, 2002.

6. W. Norton Grubb, *Working in the Middle* (San Francisco: Jossey-Bass, 1996), 2.

7. W. Norton Grubb, "Learning and Earning in the Middle, Part I: National Studies of Pre-Baccalaureate Education," *Economics of Education Review* 21, no. 4 (2002): Table 1.

8. Cynthia Engel, "Health Services Industry: Still a Job Machine?" *Monthly Labor Review* 122, no. 3 (1999); see also David R. H. Hiles, "Health Services: The Real Jobs Machine," *Monthly Labor Review* 115, no. 11 (1992).

9. Bureau of Labor Statistics, "BLS Releases 2002–12 Employment Projections" (news release, February 11, 2004), Table 3b.

10. Fiscal Policy Institute, *Health Care Industry Trends.*

11. Linda H. Aiken, "Health Professionals, Allied," in *International Encyclopedia of the Social and Behavioral Sciences* (Amsterdam: Elsevier, 2002), 6592–98. Aiken uses the term to include all health workers except physicians.

12. Maria Figueroa and Peter Lazes, *Labor-Management Participatory Projects in the Health Care Industry* (New York: Cornell University–New York State School of Industrial and Labor Relations, NYC Metropolitan District Office, 2002), 14.

13. Commission on Health Care Facilities in the Twenty-First Century and Stephen Berger, "Economic Impact: Measurement of Impact on Workforce and Workforce Retraining," *Factors Book* (New York State Department of Health, July 2005) [http://www.nyhealthcarecommission. org/factors_book.htm;last accessed January 9, 2008].

14. Christopher Rowland, "Union Looks to Organize at Hub's Top Hospitals," *Boston Globe,* August 31, 2005.

15. Christopher Rowland, "Kennedy Pushing Hospital-Union Talks," *Boston Globe,* August 19, 2006.

16. Diana Pearce with Jennifer Brooks, *The Self-Sufficiency Standard for the City of New York* (New York: Women's Center for Education and Career Advancement, 2000). This measure assumes employers provide health care but employees pay a percentage of the premiums, includes expenses for child care, and calculates rents on the basis of market prices. For a family of one adult and a school-age child in the Bronx, it estimates the following monthly costs: housing ($740), child care ($498), food ($343), transportation to and from work ($63), health care ($273), and taxes ($514).

17. W. Norton Grubb, "The Returns to Education in the Sub-Baccalaureate Labor Market, 1984–1990," *Economics of Education Review* 16, no. 3 (1997): 241, 236. Data were from the 1984, 1987, and 1990 Survey of Income and Program Participation. Other fields included in the data were business, education, engineering/computers, public service, vocational/technical subjects (e.g., cosmetology), and associate's degrees in academic subjects. In Grubb's study, sample sizes for men in health-related occupations were too small to estimate economic returns.

18. U.S. Department of Labor, Bureau of Labor Statistics, Occupational Employment Statistics (OES), www.bls.gov.

19. Paula England, Michelle Budig, and Nancy Folbre, "Wages of Virtue: The Relative Pay of Care Work," *Social Problems* 49, no. 4 (2002). *Caring labor* is defined as a "face-to-face service that develops the human capabilities of the recipient" (455).

20. Kevin J. Dougherty and Marianne F. Bakia, "Community Colleges and Contract Training: Content, Origins, and Impact," *Teachers College Record* 102, no. 1 (2000).

21. Thomas Bailey and Elliot B. Weininger, "Performance, Graduation, and Transfer of Immigrants and Natives in City University of New York Community Colleges," *Educational Evaluation and Policy Analysis* 24, no. 4 (2002).

22. For an analysis of CUNY's history and its open admissions policy, see David E. Lavin and David Hyllegard, *Changing the Odds: Open Admissions and the Life Chances of the Disadvantaged* (New Haven, CT: Yale University Press, 1996).

23. Center for an Urban Future, *CUNY on the Job: The City's New Workforce Workhorse* (New York: Center for an Urban Future, 2004), 2. Continuing education and workforce programs include adult education courses, employment and welfare-to-work programs, and business contract training.

24. U.S. Department of Labor, Bureau of Labor Statistics, Occupational Employment Statistics (OES).

25. The description of the union that follows is drawn from Leon Fink and Brian Greenberg, *Upheaval in the Quiet Zone: A History of Hospital Workers' Union, Local 1199* (Urbana: University of Illinois Press, 1989).

26. Fink and Greenberg, *Upheaval in the Quiet Zone,* 26, 16–17, 110–11, 95–96.

27. Christopher Rowland, "Union May Set Sites on Beth Israel," *Boston Globe,* August 4, 2006.

28. These studies were carried out under grants from the 1199 joint labor-management Training and Upgrading Fund to the Center for the Study of Culture, Technology and Work at the City University of New York (CUNY) Graduate Center, directed by Stanley Aronowitz.

29. Richard Sennett and Jonathan Cobb, *The Hidden Injuries of Class* (New York: Vintage Books, 1973), 45.

1. The Pull and Perils of Health Care Work

1. In 1993, African Americans accounted for 15.5% of the medical care labor force but only 10.6% of the total labor force. Health sector jobs accounted for 19.2% of African American female employment but only 4.7% for African American men. African American women held 13% of all hospital jobs, 19.6% of all nursing home jobs, and 25% of nursing home aide positions. David U. Himmelstein, James P. Lewontin, and Steffie Woolhandler, "Medical Care Employment in the United States, 1968 to 1993: The Importance of Health Sector Jobs for African Americans and Women," *American Journal of Public Health* 86, no. 4 (1996).

2. Arlie Hochschild, "The Nanny Chain," *American Prospect,* January 3, 2000.

3. Center for Health Workforce Studies (CHWS), *The Health Care Workforce in New York City, 2000* (Albany: Center for Health Workforce Studies, School of Public Health, SUNY at Albany, 2000), 29, table 13.

4. Jaber Gubrium, *Living and Dying at Murray Manor* (New York: St. Martin's Press, 1975).

5. Peter G. Fitzpatrick, "Turnover of Certified Nursing Assistants: A Major Problem for Long-Term Care Facilities," *Hospital Topics* 80, no. 2 (2002); Linda Hollinger-Smith, Anna Ortigara, and David Lindeman, "Developing a Comprehensive Long-Term Care Workforce Initiative," *Alzheimer's Care Quarterly* 2, no. 3 (2001); Robyn Stone, *Frontline Workers in Long-Term Care: A Background Paper* (Washington, DC: Institute for the Future of Aging Services, American Association of Homes and Services for the Aging, 2001).

6. Health Resources and Services Administration (HRSA), *State Health Workforce Profiles 2000: New York,* v.

7. Gordon Lafer, "Hospital Speedups and the Fiction of a Nursing Shortage," *Labor Studies Journal* 30, no. 1 (2005): 31. Nurses "potentially available for work" refers to those who are not disabled and have no young children at home. Lafer's analysis is based in part on data from Ernell Spratley et al., *The Registered Nurse Population, March 2000: Findings from the National Sample Survey of Registered Surveys* (U.S. Department of Health and Human Services, Health Resources and Services Administration, Bureau of Health Professions, Division of Nursing, 2001). For a comprehensive discussion of these issues, see Suzanne Gordon, *Nursing against the Odds* (Ithaca: Cornell University Press, 2005).

8. Linda H. Aiken et al., "Hospital Nurse Staffing and Patient Mortality, Nurse Burnout, and Job Dissatisfaction," *JAMA* 288 (2002); Jack Needleman et al., "Nurse-Staffing Levels and the Quality of Care in Hospitals," *New England Journal of Medicine* 346 (2002).

9. Thomas Edward Gass, *Nobody's Home: Candid Reflections of a Nursing Home Aide* (Ithaca: Cornell University Press, 2004), 57.

10. Steven Henry Lopez, "Culture Change Management in Long-Term Care: A Shop-Floor View," *Politics and Society* 34, no. 1 (2006): 67, 60.

11. Lopez, "Culture Change Management," 68–69.

12. Nancy Foner, *The Caregiving Dilemma: Work in an American Nursing Home* (Berkeley: University of California Press, 1994), esp. 131–40. Foner carried out her fieldwork in 1988–89.

13. Ariel Ducey, "What's the Use of Job Descriptions?" *Working USA* 6, no. 2 (2002).

14. Gass, *Nobody's Home,* 57.

15. Foner, *Caregiving Dilemma,* esp. 59–68.

16. Timothy Diamond, *Making Gray Gold: Narratives of Nursing Home Care* (Chicago: University of Chicago Press, 1992).

17. Jeff Goldsmith, David Blumenthal, and Wes Rishel, "Federal Health Information Policy: A Case of Arrested Development," *Health Affairs* 22, no. 4 (2003): 45. As the authors point out, such sophisticated financial systems are unnecessary in single-payer health systems.

18. Deborah Stone, "Care and Trembling," *American Prospect* 43 (March–April 1999).

19. Diamond, *Making Gray Gold;* Stone, "Care and Trembling."

20. In 1998, the starting salary for PAs in New York City hospitals ranged from $43,561 to $67,000, though it had likely increased by the time Steve and I spoke. CHWS, *Health Care Workforce in New York City, 2000,* 30, Table 14.

21. Bureau of Labor Statistics, U.S. Department of Labor, Bureau of Labor Statistics, Occupational Employment Statistics (OES), www.bls.gov.

22. CHWS, *Health Care Workforce in New York City, 2000,* 30, Table 14.

23. Isabel Wilkerson, "Angela Whitaker's Climb," *New York Times,* June 12, 2005.

24. Gordon, *Nursing Against the Odds,* 34.

25. Spratley et al., Registered Nurse Population, March 2000.

26. Shoshana Zuboff, *In the Age of the Smart Machine: The Future of Work and Power* (New York: Basic Books, 1988).

2. Restructuring the New York Way

1. The health policy analysts are: Stephen M. Shortell, Robin R. Gillies, and Kelly J. Devers, "Reinventing the American Hospital," *Milbank Quarterly* 73, no. 2 (1995): 131, 139; Pew Health Professions Commission, *Critical Challenges: Revitalizing the Health Professions for the Twenty-First Century* (Pew Health Professions Commission, December 1995), 10 [http://www.futurehealth.ucsf.edu/summaries/challanges.html; last accessed April 7, 2008].

2. W. Richard Scott et al., *Institutional Change and Healthcare Organizations: From Professional Dominance to Managed Care* (Chicago: University of Chicago Press, 2000), 17.

3. Milt Freudenheim, "Survey Finds Health Costs Rose in '95," *New York Times,* January 30, 1996. Growth in national health expenditures slowed to an average of about 5.5% from 1994 to 1999. In 1993 and 2000, by contrast, health expenditures grew over 7%; in 2002 they jumped by 9.1%. See Centers for Medicare and Medicaid Services (CMS), Office of the Actuary, National Health Statistics Group, Historical Estimates [http://www.cms.hhs.gov/National HealthExpendData].

4. Medicaid was the largest payer of inpatient care in the city in 1996, reimbursing 38% of hospital discharges. Medicaid also paid for 56% of outpatient clinic visits citywide. United Hospital Fund, "More New York City Hospitals Are Relying on Medicaid as a Major Source of Revenue of Eve of Mandatory Medicaid Managed Care" (press release, September 29, 1997).

5. Michael S. Sparer and Lawrence D. Brown, "Nothing Exceeds Like Success: Managed Care Comes to Medicaid in New York City," *Milbank Quarterly* 77, no. 2 (1999): 211, 214. In 1995, 18.7% of Medicaid eligibles were enrolled in managed care plans.

6. Raymond Hernandez, "Pataki Details a Shift in Managed Care and Exemptions," *New York Times,* July 16, 1997. In policy circles, the program is also known as the "1115 Federal Waiver" program. In New York City the program was implemented only in 1999, after the completion of federal reviews to ensure adequate primary care capacity existed to serve Medicaid recipients.

7. Jennifer Y. Ruzek et al., *The Hidden Health Care Workforce: Recognizing, Understanding and Improving the Allied and Auxiliary Workforce* (San Francisco: UCSF Center for the Health Professions, July 1999), 100.

8. David Weber, "At New York City's Mount Sinai, Reengineering Is a Way to Grow, Not a Special Project," *Strategies for Healthcare Excellence* 12, no. 12 (1999): 4.

9. Linda H. Aiken and Claire M. Fagin, "Evaluating the Consequences of Hospital Restructuring," *Medical Care* 35, no. 10, suppl. (1997); Stephen Bach, "Health Sector Reform and Human Resource Management: Britain in Comparative Perspective," *International Journal of Human Resource Management* 11, no. 5 (2000). Aiken and Fagin's article is the introduction to a special issue of *Medical Care* based on the 1996 Bellagio conference on Hospital Restructuring in North American and Western Europe.

10. Weber, "At New York City's Mount Sinai," 2.

11. Elisabeth Rosenthal, "Once in Big Demand, Nurses Are Targets for Hospital Cuts," *New York Times,* August 19, 1996.

12. Alice Lipowicz, "Union Victories; Led by Rivera, Health Care Workers Won Key Concessions That Blunted NY Reforms," *Crain's New York Business,* August 19, 1996.

13. Howard S. Berliner, Geoffrey Gibson, and Cyprian Devine-Perez, "Health Care Workers' Unions and Health Insurance: The 1199 Story," *International Journal of Health Services* 31, no. 2 (2001); Steven Greenhouse, "The Odd Couple That Did the Heavy Lifting on Pataki's Managed-Care Medicaid Deal," *New York Times,* July 16, 1997; Karen Pallarito, "Cashing in on Connections: N.Y.C. Hospitals' Funding Deal Angers Upstate Rivals," *Modern Healthcare,* August 4, 1997.

14. Commission on the Public's Health System, *CHCCDP: Are We Getting Our Money's Worth?* (New York: Commission on the Public's Health System, 2003).

15. "Self-pay" refers to people without insurance, and even though the vast majority of them are without insurance not by choice, the term nonetheless misleadingly evokes the image of individuals who refuse to become dependent on government or beholden to large insurers by paying for health care themselves.

16. Later in the program, the funding formula was changed so that individual hospitals receiving less than $1 million under CHCCDP were required to use only 10% of the funds for worker training. In addition, 1199 eventually agreed to allow individual hospitals to use up to 10% of the training portion of their grants for programs targeted at registered nurses—most of whom are represented by a competing union, the New York State Nurses' Association (NYSNA).

17. For a description of the Rate Adjustment Program, see Nancy M. Pindus, Patrice Flynn, and Demetra Smith Nightingale, *Improving the Upward Mobility of Low-Skill Workers: The Case of the Health Industry* (Washington, DC: The Urban Institute, 1995).

18. State funding totals for the HWRI, Rate Adjustment, and TANF programs are from Commission on Health Care Facilities, "Economic Impact," *Factors Book.*

19. Center for an Urban Future and New York Association for Training and Employment Professionals, *Seeking a Workforce System: A Graphical Guide to Employment and Training Services in New York* (New York: Center for an Urban Future, 2003).

20. Between 1981 and 2003, the number of community hospitals fell from 5,813 to 4,895, a decline of 16%; the number of hospital beds per 1,000 persons declined from 4.37 to 2.80; the average length of stay declined from 7.6 days to 5.7 days. The rate of inpatient admissions declined as well, although since 1994 that figure has remained fairly steady at around 118 admissions per 1,000 people. American Hospital Association, *Trendwatch: Chartbook 2005, Trends Affecting Hospitals and Health Systems* (American Hospital Association, April 2005), app., supp. data tables [http://www.aha.org/aha/research-and-trends/chartbook/2005chartbook.html; last accessed January 8, 2008].

21. Ibid.

22. Hospital care as a whole accounted for 40% of national health expenditures in 1980 and only 30.3% in 2003. By contrast, the proportion of spending on prescription drugs increased from 4.7% in 1980 to 10% in 2003. Centers for Medicaid and Medicare Services (CMS), Office of the Actuary, National Health Statistics Group. Author's calculations of data on CMS

web site, 2008, National Health Care Expenditures Tables, Table 2 [http://www.cms.hhs.gov/NationalHealthExpendData].

23. Greater New York Hospital Association, *Health Care Statistics 2003* (New York: Greater New York Hospital Association, 2003), tables 6, 12. In New York City, the number of hospital beds per 1,000 persons went from 4.7 to 3.6 from 1990 to 2001 and the average length of stay in hospitals declined from 10.4 days to 7.6 in the same period. Nationally, the number of hospital beds per 1,000 persons went from 3.7 to 2.9 from 1990 to 2001 and the average length of stay in hospitals declined from 7.2 days to 5.7 in the same period.

24. 2004 and New York City HMO Penetration: Kaiser Family Foundation, "Trends and Indicators in the Changing Health Care Marketplace," exhibits 2.14, 2.15. [http://www.kff.org/insurance/7031/ti2004-list.cfm; last accessed January 8, 2008]; 2000 HMO Penetration: Kaiser Family Foundation, "Trends and Indicators in the Changing Health Care Marketplace, 2002," exhibit 2.6. [http://www.kff.org/insurance/3161-index.cfm; last accessed January 8, 2008]; see also Greater New York Hospital Association, *Health Care Statistics 2003,* esp. table 58.

25. Sharon Salit, Steven Fass, and Mark Nowak, "Out of the Frying Pan: New York City Hospitals in an Age of Deregulation," *Health Affairs* 21, no. 1 (2002): 129.

26. Ibid., 133.

27. Commission on Health Care Facilities in the Twenty-First Century and Stephen Berger, "Potential Use of Converted Facilities: Conversion of Institutional Health Care Facilities to Alternate Uses," *Factors Book* (New York State Department of Health, July 2005) [http://www.nyhealthcarecommission.org/factors_book.htm; last accessed January 9, 2008]; Greater New York Hospital Association, "Testimony of Kenneth E. Raske, President, on the Reauthorization of the Health Care Reform Act, before the New York State Senate Health and Insurance Committees" (January 11, 2005), 6 [www.gnyha.org/525/File.aspx]. Those with over 100 beds were: Union Hospital of the Bronx (198 beds, closed 1998), Brooklyn Hospital Center-Caledonian Campus (190 beds, closed 2003), and Interfaith Medical Center-Jewish Hospital of Brooklyn (300 beds, closed 2003).

28. American Hospital Association, *Trendwatch, Chartbook 2005,* app., table 5.3. There were 2.87 million full-time equivalents (FTEs) working in the nation's community hospitals in 1980 and over 4.1 million in 2003. The number of FTE RNs working in hospitals increased from over 736,000 to over 1 million.

29. Ibid. Between 1980 and 2003, the number of FTE employees working in hospitals per adjusted admission peaked at 0.085 FTEs in 1993. In 2003, FTEs per adjusted admission had returned to near 1980-levels of 0.071.

30. CHWS, *Health Care Workforce in New York City, 2002,* ix.

31. For an account of why health care workforce forecasting failed during the same period in Philadelphia, where the situation was similar to New York City, see David Barton Smith, William Aaronson, and Richard L. Jones Jr., "The Perils of Healthcare Workforce Forecasting: A Case Study of the Philadelphia Metropolitan Area," *Journal of Healthcare Management* 48, no. 2 (2003).

32. Kathryn Haslanger, *Medicaid Managed Care in New York: A Work in Progress* (New York: United Hospital Fund, 2003), 21.

33. John Billings, Nina Parikh, and Tod Mijanovich, "Emergency Department Use: The New York Story" (New York: The Commonwealth Fund, Issue Brief, November 2000). Data from 1994 and 1998 show that the differences between Medicaid fee-for-service and Medicaid managed care recipients in use of emergency departments for nonemergent conditions were small or nonexistent. In 1998, for instance, 42% of visits to the emergency department by all Medicaid recipients were for nonemergent issues. The study did not test for statistical significance.

34. For a discussion of these issues, see Marilyn R. Ellwood and Leighton Ku, "Welfare and Immigration Reforms: Unintended Side Effects for Medicaid," *Health Affairs* 17, no. 3 (1998).

35. Lipowicz, "Union Victories."

36. Joel C. Cantor, Kathryn Haslanger, and Kathleen DeGuire, "Health Plan Responses to Medicaid Managed Care Policy in New York City," *Managed Care Quarterly* 8, no. 2 (2000): 42; Haslanger, *Medicaid Managed Care,* 3–4; Sparer and Brown, "Nothing Exceeds Like Success," 216–7.

37. Haslanger, *Medicaid Managed Care,* 6.

38. According to a 2000 survey of safety-net health plans, even though only 30% of the primary care providers in hospital-sponsored plans are based in hospitals, half of the members in hospital sponsored plans receive their primary care in a hospital clinic. According to the study's authors, "these plans are at least a partial success in steering Medicaid business to their sponsoring organizations." Michael K. Gusmano, Michael S. Sparer, Lawrence D. Brown, Catherine Rowe, and Bradford Gray, "The Evolving Role and Care Management Approaches of Safety-Net Medicaid Managed Care Plans," *Journal of Urban Health* 79, no. 4 (2002): 607. My assessment of provider-sponsored plans is additionally based on the following series of articles (although the authors' conclusions tend to be more optimistic than my own): Bradford H. Gray and Catherine Row, "Safety-net Health Plans: A Status Report," *Health Affairs* 19, no. 1 (2000); Michael S. Sparer, Lawrence D. Brown, "Uneasy Alliances: Managed Care Plans Formed by Saftey-Net Providers," *Health Affairs* 19, no. 4 (2000); Michael S. Sparer, Lawrence D. Brown, Michael K. Gusmano, Catherine Rowe, and Bradford H. Gray, "Promising Practices: How Leading Safety-Net Plans are Managing the Care of Medicaid Clients," *Health Affairs* 21, no. 5 (2002).

39. Haslanger, *Medicaid Managed Care,* 19. In addition, private hospitals that did make initial investments in creating community-based care settings have not necessarily sustained them. In 2002, Mount Sinai hospital, which sits at the boundary of some of New York's wealthiest and poorest neighborhoods, said it planned to make cuts to its outpatient clinics, which had become crucial sources of care for low-income and uninsured patients in communities around the hospital. See Janny Scott and Mary Williams Walsh, "Mt. Sinai on a Path Away from the Past," *New York Times,* August 25, 2002.

40. Amos Ilan and Catherine Lanier, *The Economic Impact of the Academic Medical Infrastructure on New York State and the New York City Metropolitan Region* (New York: Greater New York Hospital Association, 1999). The academic medical sector directly employed 252,000 people in New York State, of whom 216,000 were in the New York City region.

41. For an excellent analysis of the unintended consequences of the government's attempts to minimize its role in health care through the creation of a prospective payment system for Medicare in 1983, see Mary Ruggie, "The Paradox of Liberal Intervention: Health Policy and the American Welfare State," *American Journal of Sociology* 97, no. 4 (1992). Ruggie remains correct that the American welfare state continues to expand in the realm of health care even while espousing liberal and pro-market principles. For instance, public spending on health care underwent its largest increase since 1965 when President George W. Bush, a Republican, implemented a Medicare prescription drug plan in 2006. Still, it remains to be seen whether changes in state intervention might "lay the foundations for a future national health insurance system," as Ruggie speculates (921).

42. See Haslanger, *Medicaid Managed Care,* 20.

43. The role of management consultants in health care policy and reform is well known but has yet to be subjected to systematic study. One recent survey found no less than 68% of hospitals undertaking restructuring/reengineering initiatives in the 1990s employed external consultants at some point in the process. Stephen Lee Walston, Lawton Robert Burns, and John R. Kimberly, "Does Reengineering Really Work? An Examination of the Context and Outcomes of Hospital Reengineering Initiatives," *Health Services Research* 34, no. 6 (2000): 1371; see also Stephen Lee Walston, Linda D. Urden, and Patricia Sullivan, "Hospital Reengineering: An Evolving Management Innovation: History, Current Status and Future Direction," *Journal of Health and Human Services Administration* 23, no. 4 (2001). Even a major theoretical and empirical investigation of organizational change in health care has almost no mention of the role of external consultants—see Scott et al., *Institutional Change and Healthcare Organizations.*

44. Acccording to press releases from the office of Governor Pataki, Mount Sinai received over $11.2 million in aid from the first three installments of the CHCCDP program, of which about $2.8 million was designated for training. These funds, however, were not released until the beginning of 1999.

45. Katherine E. Finkelstein, "Layoffs Feared as Consultant Examines Mount Sinai's Budget," *New York Times,* November 29, 2001.

46. Katherine E. Finkelstein, "Celebrated Hospital Merger a Union in Name Only," *New York Times,* December 2, 2001.

47. Alison Leigh Cowan, "How a Venerable Hospital Helped Undermine Its Own Health," *New York Times,* April 7, 2003.

48. Center for Health Workforce Studies (CHWS), *An Assessment of the Impact of Hospital Restructuring on Nurse Staffing in New York City* (Albany, NY: Center for Health Workforce Studies, School of Public Health, State University of New York at Albany, 1998, June), 3.

49. Walston, Urden, and Sullivan, "Hospital Reengineering," 408.

3. The Promise of Training

1. Center for an Urban Future, *Rebuilding Job Training from the Ground Up: Workforce System Reform after 9/11* (New York: Center for an Urban Future, 2002), 5.

2. Commission on Health Care Facilities, "Economic Impact," *Factors Book.*

3. Center for an Urban Future, *Rebuilding Job Training,* 5.

4. The sections of these reports related to training were provided to me by the Commission for the Public's Health System (CPHS), which obtained them from the New York State Department of Health after it sued the State for access to records of how eligible public and voluntary hospitals had spent the $1.25 billion in CHCCDP grants. The Commission's own report on hospital spending is: Commission on the Public's Health System, *CHCCDP: Are We Getting Our Money's Worth?* The Commission's attempts to obtain the data are covered in Tom Robbins, "Hospital Holiday," *Village Voice,* May 28, 2003 [www.villagevoice.com/print/issues/0322/robbins.php].

5. Figueroa and Lazes, *Labor-Management Projects,* 13–14.

6. Commission on the Public's Health System, *CHCCDP: Are We Getting Our Money's Worth?,* 45.

7. Total HWRI grants for specific organizations here and in the rest of the chapter refer to years one and two of the HCRA 1996 HWRI program (disbursed in 1997 and 1998) and year one of the HCRA 2000 HWRI program (disbursed in 2001). They are calculated from press releases of the Office of Governor George Pataki, New York State: "Governor Announces $28.1 Million in Health Care Training Grants" (January 24, 2001); "Governor Announces Health Care Workforce Retraining Grants" (July 9, 1997); "Governor Announces New Health Care Workforce Retraining Grants" (February 13, 1998). The state's data on funding levels is not always consistent. According to the Governor's press releases, HWRI 1996 awarded between $42 and $43 million in years one and two, figures verified by Department of Health annual reports. However, the 2001 Annual Report of the Department of Labor states that "according to the Department of Health," HWRI 1996 awarded close to $59 million. It also says HWRI 2000 awarded $41 million in its first year, while the January 24, 2001 press release from the governor's office indicates just over $28 million was awarded in the first year of HWRI 2000. See State of New York Department of Health, "1998 Annual Report"; State of New York Department of Health, "1999–2000 Annual Report"; State of New York Department of Labor, "2001 Annual Report," 19.

8. 2004 Training and Upgrading Fund vendor payments, here and in the rest of the chapter, are from Internal Revenue Service, Form 5500, Schedule C, in possession of the author.

9. Center for an Urban Future, *CUNY on the Job,* 2.

10. Niev Duffy, William Ebenstein, and Deniz Kurtel, "A Preliminary Profile of Enrollment Patterns, Graduation Rates and Demographics of 1199 Represented Workers at the City University of New York" (New York: The John F. Kennedy, Jr. Institute for Worker Education, 2003). Statistics refer only to 1199 members in the National Benefit Fund database, which may not be an exhaustive list of all 1199 members.

11. Office of the Governor, New York State, "Governor Opens Bronx Health Training and Childcare Center" (press release, October 22, 2002); Steven Greenhouse, "CUNY and Union Join in a Bronx Program to Train Nurses and Improve Health Care Skills" *New York Times,* February 17, 2002.

12. Office of the Governor, New York State, "Governor Announces Health Care Workforce Retraining Grants" (press release, July 8, 1997).

13. "Training Fund in Transition," *1199 News* 15, no. 11–12 (Nov.-Dec. 1997): 6.

14. State of New York Department of Health, "1999–2000 Annual Report," 47–48.

15. "Training Fund to Reach Many More Members," *1199 News* 16, no. 2 (March-April 1998): 21.

16. Commission on Health Care Facilities, "Economic Impact," *Factors Book,* 5. Author's calculations for New York City region.

17. According to the CHCCDP reports, the thirty hospitals had together spent about $25 million of the $75.4 million they had been allotted for training in the first three cycles. My analysis of how they spent those funds is limited to the top five reported programs at each hospital (in terms of dollars spent). The top five programs accounted for 69% of spending, on average, at the hospitals. Note that the $25 million is only 13.9% of the $180 million allotted to hospitals statewide in the first three cycles, but there are no available reports of how other hospitals spent their allotments (of particular interest would be the $65 million granted to public hospitals in New York City) or of how the thirty voluntary hospitals spent the remaining funds from the first three cycles.

The number of training "encounters" in customer service was calculated by the Commission on the Public's Health System. See, *CHCCDP: Are We Getting Our Money's Worth?* Employees may participate in multiple training courses, and some courses have multiple sessions. The number cited reflects each of these encounters, not the number of individual employees trained.

18. I am grateful to the 1199/League Training and Upgrading Fund for supplying me with the summary of this report.

19. In 1999, the United States spent $1,059 per capita on health administration, as compared with $307 per capita in Canada. Steffie Woolhandler, Terry Campbell, and David Himmelstein, "Costs of Health Care Administration in the United States and Canada," *New England Journal of Medicine* 349, no. 8 (2003): 768.

20. American Hospital Association (AHA), *In Our Hands: How Hospital Leaders Can Build a Thriving Workforce* (American Hospital Association Commission on Workforce for Hospitals and Health Systems, April, 2002), 13. The other keys were to "improve the workplace partnership," "broaden the base," "collaborate with others," and "build societal support."

4. Too Skilled to Care: Multiskilling

1. Elisabeth Rosenthal, "Once in Big Demand, Nurses Are Targets for Hospital Cuts," *New York Times,* August 19, 1996.

2. President's column, *1199 News* 12, no. 7–8 (July-August 1994): 4; *1199 News* 12, no. 3 (March 1994): 8.

3. CHWS, Impact of Hospital Restructuring.

4. Ibid., 29.

5. J. Philip Lathrop, *Restructuring Health Care* (San Francisco: Jossey-Bass, 1993), 12, 64.

6. Michael Hammer and James Champy, *Reengineering the Corporation: A Manifesto for Business Revolution* (New York: HarperCollins, 1993), 42, 48.

7. Julie Sochalski, Linda H. Aiken, and Claire M. Fagin, "Hospital Restructuring in the United States, Canada, and Western Europe—an Outcomes Research Agenda," *Medical Care* 35, no. 10 (1997): OS18.

8. Quoted in Weber, "At New York City's Mount Sinai," 4.

9. Weber, "At New York City's Mount Sinai," 5, inset box.

10. In New York, for instance, standard data sources that workforce planners use to track staffing levels and patterns contain a number of limitations: They do not distinguish between all hospital personnel and those assigned to inpatient units; they make no distinctions between RNs who are managers and those who are providing direct care; and the Bureau of Labor Statistics category for "nursing aides, orderlies, and attendants" lumps together a diverse group of workers in diverse settings.

11. Robert Brannon, "Restructuring Hospital Nursing: Reversing the Trend Toward a Professional Work Force," *International Journal of Health Services* 26, no. 4 (1996).

12. Sochalski, Aiken, and Fagin, "Hospital Restructuring"; Dana Beth Weinberg, *Code Green: Money-Driven Hospitals and the Dismantling of Nursing* (Ithaca: Cornell University Press, 2003).

13. Although nursing leaders have argued that both team nursing and primary nursing (depending on which model is in the ascendant) improve the professional status of RNs, Robert Brannon argues that neither form of nursing work organization made a substantial difference in RN's status: "Professionalization and Work Intensification: Nursing in the Cost Containment Era," *Work and Occupations* 21, no. 2 (1994). The fact that some nursing leaders also argued that the status of the profession would improve as a result of reengineering and managed care suggests a problematic willingness to go with the flow of the latest managerial tactics and a disregard for the implications of such tactics for staff nurses. See Suzanne Gordon, *Nursing Against the Odds* (Ithaca: Cornell University Press, 2005), esp. 245–52.

14. Sharon Bergman Schweikhart and Vicki Smith-Daniels, "Reengineering the Work of Caregivers: Role Definition, Team Structures, and Organizational Redesign," *Hospital and Health Services Administration* 41, no. 1 (1996): 24.

15. Harry Braverman, *Labor and Monopoly Capital: The Degradation of Work in the Twentieth Century* (New York: Monthly Review Press, 1975).

16. CHWS, Impact of Hospital Restructuring.

17. Linda H. Aiken et al., "An International Perspective on Hospital Nurses' Work Environments: The Case for Reform," *Policy, Politics, & Nursing Practice* 2, no. 4 (2001): 259.

18. Weinberg, *Code Green,* 94–95.

19. Hammer and Champy, *Reengineering the Corporation,* 42, 48.

20. Braverman, *Labor and Monopoly Capital.* For criticisms of deskilling theory, see Paul Attewell, "The Deskilling Controversy," *Work and Occupations* 14, no. 3 (1987); Stephen R. Barley, "Technology, Power, and the Social Organization of Work: Towards a Pragmatic Theory of Skilling and Deskilling," *Research in the Sociology of Organizations* 6 (1988).

21. State funding under HWRI was to prepare workers for specific jobs, not general education.

22. For a classic account of this process, see Randall Collins, *The Credential Society: An Historical Sociology of Education and Stratification* (New York: Academic Press, 1979).

23. Lynn McCormick, "Reshuffling of Immigrant Nursing Aide Ladders in New York City" (Unpublished paper, Hunter College, City University of New York, n.d.), table 6.

24. Ibid.

25. Ibid., table 2.

26. McCormick found, for instance, that in 1990, 33.5% of all recent immigrants (arriving within the last five years) who had become aides went into home care positions. 66.8% and 47.1%

of aides recently arrived from the Dominican Republic and Haiti, respectively, went into home care. Ibid., table 3.

27. Policy makers and administrators always justify this shift by making some legitimate points about patient care: It is better for patients to remain at home whenever possible; it is a waste of resources for patients who do not need acute care services to be in expensive hospital beds. But recent health care policy has ultimately been driven by concern over costs, not concern over care, and it is inarguably the case that employers and payers have sought ways to pay health care workers less.

28. As mentioned in the introduction, according to England, Budig, and Folbre, the wages of those who do caring labor are subject to a penalty of 5–6% for both men and women, though certain health care occupations are an exception to this finding. They speculate, as does Norton Grubb in his research on education and income, that this exception could be accounted for by the predominance of licensed or certified occupations in health care. This is one aspect of what Weeden calls a "social closure" effect. See England, Budig, and Folbre, "Wages of Virtue"; Grubb, *Working in the Middle,* 39; Kim A. Weeden, "Why Do Some Occupations Pay More Than Others? Social Closure and Earnings Inequality in the United States," *American Journal of Sociology* 108, no. 1 (2002).

29. Karen Brodkin Sacks, *Caring by the Hour: Women, Work, and Organizing at Duke Medical Center* (Urbana: University of Illinois Press, 1988), 199, 207; see esp. 169–216.

30. One study of restructuring in New York City reported the main purpose of restructuring was to improve the quality of care and that restructuring "was generally viewed positively." However, the researchers only interviewed nurse managers and nurses whom had been selected by nurse managers to participate. CHWS, *Impact of Hospital Restructuring.*

31. Gordon, *Nursing against the Odds.*

32. Lathrop, *Restructuring Health Care,* 167.

33. Hammer and Champy, *Reengineering the Corporation,* 70.

34. Center for Health Workforce Studies (CHWS), *The Health Care Workforce in New York State, 2004: Trends in the Supply and Demand for Health Workers* (Albany, NY: Center for Health Workforce Studies, School of Public Health, State University of New York at Albany, May 2005), 47, 42, 19.

35. CHWS, *Health Care Workforce in New York City, 2000,* 8.

36. Ibid., 34, fig. 20. The figure includes an unknown number of workers who were later recalled to their jobs. The Center for Health Workforce Studies, to which 1199 provided this data, furthermore notes that no job profile of 1199 membership exists.

37. Fiscal Policy Institute, *Health Care Industry Trends.* Different periods yield different results: between 1995 and 2000, the number of staff in HHC hospitals declined by 7,296 workers, or almost 23% of the workforce, see Howard S. Berliner, Christine T. Kovner, and Cordelia Reimers, "The Health Care Workforce in Los Angeles County and New York City: A Comparison and Analysis," *International Journal of Health Services* 32, no. 2 (2002): table 7. From 1994 to 1998, employment in public hospitals declined by 16,037 jobs, or by almost 25%, see CHWS, *Health Care Workforce in New York City, 2000,* 8, table 2. Between 1995 and 2004, public-sector hospital jobs decreased by 26%, see CHWS, *The Health Care Workforce in New York State, 2004,* 47.

38. Salit, Fass, and Nowak, "Out of the Frying Pan," 131.

39. "Mission Possible? New York City's Municipal Hospitals in an Era of Declining Resources," *Hospital Watch* 13, no. 1 (2002): 4.

40. Salit, Fass, and Nowak, "Out of the Frying Pan."

41. Greater New York Hospital Association, *Health Care Statistics 2003,* tables 5, 7. Data are from the American Hospital Association (AHA) Annual Survey of Hospitals. The number of community hospital beds in New York City declined between 1990 and 1997, from 34,148 to 30,223, but they stabilized thereafter, numbering 29,032 in 1998 and 29,058 in 2001. In the AHA

survey, "community" hospitals includes public and private hospitals, so it is likely that New York City private hospitals lost few (if any) beds in the period, since most of the cuts to the hospital system occurred at public hospitals in the 1990s. The data also show the number of total hospital admissions in New York City increased over the decade, from 1,062,000 in 1990 to 1,154,000 in 2001.

42. Peter Lazes et al., "The Use and Impact of Re-Engineering and Restructuring in Acute Care Hospitals" (research report, Cornell and Indiana Universities, 2003), 5.

43. Ibid., 5.

44. Hammer and Champy, *Reengineering the Corporation,* 5, 2.

45. Commission on the Public's Health System, *CHCCDP: Are We Getting Our Money's Worth?* The effects of the clinics on access to and utilization of the health care system are basically undocumented. In addition, as discussed in chapter 2, hospital-based clinics and out-patient departments were not necessarily the best method of getting care into underserved communities.

46. Steven Greenhouse, "Union Boss Says Even Democrats Can Err," *New York Times,* January 20, 2002.

47. Lathrop, Restructuring Health Care, 2.

5. "It All Comes Down to You": Self-Help and Soft Skills

1. I observed this course as part of a research team evaluating it. See the appendix for further details of the study; see also Ariel Ducey, Heather Gautney, and Dominic Wetzel, "Regulating Affective Labor: Communication Skills Training in the Health Care Industry," *Research in the Sociology of Work* 12 (2003).

2. Lathrop, *Restructuring Health Care,* 166–67.

3. David McNally, *Even Eagles Need a Push* (New York: Dell, 1994), 141, 21. Micki McGee, in her analysis of self-help literature more broadly, calls this "Imagineering." See *Self-Help, Inc.: Makeover Culture in American Life* (New York: Oxford University Press, 2005), 162–67.

4. See http://www.thericks.com/ricks/ricks-index.htm [last accessed April 15, 2008].

5. Ray Bingham, "Leaving Nursing: Hospital Staffing Cuts Have Created Conditions under Which This Dedicated Nurse Can No Longer Work," *Health Affairs* 21, no. 1 (2002).

6. Burton R. Clark, "The Cooling-out Function in Higher Education," *American Journal of Sociology* 65, no. 6 (1960).

7. Arlie Russell Hochschild, *The Managed Heart: Commercialization of Human Feeling* (Berkeley: University of California Press, 1983). John Van Maanen and Gideon Kunda, "'Real Feelings': Emotional Expression and Organizational Culture," *Research in Organizational Behavior* 11 (1989).

8. As a "face-to-face service that develops the human capabilities of the recipient," caring labor is more specific than either "interactive service work" or "emotional labor," which have also been used to describe the kind of work more and more Americans do in the current labor market. Both of the latter can extend to occupations such as stewardesses, retail clerks, taxi drivers, receptionists, and so forth—occupations that require interpersonal and emotional skills and abilities, but which do not promote the "development, learning, skill acquisition, or physical and psychological health of the recipient" of services. England, Budig, and Folbre, "Wages of Virtue," 455, 459.

9. Commission on Health Care Facilities, "Economic Impact," *Factors Book,* 5.

10. Lazes et al., "The Use and Impact of Re-Engineering."

11. Conference Board of Canada, *Success by Design: What Works in Workforce Development* (Ottawa, Ontario: Conference Board of Canada, 2002), 3.

12. 1199 SEIU, "Annual Review" (New York: Employment, Training & Job Security Program, 2003), 2.

13. The figure is taken from an internal analysis of the reports by the Commission for the Public's Health System. See Commission on the Public's Health System, *CHCCDP: Are We Getting Our Money's Worth?* Cycle two and three funds were released to hospitals in 2001.

14. Unlike many registered nurses and most nursing assistants in other parts of the country, these women were less likely to show their discontent with the conditions of their work by quitting—they had unionized jobs with benefits. But their discontent was nonetheless apparent in their layered responses to the training and in tactics such as calling in sick, refusing to come out of description, and taking extra time to talk to patients.

15. Rick Fantasia, in his case studies of workers' collective action, shows the "cultures of solidarity" that emerge in instances of conflict between labor and management do not generally respect the boundaries of existing institutional forms, such as labor unions, occupational groups, or organizations, though they may take advantage of such forms as the basis for mobilization. Such cultures are neither borne out of abstract consciousness nor, at least in the United States, directed at general targets, such as class inequality; they are practices and relationships created of necessity when workers' rights and sense of dignity are violated in concrete and tangible ways. Then workers seek, or are often forced, to take action beyond the narrow limits imposed by institutionalized trade unionism. Often, these forms of collective action are not only an attempt to overcome managerial attacks on workers' rights but also are forged by such attacks. Therefore, it is worth considering that soft skills training was the product of a new era of management-union "jointness," so to the extent workers resisted such courses or found them wanting, they might blame their union as much as their employers. Rick Fantasia, *Cultures of Solidarity: Consciousness, Action, and Contemporary American Workers* (Berkeley: University of California Press, 1988).

6. Training without End: Upgrading

1. Health/PAC Bulletin, "What Course for Health Workers?" in *Prognosis Negative: Crisis in the Health Care System,* ed. David Kotelchuck (New York: Vintage Books, 1976), 251.

2. In this chapter, to protect the confidentiality of the workers interviewed, the names of hospitals where they work have been replaced by pseudonyms. As throughout the book, the names of the health care workers are also pseudonyms.

3. This description perhaps contained a bit of posturing, but regardless, as more men go into health care, they may find themselves in jobs that are more difficult to depict as masculine, a phenomenon that may entail changes in the culture, values, and lifestyle of working-class families in a service economy.

4. American Medical Association, *Health Professions Education Data Book 2003–2004* (Chicago: American Medical Association, 2003).

5. According to the Bureau of Labor Statistics, the annual median wage for physical therapy assistants in the New York City metropolitan area was $42,590 in 2001. Bureau of Labor Statistics, U.S. Department of Labor, Bureau of Labor Statistics, Occupational Employment Statistics (OES), www.bls.gov.

6. To get a sense of the Bronx—and the Grand Concourse—before and after Robert Moses sliced it in two with the Cross-Bronx Expressway, see Marshall Berman, *All That Is Solid Melts into Air: The Experience of Modernity* (New York: Simon and Schuster, 1982), section V.

7. As Stanley Aronowitz has noted, "This is a time of work without end for many Americans and a work-shortage for many others." "The Last Good Job in America," in *Post-Work: The Wages of Cybernation,* ed. Stanley Aronowitz and Jonathan Cutler (New York: Routledge, 1998), 213.

8. U.S. Department of Labor, Bureau of Labor Statistics, Occupational Employment Statistics (OES).

9. Stanley Aronowitz, *False Promises: The Shaping of American Working Class Consciousness* (New York: McGraw-Hill, 1973).

7. From Skills to Meaning

1. Figueroa and Lazes, *Labor-Management Projects,* 8–9. I would contend that equally important to evaluations of "quality and performance," even necessary precursors to them, are descriptions of the conditions of health care work and the experiences of health care workers.

2. Gordon Lafer, *The Job Training Charade* (Ithaca: Cornell University Press, 2002).

3. Ivar E. Berg, *Education and Jobs: The Great Training Robbery* (New York: Published for the Center for Urban Education by Praeger Publishers, 1970), see esp. chap. 4.

4. Collins, *Credential Society.*

5. Louis Uchitelle, *The Disposable American: Layoffs and Their Consequences* (New York: Alfred A. Knopf, 2006), 67, and chap. 3.

6. Michael J. Handel, "Skills Mismatch in the Labor Market," *Annual Review of Sociology* 29 (2003): 138.

7. Center for an Urban Future, *Labor Gains: How Union-Affiliated Training Is Transforming New York's Workforce Landscape* (New York: Center for an Urban Future, 2003).

8. See, e.g., Beverly Takahashi and Edwin Meléndez, "Union-Sponsored Workforce Development Initiatives," in *Communities and Workforce Development,* ed. Edwin Meléndez (Kalamazoo, MI: W.E. Upjohn Institute for Employment Research, 2004).

9. W. Norton Grubb, "Evaluating Job Training Programs in the United States: Evidence and Explanations" (Berkeley: National Center for Research in Vocational Education, Graduate School of Education, University of California, 1995); Lafer, *Job Training Charade.*

10. Perhaps the theory that best captures the way in which the division of labor can be unrelated to the requirements of the work itself is Andrew Abbott's work on "jurisdictional conflicts" among the professions: Andrew Delano Abbott, *The System of Professions: An Essay on the Division of Expert Labor* (Chicago: University of Chicago Press, 1988).

11. Gordon, *Nursing against the Odds.*

12. In *Even Eagles Need a Push,* David McNally himself acknowledges that his readers may feel that they are being underutilized. He asks whether "you had far more to offer than was either being asked of you or you were asking of yourself"? Citing Dick Leider, McNally reports the major problem facing the American worker may not be burnout, but "rust-out," the "gross underutilization of an individual's potential." McNally, however, ascribes this problem to the desire to play it safe, the fear of risk. "In a nation that has produced some of the most brilliant achievers, many of us will suppress or deny our capabilities for the illusion of security. The trade-off for this choice is soul-destroying. Those who have a zest for life are willing to take the risk of pitting their skills and talents against the unknown." McNally, *Even Eagles Need a Push,* 91. Making $7 an hour as a home health aide, or even $14 an hour as a nursing assistant, is not a choice people make to play it safe, to be secure. It hardly qualifies as an "illusion of security."

13. David W. Livingstone, "Lifelong Learning and Underemployment in the Knowledge Society: A North American Perspective," *Comparative Education* 35, no. 2 (1999): 163–86.

14. David W. Livingstone, *The Education-Jobs Gap: Underemployment or Economic Democracy* (Aurora, Ontario: Garamond Press, 2004), esp. cap. 2.

15. Philip Moss and Chris Tilly, *Stories Employers Tell: Race, Skill, and Hiring in America* (New York: Russell Sage Foundation, 2001).

16. Handel, "Skills Mismatch," 150, 157.

17. Conference Board of Canada, *Success by Design.*

18. Gordon Lafer, "What Is 'Skill'? Training for Discipline in the Low-Wage Labour Market," in *The Skills That Matter,* ed. Chris Warhurst and Irena Grugulis (New York: Palgrave MacMillan, 2004), 118.

19. And even if communication skills are "skills" that these workers don't have and that would be beneficial to their chances of escaping the world of low-wage work, those are skills that people learn in education programs, by reading, writing, and thinking critically, and from their friends and family members who have themselves escaped the world of low-wage work, not in the kind of two-day in-services I have observed.

20. Steven Brint and Jerome Karabel, *The Diverted Dream: Community Colleges and the Promise of Educational Opportunity in America, 1900–1985* (New York: Basic Books, 1989); Joe Kincheloe, *How Do We Tell the Workers? The Socioeconomic Foundations of Work and Vocational Education* (Boulder, CO: Westview Press, 1999); Fred Pincus, "The False Promises of Community Colleges: Class Conflict and Vocational Education," *Harvard Educational Review* 50, no. 3 (1986): 332–61.

21. 2000 U.S. Census, State and County QuickFacts, http://quickfacts.census.gov; David Leonhardt, "U.S. Poverty Rate Was Up Last Year," *New York Times,* August 31, 2005. Official government statistics may underestimate poverty in New York City because they are not adjusted for the higher costs of living (especially for housing) in urban areas.

22. Paul Willis, "Labor Power, Culture, and the Cultural Commodity," in *Critical Education in the New Information Age* (Lanham, MD: Rowman & Littlefield, 1999), 139.

23. Writing about the legacy of slavery, Paul Gilroy has said, "in the critical thoughts of blacks in the West, social self-creation through labor is not the center-piece of emancipatory hopes." *The Black Atlantic: Modernity and Double Consciousness* (Cambridge, MA: Harvard University Press, 1993), 40.

24. Bureau of Labor Statistics, U.S. Department of Labor, Bureau of Labor Statistics, Occupational Employment Statistics (OES), www.bls.gov. In the same year, the official poverty threshold for a family of four was $18,104 as determined by the U.S. Census. Such thresholds do not account for differences in the cost of living in various regions.

25. Robert B. Reich, *The Work of Nations: Preparing Ourselves for 21st Century Capitalism,* 1st ed. (New York: Alfred A. Knopf, 1991), 176. This account of Reich's policies is derived in part from Uchitelle, *The Disposable American,* chap. 7.

26. Lawrence Mishel, Jared Bernstein, and Heather Boushey, *The State of Working America 2002/2003* (Ithaca: Cornell University Press, 2003), 158–63.

8. A Common Cause

1. Fink and Greenberg, *Upheaval in the Quiet Zone,* 178–9.

2. Theresa Agovino, "Hospital Workers' Union at an Impasse," *Crain's New York Business,* June 26, 1989.

3. In the early 1990s the Fund placed regular notices and calls for applications in the pages of the union newsletter, *1199 News,* some for more organized programs such as remedial and college prep courses, nascent stipend and "forgivable loan" programs for upgrading, and part-time programs in medical terminology, coding, computer training, among others. Nonetheless, the $16 million dollars the Fund expected from the state for such programs as a result of the 1989 contract paled in comparison to the funding received in late 1990s.

4. "Training Fund to Reach Many More Members," *1199 News* 16, no. 2 (March-April 1998): 21.

5. 1199 SEIU, "Annual Review."

6. Doris Turner, long mentored by Davis, was elected as his first successor. During her presidency, 1199 separated from the national union it had itself established (based in Philadelphia) and was overtaken by racial and political conflict. Turner was eventually found guilty of vote tampering in her election campaign and presided over a disastrous 1984 strike, in which workers never received the full wage increase they were promised because Turner refused to acknowledge or honor give-backs she had secretly made to hospitals. An oppositional slate, which included Dennis Rivera, elected Giorgeanna Johnson as president in 1986, and although her presidency too became

contentious on the basis of race, contract negotiations under her tenure were more successful; hospitals welcomed stability in the union leadership, and the League agreed to a one-time 5% bonus (to make up for raises never paid under the previous contract) and a 13% raise over three years. In return, the union allowed employers to reduce contributions to the Pension and Training and Upgrading Funds, the latter of which was becoming financially unstable. Fink and Greenberg, *Upheaval in the Quiet Zone,* 230, see chap. 10.

7. Agovino, "Hospital Workers' Union at an Impasse."

8. Howard W. French, "High-Stakes Strike Looms for Hospitals," *New York Times,* October 1, 1989; Howard W. French, "The Hospital Workers Are the Envy of Labor Now," *New York Times,* October 8, 1989; Sam Roberts, "As Hospital Agreement Is Reached, a Strong Union and Leader Emerge," *New York Times,* October 5, 1989. There is reason to believe, though it is not entirely clear, that the state did, in the end, underwrite the wage increases. In his column in the September 1989 issue of *1199 News* (7, no. 8), Dennis Rivera wrote, "the state of New York has increased its reimbursement to hospitals to pay for higher labor costs by 7.3%. And yet management has actually said the problem is not their ability to pay but rather their refusal to give more than they think is 'fair'" (p. 2). However, this increased reimbursement was not mentioned in subsequent articles that celebrated the contract. This could have been for several reasons: (1) the increased reimbursement was not necessarily for higher labor costs and the union had to fight in any case to have them allotted to wages; (2) the increased funds did not in fact transpire; or (3) the union chose not to mention these funds again in order to maintain images of the 1989 contract campaign as one in which it had thoroughly defeated management.

9. Dr. Robert Newman was president. Sam Roberts, "Beth Israel Reaches Pact with Union," *New York Times,* February 20, 1992.

10. Sam Roberts, "Private Hospitals in New York Reach Accord on Job Security," *New York Times,* June 11, 1992.

11. Figueroa and Lazes, *Labor-Management Projects,* 15.

12. Melinda Henneberger, "Hospitals Swap Job Guarantees for Pay Limits," *New York Times,* September 20, 1994.

13. An article in the March 1994 issue (12, no. 3) of *1199 News,* which was devoted to the issue of health care restructuring, contains the first mention of the term "cross-training."

14. Rivera explicitly drew this link in his November 1993 column in *1199 News,* though evidence from the newsletter also suggests that restructuring was underway before the Clinton plan was in full swing (President's column, *1199 News* 11, no. 11 [November 1993]). The July-August, 1993 issue, for instance, had already raised the issue of restructuring, but in the context of broader upheaval in health care, not the Clinton plan in particular (11, no. 7–8 [July-August 1993]).

15. The November 1993 issue of *1199 News* was devoted to analyzing the Clinton Health Plan and presenting 1199's concerns (11, no. 11).

16. Ian Fisher, "Pressure on All Sides in the Battle of the Budget," *New York Times,* March 14, 1995; Steven Lee Myers, "Guiliani's Spending Plan: The Overview; Giuliani Seeks Deepest Cuts in City Spending since 1930's," *New York Times,* February 15, 1995.

17. Henneberger, "Hospitals Swap Job Guarantees."

18. "We're Not Accepting Layoffs," *1199 News* 11, no. 7–8 (July–August 1993): 5.

19. *1199 News* 12, no. 3 (March 1994): 8.

20. "Preparing for Tomorrow," *1199 News* 12, no. 9 (September 1994): 17.

21. Though the contract was ratified by 93% of those voting in October (12,920 to 835), only about one-third of those covered by the contract voted. "Members Say 'Yes!' to Job Security," *1199 News* 12, no. 11 (November 1994): 3.

22. "Our Groundbreaking Agreement," president's column, *1199 News* 12, no. 10 (October 1994): 4.

23. *1199 News* 12, no. 11 (November 1994): 7–11.

24. Barbara Benson, "Layoffs Split 3 Local Unions," *Crain's New York Business* 10, no. 47 (1994).

25. Bob Master, in Steve Early et al., "An Exchange of Views: Will Endorsing Republicans Teach Turncoat Dems the Right Lesson?" *Labor Notes* 279 (June 2002): 8. See also James Dao, "Poll Finds Pataki's Ratings Are Low over Budget Cuts," *New York Times,* May 4, 1995; Ian Fisher, "Pataki Getting Low Marks for Job Performance, Poll Shows," *New York Times,* March 7, 1995.

26. "N.Y. to Cut Medicaid Spending by 9% or $2.1 Billion," *Inside Health Care Reform* 3, no. 11 (June 15, 1995).

27. DC37 Leader Stanley Hill took a different approach in the period. Even though DC37 members included public hospital workers in Local 420, Hill and several other city union leaders signed on to a letter from Mayor Giuliani to the governor and state legislative leaders asking for state actions that would allow the city to reduce Medicaid (as well as welfare) benefits. Such cuts would negatively impact many city hospitals. Rivera "was said by those close to him to be outraged" by the letter and his fellow union leader's capitulation. Wayne Barrett, "Solidarity Whenever: Union Leaders Find It Useful to Shun the Poor, for the Moment," *Village Voice,* May 30, 1995. A year later, Hill was forced to resign after allegations of voting fraud at the union during the vote that ratified DC37's 1996 contract—a contract that called for a two-year pay freeze. Hill was never convicted in relation to the fraud, but several leaders of DC37 Local 1549, where the fraud occurred, were. Ray Sanchez, "Calls for New Chief, Contracts," *Newsday,* November 25, 1998.

28. Steven Greenhouse, "Contract Offers Job Security for 50,000 in Hospitals," *New York Times,* June 22, 1998; Steven Greenhouse, "Nursing Homes and Hospitals Hit by Strike," *New York Times,* June 26, 1996. The lay-off figure was also cited in the president's column and an article on contract negotiations in *1199 News* 15, no. 7–8 (July-August 1997).

29. "Without Members It Doesn't Mean a Thing," *1199 News* 15, no. 7–8 (July-August, 1997): 7.

30. Center for Health Workforce Studies (CHWS) and New Century Concepts, *The Changing Health Care System in New York City: Implications for the Workforce* (Albany: Center for Health Workforce Studies, School of Public Health, State University of New York at Albany, 1997).

31. Steven Greenhouse, "Workers Plan to Rally to Pressure Hospitals for a Contract by June 30," *New York Times,* June 18, 1998; David Rohde, "At Rally, Hospital Workers Vow to Strike to Protect Jobs," *New York Times,* June 19, 1998; Neil MacFarquhar, "Contract Protects Jobs for Workers at 6 Hospitals," *New York Times,* December 2, 1998.

32. CHWS, *Changing Health Care System,* 1, 6, 35, 51.

33. Steven Greenhouse, "Union Plan Sees Buyouts Saving Jobs," *New York Times,* July 12, 1997.

34. "In Their Face: Time to Show Management We're Not Disposable," president's column, *1199 News* 15, no. 5–6 (May-June 1997): 4.

35. "Day One of a Nine-month Campaign," president's column, *1199 News* 15, no. 9–10 (Sept.-Oct. 1997): 11.

36. Steven Greenhouse, "Health Care Union Votes to Merge, Creating Giant," *New York Times,* March 8, 1998; Steven Greenhouse, "Service Unions to Merge in Bid for More Clout," *New York Times,* January 7, 1998; Michael Hirsch, "Titanic," *Village Voice,* January 20, 1998. Some suggested privately that accusations against 144's leader were trumped up to enable 1199's hostile takeover.

37. Greenhouse, "Contract Offers Job Security."

38. The contract was ratified by 98% in late June (22,969 in favor, 391 against). About half of those under the contract voted. "Contract '98: We Won!," *1199 News* 16, no. 4 (July-August 1998): 3.

39. Figueroa and Lazes, *Labor-Management Projects,* 14.

40. Greenhouse, "Contract Offers Job Security."

41. Rima Cohen, "From Strategy to Reality: The Enactment of New York's Family Health Plus Program," *Journal of Health Politics, Policy, and Law* 26, no. 6 (2001): 1388.

42. Steve Malanga, "City Work: The State Wastes Health-Care Dollars," *Newsday,* February 20, 2001.

43. "New York Opts for Quick Cash in Tobacco Deal," *Wall Street Journal,* September 25, 2000; Richard Pérez-Peña, "The Mayor's Budget Plan: Proposals; New York Officials See Tobacco Funds as Fiscal Solution," *New York Times,* November 21, 2002; Joel Stashenko, "Spitzer: Tobacco Payments Will Be Lower Than Projections," *Associated Press Newswire,* December 27, 2000.

44. Steven Greenhouse, "Health Care Workers Extend Contract in Wake of Attacks," *New York Times,* October 9, 2001.

45. Richard Pérez-Peña, "Clamor Grows for Fiscal Aid to Hospitals," *New York Times,* December 1, 2001.

46. James C. Robinson, "The Curious Conversion of Empire Blue Cross," *Health Affairs* 22, no. 4 (2003): 101.

47. In New York State, authority in the legislature is "more centralized than in almost any other legislature in America." Terms of the state budget, for instance, are typically determined by three people—the governor, Senate majority leader, and Assembly speaker. Rivera cultivated relationships with all three and was sometimes considered a fourth member of the group when health care issues were on the table. For a summary of the issues, see James Dao, "Rank and File of Albany Chafing at Their Bit Parts," *New York Times,* January 3, 1998.

48. Kenneth Lovett, "The $750m Handshake—Gov Gives Health Workers a Boost," *New York Post,* January 16, 2002; Kenneth Lovett and Fredric U. Dicker, "Union Gets Healthy Payback on 76g Gift," *New York Post,* January 19, 2002; James C. McKinley Jr., "Albany Deal Would Raise Hospital Pay," *New York Times,* January 16, 2002.

49. Steven Greenhouse, "Hospital Agreement Provides State-Financed Raises," *New York Times,* January 12, 2002.

50. In February, the governor announced the receipt of $508 million in additional Medicaid funding from the feds to which the state was entitled through existing federal regulations, which could be used to pay county-operated public hospitals, but these funds were not the hoped-for increased in the federal share of the Medicaid tab.

51. See, e.g., Tom Robbins, "Blue Cross Hijacked," *Village Voice,* February 13, 2002; Tom Robbins, "Labor's Cheap Date with Pataki," *Village Voice,* September 10, 2002.

52. Alison L. Cowan and James C. McKinley Jr., "Critics Say Albany Is Wasting Insurance Windfall," *New York Times,* February 1, 2003; Joyce Purnick, "Flying Shoes, Health Care and Politics," *New York Times,* April 4, 2002. Indeed, in late 1997, union and voluntary hospitals had proposed taking over Blue Cross and Blue Shield themselves, which would have made them the biggest health insurer in the state. Ian Fisher, "Hospitals and Unions Propose Takeover of Empire Blue Cross," *New York Times,* December 13, 1997.

53. Master, in Early et al., "An Exchange of Views," 8.

54. Quoted in Kim Phillips-Fein, "Does That Elephant Bite? Union Alliances with the GOP," *New Labor Forum* 12, no. 1 (2003): 14.

55. Ibid., 15.

56. New York State, Office of the Governor, "Governor Pataki, Majority Leader Bruno, Speaker Silver Announce Signing of Historic Health Care Legislation" (press release, January 25, 2002).

57. Fredric Dicker, "Pataki Says: Burn Off Deficit with Tobacco $$," *New York Post,* December 11, 2002; James C. McKinley Jr., "Pataki Seeks to Tap Health Fund in Budget Crisis," *New York Times,* February 26, 2003.

58. Joyce Purnick, "Reality Versus Albany," *New York Times,* April 3, 2003.

59. Alison L. Cowan and James C. McKinley Jr., "Critics Say Albany Is Wasting Insurance Windfall," February 1, 2003. See also Al Baker, "Budget Counts on a Windfall to Ease a Gap," *New York Times,* February 22, 2005. This idea seemed less than wise because even the Blue Cross proceeds, which actually amounted to close to $2 billion dollars when the stocks were issued, were tied up in a lawsuit and were not released for several years.

60. Al Baker, "In Battle over the State Budget, Pataki Is Assailed on All Sides," *New York Times,* March 19, 2003.

61. Quote from Purnick, "Reality Versus Albany." See also Fredric Dicker, "Layoff-Wary Hosp Union: Time to Raise Taxes," *New York Post,* April 2, 2003; Winnie Hu and Jr. James C. McKinley, "Health Workers, 2002 Pataki Allies, Jam into Albany to Denounce His Cuts," *New York Times,* April 2, 2003.

62. Al Baker, "State Legislature Overrides Pataki on Budget Vetoes," *New York Times,* May 16, 2003; James C. McKinley Jr., "Pataki Says Legislators' Budget Is Sure to Unravel," *New York Times,* May 7, 2003; James C. McKinley Jr., "Who Blinked on Budget? That Depends on Source," *New York Times,* May 25, 2003.

63. Steven Greenhouse, "Health Union to Give up Part of Raise," *New York Times,* May 8, 2004.

64. Fink and Greenberg, *Upheaval in the Quiet Zone,* 202.

65. Elinor Langer, "The Hospital Workers: 'The Best Contract Anywhere'?" in *Prognosis Negative: Crisis in the Health Care System,* ed. David Kotelchuck (New York: Vintage Books, 1976), 266.

66. *1199 News* 9, no. 4 (April 1991): 10.

67. Perhaps because the sickest and most difficult to treat patients were excluded from Medicaid managed care plans.

68. United Hospital Fund, "Trends through December 1997," *Hospital Watch: A Quarterly Report on Hospitals in New York City* 9, no. 3 (1998); United Hospital Fund, "Operating Margins Drop for Second Consecutive Year," *Hospital Watch: A Quarterly Report on Hospitals in New York City,* 10, no. 3 (1999).

69. "What's Happening to Health Care? Why Our Jobs Are Changing and What We Can Do About It," *1199 News* 15, no. 1–2 (January-February 1997): 6–14.

70. Robert J. Blendon et al., "Understanding the Managed Care Backlash," *Health Affairs* 17, no. 4 (1998).

71. Lisa Clemans-Cope and Bowen Garrett, *Changes in Employer-Sponsored Health Insurance Sponsorship, Eligibility, and Participation: 2001 to 2005* (Washington, DC: Henry J. Kaiser Family Foundation, Kaiser Commission on Medicaid and the Uninsured, 2006).

72. Malanga, "City Work."

73. Alice Lipowicz, "Health Care's Big Layoff Payoff: Cash for Retraining Left Unspent as Employment Grows," *Crain's New York Business,* September 6, 1999.

74. Richard Pérez-Peña, "Ads Attack Pataki's Plan on Hospitals," *New York Times,* March 13, 1999.

75. Marty Rosen, "Hosps Too Broke to Insure Workers," *Daily News,* June 23, 1999. See also Pérez-Peña, "Ads Attack Pataki's Plan on Hospitals."

76. Jennifer Steinhauer, "Worker Shortage in Health Fields Worst in Decades," *New York Times,* December 25, 2000; Jennifer Steinhauer, "Workers Cut as Hospitals Tighten Belts," *New York Times,* June 17, 2000.

77. New York State, Office of the Governor, "Governor Announces $28.1 Million in Health Care Training Grants" (press release, January 24, 2001); New York State, Office of the Governor, "Governor Pataki Announces $500 Million in Aid to Hospitals," (press release, January 9, 2001).

78. A 1999 study of academic health centers (AHCs) nationwide noted that operating margins are only one measure of financial viability and "on most indicators the financial position of

AHCs improved during the period 1993–1997." Such measures include days cash on hand, long-term debt-to-equity ratio, and net assets per bed. The study also noted that the data on AHCs and their financial performance is inadequate. Gerard F. Anderson, George Greenberg, and Craig K. Lisk, "Academic Health Centers: Exploring a Financial Paradox," *Health Affairs* 18, no. 2 (1999): 160, exhibit 1.

79. Pérez-Peña, "Ads Attack Pataki's Plan on Hospitals."

80. Consumer Price Index (CPI) calculations by author, based on data from the Bureau of Labor Statistics, www.bls.gov/CPI. Data are for the "New York–Northern New Jersey–Long Island" metropolitan statistical area and based on the annual average CPI for all urban consumers, on all consumer items, not seasonally adjusted. The figure for hospital services is based on the annual average CPI for U.S. cities (not seasonally adjusted) because data on the CPI for hospital services is not available for the "New York–Northern New Jersey–Long Island" metropolitan statistical area alone. However, the CPI for "medical care"—which includes hospital services—in that metropolitan area increased by 110% in the period under consideration.

81. Figueroa and Lazes, *Labor-Management Projects,* 5.

82. Ibid., section I.

83. Bruce Nissen has nicely defined the difference between "value added" and "social movement" unionism. 1199 is a complex mixture of both, displaying both a cooperative impulse toward employers and a commitment to larger issues of social and working class justice. Yet, Nissen argues both types of unionism—and 1199—neglect what has long been central to U.S. unionism, according to David Brody, a labor historian: *industrial justice*—that is, justice on the job. Bruce Nissen, "Alternative Strategic Directions for the U.S. Labor Movement: Recent Scholarship," *Labor Studies Journal* 28, no. 1 (2003): esp. 146–7.

84. Chuck Idelson, in Early et al., "An Exchange of Views," 11.

85. Figueroa and Lazes, *Labor-Management Projects,* 31.

86. www.techleadersconsult.com/services.htm [last accessed April 30, 2008].

87. Ruzek et al., *Hidden Health Care Workforce,* 130.

88. Nancy Folbre, "Demanding Quality: Worker/Consumer Coalitions and 'High Road' Strategies in the Care Sector," *Politics and Society* 34, no. 1 (2006): 19.

89. Bruce Herman, "How High-Road Partnerships Work," *Social Policy* (Spring 2001): 11–19.

90. Julie Connelly, "As Industrial Jobs Decline, Training Programs Grow," *New York Times,* January 30, 2001.

91. Langer, "The Hospital Workers: 'The Best Contract Anywhere'?" 284–85, 71–73.

9. Education as a Benefit

1. As Jacob Hacker points out, in the United States one of the key policy decisions that "re-shaped the politics of health policy" in "fundamental and irreversible ways," was that the initial populations targeted by public programs (Medicare and Medicaid) were the elderly, disabled and the very poor, which are the most difficult and costly groups to insure. "Covering them under public auspices has greatly increased the strain on public budgets while freeing the private sector to focus on those populations for which private insurance is most viable." Other developed countries like the United Kingdom and Germany, by contrast, first targeted the *working* population under public programs, which created an "expansionary political dynamic." Moreover, U.S. public programs were implemented after private insurance plans, largely controlled by the medical profession, had already gained a firm foothold in the market for health care services. Jacob S. Hacker, "The Historical Logic of National Health Insurance: Structure and Sequence in the Development of British, Canadian, and U.S. Medical Policy," *Studies in American Political Development* 12, no. 1 (Spring 1998): 82.

2. Jennifer Klein, "The Politics of Economic Security: Employee Benefits and the Privatization of New Deal Liberalism," *The Journal of Policy History* 16, no. 1 (2004): 42.

3. Rick Fantasia and Kim Voss, *Hard Work: Remaking the American Labor Movement* (Berkeley: University of California Press, 2004), 46. See also Fantasia, *Cultures of Solidarity*, chap. 2.

4. Michael K. Brown, "Bargaining for Social Rights: Unions and the Reemergence of Welfare Capitalism, 1945–1952," *Political Science Quarterly* 12, no. 4 (1997–98): 651.

5. Klein, "Politics of Economic Security," esp. 40–42.

6. In exchange for "membership maintenance clauses" from the NWLB.

7. Fantasia and Voss, *Hard Work*, 47–48.

8. Beth Stevens, "Labor Unions, Employee Benefits, and the Privatization of the American Welfare State," *Journal of Policy History* 2, no. 3 (1990): 239.

9. Alan Derickson, "Health Security for All? Social Unionism and Universal Health Insurance, 1935–1958," *The Journal of American History* 80, no. 4 (1994): 1345–46; see also Ivana Krajcinovic, *From Company Doctors to Managed Care: The United Mine Worker's Noble Experiment* (Ithaca, NY: Cornell University Press, 1997).

10. Klein, "The Politics of Economic Security," 48.

11. Brown, "Bargaining for Social Rights," 660. See also Stevens, "Privatization of the American Welfare State," 246.

12. Nelson Lichtenstein, "From Corporatism to Collective Bargaining: Organized Labor and the Eclipse of Social Democracy in the Postwar Era," in *The Rise and Fall of the New Deal Order, 1930–1980,* ed. Steve Fraser and Gary Gerstle (Princeton, NJ: Princeton University Press, 1989), 132–33. Retail prices rose 26% between December 1943 and June 1947: Stevens, "Privatization of the American Welfare State," 239–41.

13. Fantasia and Voss, *Hard Work*, 50–51.

14. Lichtenstein, "From Corporatism to Collective Bargaining," 134.

15. Stevens, "Privatization of the American Welfare State," esp. 244–46, 38–39, 52.

16. Brown, "Bargaining for Social Rights," 653.

17. David J. Rothman, "A Century of Failure: Health Care Reform in America," *Journal of Health Politics, Policy, and Law* 18, no. 2 (1993).

18. Raymond Munts, *Bargaining for Health: Labor Unions, Health Insurance and Medical Care* (Madison: University of Wisconsin Press, 1967), esp. chap. 8.

19. Gerald Markowitz and David Rosner argue that in handing over the administration of health plans to third parties, even nonprofit parties, "organized labor generally forfeited any semblance of control over the actual delivery and distribution of health care services." 1199, however, controls its own health plan today and there is little to suggest that it uses this control to change the delivery of services or organization of health care work. Markowitz and Rosner also argue that, more profoundly, labor unions lost control over the definitions of health and sickness, so that health became an individual, medical problem rather than a class problem linked to the conditions of work. Any abdication of control over health and health services is doubly problematic for a health care workers' union, whose members' quality of daily life hinges on the definition of health and the organization of health services. David Rosner and Gerald Markowitz, "The Struggle over Employee Benefits: The Role of Labor in Influencing Modern Health Policy," *Milbank Quarterly* 81, no. 1 (2003): 65; Gerald Markowitz and David Rosner, "Seeking Common Ground: A History of Labor and Blue Cross," *Journal of Health Politics, Policy, and Law* 16, no. 4 (1991).

20. Paul Starr, *The Social Transformation of American Medicine* (New York: Basic Books, 1982), 313.

21. Andrew L. Stern, "Labor Rekindles Reform," *American Journal of Public Health* 93, no. 1 (2003): 96, 97.

22. Brown, "Bargaining for Social Rights," 649; Derickson, "Health Security for All?" 1351; Klein, "The Politics of Economic Security," 49.

23. Brown, "Bargaining for Social Rights," 654–55, fig. 1.

24. In 1946, conservative senator Robert Taft told democrat James Murray (MT) that the universal health insurance bill of which Murray was a cosponsor was "the most socialistic measure that this Congress has ever had before it, seriously" (quoted in Derickson, "Health Security for All?" 1342). See also Alan Derickson, "'Take Health from the List of Luxuries': Labor and the Right to Health Care, 1915–1949," *Labor History* 41, no. 2 (2000). While arguing for a union role in negotiating and managing voluntary benefit plans during the Taft-Hartley debate a few years later, Murray found himself claiming that voluntary plans would "decrease the responsibility and burdens of the State." In the face of the conservative upsurge he was forced, like other Democrats, to adopt rhetoric contrary to his own belief the state had an obligation to provide its citizens with health security. Brown, "Bargaining for Social Rights," 647, 668.

25. Derickson, "Health Security for All?"

26. Brown, "Bargaining for Social Rights," 658.

27. Derickson, "Health Security for All?" 1351.

28. For instance, Nelson Cruikshank, in Brown, "Bargaining for Social Rights," 649; and Burns, in Stevens, "Privatization of the American Welfare State," 243.

29. Brown, "Bargaining for Social Rights," 648.

30. Ibid., 657; Jill S. Quadagno, *One Nation, Uninsured: Why the U.S. Has No National Health Insurance* (New York: Oxford University Press, 2005), 49.

31. Brown, "Bargaining for Social Rights," 665.

32. Marie Gottschalk, *The Shadow Welfare State: Labor, Business, and the Politics of Health Care in the United States* (Ithaca, NY: ILR Press, 2000), 51, see chap. 2.

33. Brown, "Bargaining for Social Rights," 672–73.

34. Derickson, "Health Security for All?" 1356.

35. Gottschalk, *Shadow Welfare State*.

36. "No More Lip Service. It's Time for Action!" president's column, *1199 News* 8, no. 6 (June 1990): 2. In 1990, the Benefit Fund trustees proposed reductions in benefits because of rising costs, though they eventually withdrew the proposal when it went to arbitration.

37. Sam Roberts, "A New Face for American Labor," *New York Times Magazine,* May 10, 1992.

38. In May 1993, the union's Executive Council voted to support a single-payer health care system, but a November *1199 News* article on the Clinton reform plan described several single-payer alternatives in Congress without endorsing them. "Time for Real Reform," *1199 News* 11, no. 6 (June 1993): 3; *1199 News* 11, no. 11 (November 1994).

39. Doug Henwood, "Old Party, New Bottle," *Left Business Observer,* April 1993.

40. Ibid.

41. Jack Newfield, "Rivera Rules (Interview with Union Leader Dennis Rivera)," *Tikkun* 12, no. 6 (1997).

42. President's column, *1199 News* 12, no. 1–2 (Jan.-Feb. 1994): 3.

43. Ibid., 6.

44. *1199 News* 11, no. 12 (December 1993): 20; President's column, *1199 News* 15, no. 1–2 (Jan.-Feb. 1997).

45. Newfield, "Rivera Rules."

46. Stern, "Labor Rekindles Reform," 97.

47. Roberts, "Beth Israel Reaches Pact with Union," *New York Times,* February 20, 1992.

48. *1199 News* 15, no. 7–8 (July-August 1997): 7.

49. "Ready for Take-Off," President's column, *1199 News* 16, no. 2 (March-April 1998): 6.

50. Steven Greenhouse, "Union Will Steer Members to Rite Aid in Return for Promise Not to Fight Organizing Drives," *New York Times,* September 16, 1998. In *1199 News,* the story was presented somewhat differently. A short notice buried on p. 27 of the September-October 1998 issue

(vol. 16, no. 5) informed members that the Benefit Fund had changed drug vendors, to Rite Aid's Eagle division, "based on Rite Aid's agreement to save the Fund almost $8 million." The cover of the next issue (16, no. 6, Nov. 1998) declared proudly, "Organize! Rite Aid Drive nets 1,500 new members." No connection was made between the Benefit Fund deal and organizing in the newsletter articles. In June 1999, however, the newsletter published a brief letter from a member, who wrote, "I understand that the Benefit Fund contracted with Rite Aid pharmacies in order to promote or facilitate Rite-Aid workers in joining 1199…The fact that no pharmacy can join the 1199 program if they are located within a one-mile radius of a Rite Aid pharmacy is totally unfair. 1199 is destroying the small drug stores…I am shocked and dismayed that the 1199 Benefit Fund would do such a thing." (Letters, *1199 News* 17, no. 5: 8).

51. I am indebted to conversations with Joel Vandevusse on this point.

52. Physicians for a National Health Program, "Dr. Martin Luther King, Jr.'s Favorite Union Endorses Hr 676" (press release, February, 2006), www.pnhp.org/news/2006/february/dr_martin_luther_ki.php.

53. Fink and Greenberg report that long-time president Leon Davis once said of the city's Health and Hospitals Corporation, "in a typically acerbic moment," that the city "can't run a shit-house." Fink and Greenberg, *Upheaval in the Quiet Zone,* 203.

54. Teresa A. Coughlin and Amy Westpfahl Luztky, *Recent Changes in Health Policy for Low-Income People in New York* (Washington, DC: The Urban Institute, State Update, no. 22, 2002), 13. Parents with incomes up to 150% of the federal poverty level and single adults and childless couples with incomes up to 100% of the FPL are eligible for Family Health Plus.

55. See Kirsten L. Aspengren, Denise Soffel, and David Wunsch, "Lost in the Medicaid Maze: Voices from the Frontlines of New York City's Public Insurance Programs" (New York City Task Force on Medicaid Managed Care, 2003); Kathryn Haslanger, "Radical Simplification: Disaster Relief Medicaid in New York City," *Health Affairs* 22, no. 1 (2003).

56. See Joshua Green, "The New War over Wal-Mart," *Atlantic Monthly* (June 2006).

57. In the same period, the share of all businesses offering health benefits declined from 69% in 2000 to 60% by 2005. Most of this decline was concentrated in smaller firms, but even at large firms (over 100 employees) the percentage of employees covered by employer-sponsored insurance dropped from 88.2% to 85.1%. Lisa Clemans-Cope and Bowen Garrett, *Changes in Employer-Sponsored Health Insurance.*

58. The legislation is the Employment Retirement Income Security Act (ERISA). For background, see Daniel M. Fox and Daniel C. Schaffer, "Health Policy and ERISA: Interest Groups and Semipreemption," *Journal of Health Politics, Policy, and Law* 14, no. 2 (1989). An interesting note is that joint labor-management Taft-Hartley Funds are also self-insured and exempt from state regulations under ERISA legislation. The 1199/League health plan is therefore exempt from the taxes New York State imposed on commercial insurers to finance HCRA pools.

59. See the moving stories in Susan Starr Sered and Rushika J. Fernandopulle, *Uninsured in America: Life and Death in the Land of Opportunity* (Berkeley: University of California Press, 2005).

60. Greenhouse, "Unions Merge in Bid."

61. The Commission on the Public's Health System permitted me to view the few (and skeletal) site reports they had obtained from the state.

62. Christopher Rowland, "Bay State Medical Workers Gain Allies," *Boston Globe,* October 17, 2005.

63. Christopher Rowland, "SEIU May Want to Organize Beth Israel Deaconess," *Boston Globe,* August 4, 2006.

64. "Making Changes in Massachusetts," *Our Life and Times Magazine,* New York: 1199 SEIU (January 2006).

65. Stanley Aronowitz, "Unions as Counter-Public Spheres," in *Masses, Classes, and the Public Sphere,* ed. Mike Hill and Warren Montag (London: Verso, 2000), 96.

66. The Association of Joint Labor/Management Educational Programs, www.workplace learning.org (site last accessed August 15, 2007).

67. Elaine Butler, "Knowing 'Now,' Learning Futures. The Politics of Knowledge Practices of Vocational Education and Training," *International Journal of Lifelong Education* 19, no. 4 (2000): 329.

68. Moe Foner and Dan North, *Not for Bread Alone: A Memoir* (Ithaca: Cornell University Press, 2002), 57–58.

69. Ibid., 86.

70. Ibid., 101.

71. Ruth Needleman has argued, however, that union education departments now focus mostly on "the dissemination of the practices and policies of the international union," rather than the building of class consciousness and solidarity. "Going Back to School: What Should Union Education Be About?" *New Labor Forum* 13, no. 2 (2004): 103. See also Jojo Geronimo, "Reclaiming Education's Role: A Response to Ruth Needleman," *New Labor Forum* 13, no. 3 (2004).

72. Al Nash, "Local 1199, Drug and Hospital Union: An Analysis of the Normative and Institutional Orders of a Complex Organization," *Human Relations* 27, no. 6 (1974).

73. Aronowitz, *False Promises,* 15.

74. Nash, "Local 1199, Drug and Hospital Union," 551.

75. Aronowitz, "Unions as Counter-Public Spheres"; John Ehrenreich, "Hospital Unions: A Long Time Coming," in *Prognosis Negative: Crisis in the Health Care System,* ed. David Kotelchuck (New York: Vintage Books, 1976).

76. This is a perspective voiced by many right-wing critics, many of whom are supported by the Manhattan Institute. See in particular the Institute's affiliated publication, *City Journal,* and articles by Steven Malanga (www.city-journal.org).

77. Derickson, "Take Health from the List of Luxuries."

78. Jennifer Klein, *For All These Rights: Business, Labor and the Shaping of America's Public-Private Welfare State* (Princeton, NJ: Princeton University Press, 2003), 269–70.

79. Klein, "The Politics of Economic Security," esp. 39.

80. Derickson, "Health Security for All?" 1338–39.

81. Munts, *Bargaining for Health,* 5.

82. Klein, "The Politics of Economic Security."

83. Newfield, "Rivera Rules."

84. Krajcinovic, *From Company Doctors to Managed Care,* 41–42.

85. Munts, *Bargaining for Health,* 47.

Conclusion: A Dose of Idealism

1. Under the Nursing Home Reform Act of the Omnibus Budget Reconciliation Act of 1987 (OBRA 1987), nursing assistants working in certified home health agencies or Medicare-and/or Medicaid-certified nursing homes must complete a minimum of 75 hours of training and/or pass a competency exam. There are no federal minimum training requirements for home care workers or personal care workers employed by other types of agencies, in assisted living facilities, or directly by clients in their homes. In the absence of federal requirements, individual states have established vastly different training requirements for direct care providers. See Paraprofessional Healthcare Institute, "The Role of Training in Improving the Recruitment and Retention of Direct-Care Workers in Long-Term Care," *Workforce Strategies,* no. 3 (January 2005).

2. Paraprofessional Healthcare Institute, *Training Quality Home Care Workers* (New York: PHI Technical Series Publication, August 2003).

3. Separating the two types of motives is difficult; it is largely an analytical exercise because they are rarely separated in experience. In her seminal work on emotional labor, Arlie Hochschild documented how airline stewardesses are expected to manage the emotions of passengers as part of the "service" the airline provides. Her perspective was that private feelings are "transmuted" into public displays according to an increasingly engineered and administered logic. The training for stewardesses she observed is not unlike some of the training I have observed for health care providers, in which they are encouraged to treat patients as "clients" or "customers," to never say "no," to think of clients/patients as family members and the hospital as a business and themselves as advertisements for it. But Hochschild was more confident than I think is warranted about the line between emotions motivated by commercial ends and those motivated by genuine, or "real" attachment and affection. Hochschild, *The Managed Heart*. For similar criticisms, see Nicky James, "Emotional Labour: Skill and Work in the Social Regulation of Feelings," *Sociological Review* 37, no. 1 (1989); Cas Wouters, "The Sociology of Emotions and Flight Attendants: Hochschild's Managed Heart," *Theory, Culture & Society* 6 (1989).

4. Viviana A. Zelizer, "Intimate Transactions," in *The New Economic Sociology,* ed. Mauro F. Guillen et al. (New York: Russell Sage Foundation, 2002), 276. Even if there is an element of truth in the "hostile-worlds" view that the integration of caregiving with markets or emotions with commerce undermines care, we have not organized our society to make unpaid caregiving a viable alternative—most people cannot sacrifice the income to stay at home and care for their friends or family members (though they often do) and the government provides little to no support for those activities. Such caregiving needs to be supported—perhaps through paying even familial caregivers (long the aim of certain feminist movements) or indirect tactics that make voluntary caregiving and economic security compatible. Nonetheless, attention and creativity would also be required to respond to the fact that such care would be disproportionately provided by women, many of whom have never, ultimately, "chosen" to be the primary caregivers but do so (and do so well) because gender roles in our society have made caregiving a primarily feminine activity. Though such roles may be ingrained and dear to many of us, they are often neither wholly chosen nor justly assigned.

5. American Hospital Association (AHA), *In Our Hands.*

6. Note that there are different types of caregiving, not all of which are held in such low esteem. Joan Tronto, *Moral Boundaries: A Political Argument for an Ethic of Care* (New York: Routledge, 1993).

7. Anthony Heyes, "The Economics of Vocation or 'Why Is a Badly Paid Nurse a Good Nurse'?" *Journal of Health Economics* 24, no. 3 (2005). For a rebuttal, see Julie A. Nelson and Nancy Folbre, "Why a Well-Paid Nurse Is a Better Nurse," *Nursing Economics* 24, no. 3 (2006).

8. The growing number of "technicians" in health care—many of whom rightly recognize that caregiving work is not a path to greater status and pay—find that they are subject to another kind of slight, that they are "just" technicians who carry out but don't understand various tests and procedures.

9. Gabrielle Meagher has argued that the basis of good care in situations of paid caregiving need not be feelings of affection, like those we typically expect in familial and unpaid caring relationships (though, of course, those relationships too are more complex than is often acknowledged). There are a number of other possible motivations to care, such as the bond of a contract, a sense of professional duty, or compassion, which are neither feelings of affection nor faked and superficial displays of emotion, but which nonetheless enable "good enough" care. Feelings of affection may very well arise between paid caregivers and those for whom they care, but "these feelings are not—or even cannot be—a necessary basis for good quality care." Moreover, the expectation—which can shade at times into an unvoiced dictum—that paid caregivers should be motivated by personal feelings of affection places upon them a nearly impossible burden. When caregivers fail to meet such an unreasonable demand, the personal and emotional consequences for them, as well

as the care they provide, are potentially damaging. Gabrielle Meagher, "What Can We Expect from Paid Carers?" *Politics and Society* 34, no. 1 (2006): 48. Meagher's argument is compelling, though she still retains the focus on these workers' motivations, rather than the external conditions of their work.

10. Robert A. Scott et al., "Organizational Aspects of Caring," *Milbank Quarterly* 73, no. 1 (1995): 84. See also Daniel F. Chambliss, *Beyond Caring: Hospitals, Nurses, and the Social Organization of Ethics* (Chicago: University of Chicago Press, 1996).

11. Ellen Willis, "The Writer's Voice: Intellectual Work in the Culture of Austerity," in *Post-Work: The Wages of Cybernation,* ed. Stanley Aronowitz and Jonathan Cutler (New York: Routledge, 1998), 259. Willis explains that the counterculture of the 1960s made demands for expansion of the welfare state and criticisms of inequality part of mainstream debate. This counterculture, however, depended on the postwar prosperity that reached many (though not all) Americans and allowed them the freedom and time for political, artistic, and creative expression. Suppressing the counterculture therefore required a systematic attack on prosperity, which the "economic elite" began as early as the late 1960s. Their "objective was convincing the middle class that the money simply wasn't there, whether for high wages or for social benefits." Calls for higher wages or better benefits were successfully framed as irresponsible and wasteful, the product of a lack of personal discipline. "This brand of moralism," writes Willis, "served a practical function: in diverting people's attention from the corporate agenda to their own alleged lack of social discipline and unrealistic expectations, it discouraged rebellion in favor of guilty, resigned acquiescence."

Appendix: A Note on Methods

1. Ariel Ducey, Heather Gautney, and Dominic Wetzel, "Regulating Affective Labor."

BIBLIOGRAPHY

1199 SEIU. "Annual Review." New York: Employment, Training & Job Security Program, 2003.

Abbott, Andrew Delano. *The System of Professions: An Essay on the Division of Expert Labor.* Chicago: University of Chicago Press, 1988.

Aiken, Linda H. "Health Professionals, Allied." In *International Encyclopedia of the Social and Behavioral Sciences,* 6592–98. Elsevier, 2002.

Aiken, Linda H., Sean P. Clarke, Douglas M. Sloane, and Julie A. Sochalski. "An International Perspective on Hospital Nurses' Work Environments: The Case for Reform." *Policy, Politics, & Nursing Practice* 2, no. 4 (2001): 255–63.

Aiken, Linda H., Sean P. Clarke, Douglas M. Sloane, Julie Sochalski, and Jeffrey H. Silber. "Hospital Nurse Staffing and Patient Mortality, Nurse Burnout, and Job Dissatisfaction." *JAMA* 288 (2002): 1987–93.

Aiken, Linda H., and Claire M. Fagin. "Evaluating the Consequences of Hospital Restructuring." *Medical Care* 35, no. 10 (1997): OS1–OS4.

American Hospital Association. *Trendwatch Chartbook 2005: Trends Affecting Hospitals and Health Systems.* American Hospital Association, May 2005. http://www.ahapolicy forum.org/ahapolicyforum/trendwatch/chartbook2005.html (accessed June 5,2005).

American Medical Association. *Health Professions Education Data Book 2003–2004.* Chicago: American Medical Association, 2003.

Anderson, Gerard F., George Greenberg, and Craig K. Lisk. "Academic Health Centers: Exploring a Financial Paradox." *Health Affairs* 18, no. 2 (1999): 156–67.

Aronowitz, Stanley. *False Promises: The Shaping of American Working Class Consciousness.* New York: McGraw-Hill, 1973.

——. "The Last Good Job in America." In *Post-Work: The Wages of Cybernation,* edited by Stanley Aronowitz and Jonathan Cutler, 203–24. New York: Routledge, 1998.

——. "Unions as Counter-Public Spheres." In *Masses, Classes, and the Public Sphere,* edited by Mike Hill and Warren Montag, 83–104. London: Verso, 2000.

Aspengren, Kirsten L., Denise Soffel, and David Wunsch. "Lost in the Medicaid Maze: Voices from the Frontlines of New York City's Public Insurance Programs." New York City Task Force on Medicaid Managed Care, 2003.

Attewell, Paul. "The Deskilling Controversy." *Work and Occupations* 14, no. 3 (1987): 323–46.

Bach, Stephen. "Health Sector Reform and Human Resource Management: Britain in Comparative Perspective." *International Journal of Human Resource Management* 11, no. 5 (2000): 925–42.

Bailey, Thomas, and Elliot B. Weininger. "Performance, Graduation, and Transfer of Immigrants and Natives in City University of New York Community Colleges." *Educational Evaluation and Policy Analysis* 24, no. 4 (2002): 359–77.

Barley, Stephen R. "Technology, Power, and the Social Organization of Work: Towards a Pragmatic Theory of Skilling and Deskilling." *Research in the Sociology of Organizations* 6 (1988): 33–80.

Berg, Ivar E. *Education and Jobs: The Great Training Robbery.* New York: Published for the Center for Urban Education by Praeger Publishers, 1970.

Berliner, Howard S., Geoffrey Gibson, and Cyprian Devine-Perez. "Health Care Workers' Unions and Health Insurance: The 1199 Story." *International Journal of Health Services* 31, no. 2 (2001): 279–89.

Berliner, Howard S., Christine T. Kovner, and Cordelia Reimers. "The Health Care Workforce in Los Angeles County and New York City: A Comparison and Analysis." *International Journal of Health Services* 32, no. 2 (2002): 299–311.

Berman, Marshall. *All That Is Solid Melts into Air: The Experience of Modernity.* New York: Simon and Schuster, 1982.

Billings, John, Nina Parikh, and Tod Mijanovich. "Emergency Department Use: The New York Story" (issue brief). New York: The Commonwealth Fund, 2000.

Bingham, Ray. "Leaving Nursing: Hospital Staffing Cuts Have Created Conditions under Which This Dedicated Nurse Can No Longer Work." *Health Affairs* 21, no. 1 (2002): 211–17.

Blendon, Robert J., Mollyann Brodie, John M. Benson, Drew E. Altman, L. Levitt, T. Hoff, and L. Hugick. "Understanding the Managed Care Backlash." *Health Affairs* 17, no. 4 (1998): 80–95.

Brannon, Robert. "Restructuring Hospital Nursing: Reversing the Trend Toward a Professional Work Force." *International Journal of Health Services* 26, no. 4 (1996): 643–54.

Brannon, Robert L. "Professionalization and Work Intensification: Nursing in the Cost Containment Era." *Work and Occupations* 21, no. 2 (1994): 157–78.

Braverman, Harry. *Labor and Monopoly Capital: The Degradation of Work in the Twentieth Century.* New York: Monthly Review Press, 1975.

Brint, Steven, and Jerome Karabel. *The Diverted Dream: Community Colleges and the Promise of Educational Opportunity in America, 1900–1985.* New York: Basic Books, 1989.

Brodkin Sacks, Karen. *Caring by the Hour: Women, Work, and Organizing at Duke Medical Center.* Urbana: University of Illinois Press, 1988.

Brown, Michael K. "Bargaining for Social Rights: Unions and the Reemergence of Welfare Capitalism, 1945–1952." *Political Science Quarterly* 12, no. 4 (1997–98): 645–74.

Butler, Elaine. "Knowing 'Now,' Learning Futures: The Politics of Knowledge Practices of Vocational Education and Training." *International Journal of Lifelong Education* 19, no. 4 (2000): 322–42.

Cantor, Joel C., Kathryn Haslanger, and Kathleen DeGuire. "Health Plan Responses to Medicaid Managed Care Policy in New York City." *Managed Care Quarterly* 8, no. 2 (2000): 39–47.

Center for an Urban Future. *CUNY on the Job: The City's New Workforce Workhorse.* New York: Center for an Urban Future, 2004.

——. *Labor Gains: How Union-Affiliated Training Is Transforming New York's Workforce Landscape.* New York: Center for an Urban Future, 2003.

——. *Rebuilding Job Training from the Ground Up: Workforce System Reform after 9/11.* New York: Center for an Urban Future, 2002.

Center for an Urban Future, and New York Association for Training and Employment Professionals. *Seeking a Workforce System: A Graphical Guide to Employment and Training Services in New York.* New York: Center for an Urban Future, 2003.

Center for Health Workforce Studies. *An Assessment of the Impact of Hospital Restructuring on Nurse Staffing in New York City.* Albany: Center for Health Workforce Studies, School of Public Health, State University of New York (SUNY) at Albany, June 1998.

——. *The Health Care Workforce in New York City, 2000.* Albany: Center for Health Workforce Studies, School of Public Health, SUNY at Albany, 2000.

——. *The Health Care Workforce in New York City, 2002.* Albany: Center for Health Workforce Studies, School of Public Health, SUNY at Albany, 2002.

——. *The Health Care Workforce in New York State, 2004: Trends in the Supply and Demand for Health Workers.* Albany: Center for Health Workforce Studies, School of Public Health, SUNY at Albany, May 2005.

Center for Health Workforce Studies, and New Century Concepts. *The Changing Health Care System in New York City: Implications for the Workforce.* Albany: Center for Health Workforce Studies, School of Public Health, SUNY at Albany, 1997.

Chambliss, Daniel F. *Beyond Caring: Hospitals, Nurses, and the Social Organization of Ethics.* Chicago: University of Chicago Press, 1996.

CHWS. See Center for Health Workforce Studies.

Clark, Burton R. "The Cooling-out Function in Higher Education." *American Journal of Sociology* 65, no. 6 (1960): 569–76.

Clemans-Cope, Lisa, and Bowen Garrett. *Changes in Employer-Sponsored Health Insurance Sponsorship, Eligibility, and Participation: 2001 to 2005.* Washington, DC: Henry J. Kaiser Family Foundation, Kaiser Commission on Medicaid and the Uninsured, 2006.

Cohen, Rima. "From Strategy to Reality: The Enactment of New York's Family Health Plus Program." *Journal of Health Politics, Policy and Law* 26, no. 6 (2001): 1375–93.

Collins, Randall. *The Credential Society: An Historical Sociology of Education and Stratification.* New York: Academic Press, 1979.

Commission on Health Care Facilities in the Twenty-First Century, and Stephen Berger. 2005. *Factors Book.* New York State Department of Health, http://www.nyhealthcarecommission.org/factors_book.htm. (accessed January 9, 2008).

Commission on the Public's Health System. *CHCCDP: Are We Getting Our Money's Worth?* New York: Commission on the Public's Health System, 2003.

Conference Board of Canada. *Success by Design: What Works in Workforce Development.* Ottawa, Ontario: Conference Board of Canada, Report 380–02, December 2002.

Coughlin, Teresa A., and Amy Westpfahl Luztky. *Recent Changes in Health Policy for Low-Income People in New York.* Washington, DC: The Urban Institute, State Update, no. 22, 2002.

Derickson, Alan. "Health Security for All? Social Unionism and Universal Health Insurance, 1935–1958." *The Journal of American History* 80, no. 4 (1994): 1333–56.

———. " 'Take Health from the List of Luxuries': Labor and the Right to Health Care, 1915–1949." *Labor History* 41, no. 2 (2000): 171–87.

Diamond, Timothy. *Making Gray Gold: Narratives of Nursing Home Care.* Chicago: University of Chicago Press, 1992.

Dougherty, Kevin J., and Marianne F. Bakia. "Community Colleges and Contract Training: Content, Origins, and Impact." *Teachers College Record* 102, no. 1 (2000): 197–243.

Ducey, Ariel. "What's the Use of Job Descriptions?" *Working USA* 6, no. 2 (2002): 40–55.

Ducey, Ariel, Heather Gautney, and Dominic Wetzel. "Regulating Affective Labor: Communication Skills Training in the Health Care Industry." *Research in the Sociology of Work* 12 (2003): 49–72.

Duffy, Niev, William Ebenstein, and Deniz Kurtel. "A Preliminary Profile of Enrollment Patterns, Graduation Rates and Demographics of 1199 Represented Workers at the City University of New York." New York: The John F. Kennedy, Jr. Institute for Worker Education, 2003.

Early, Steve, Bob Master, Hetty Rosenstein, Ellen David Friedman, and Chuck Idelson. "An Exchange of Views: Will Endorsing Republicans Teach Turncoat Dems the Right Lesson?" *Labor Notes* 279 (June 2002): 7–11.

Ehrenreich, John. "Hospital Unions: A Long Time Coming." In *Prognosis Negative: Crisis in the Health Care System,* edited by David Kotelchuck, 255–66. New York: Vintage Books, 1976.

Ellwood, Marilyn R., and Leighton Ku. "Welfare and Immigration Reforms: Unintended Side Effects for Medicaid." *Health Affairs* 17, no. 3 (1998): 137–51.

Engel, Cynthia. "Health Services Industry: Still a Job Machine?" *Monthly Labor Review* 122, no. 3 (1999): 3–14.

England, Paula, Michelle Budig, and Nancy Folbre. "Wages of Virtue: The Relative Pay of Care Work." *Social Problems* 49, no. 4 (2002): 455–73.

Fantasia, Rick. *Cultures of Solidarity: Consciousness, Action, and Contemporary American Workers.* Berkeley: University of California Press, 1988.

Fantasia, Rick, and Kim Voss. *Hard Work: Remaking the American Labor Movement.* Berkeley: University of California Press, 2004.

Figueroa, Maria, and Peter Lazes. *Labor-Management Participatory Projects in the Health Care Industry.* New York: Cornell University–New York State School of Industrial and Labor Relations, NYC Metropolitan District Office, 2002.

Fink, Leon, and Brian Greenberg. *Upheaval in the Quiet Zone: A History of Hospital Workers' Union, Local 1199.* Urbana: University of Illinois Press, 1989.

Fiscal Policy Institute. *Health Care Industry Trends and Issues.* Albany, NY: Fiscal Policy Institute, 2002.

Fitzpatrick, Peter G. "Turnover of Certified Nursing Assistants: A Major Problem for Long-Term Care Facilities." *Hospital Topics* 80, no. 2 (2002): 21–26.

Folbre, Nancy. "Demanding Quality: Worker/Consumer Coalitions and 'High Road' Strategies in the Care Sector." *Politics and Society* 34, no. 1 (2006): 11–31.

Foner, Moe, and Dan North. *Not for Bread Alone: A Memoir.* Ithaca: Cornell University Press, 2002.

Foner, Nancy. *The Caregiving Dilemma: Work in an American Nursing Home.* Berkeley: University of California Press, 1994.

Fox, Daniel M., and Daniel C. Schaffer. "Health Policy and ERISA: Interest Groups and Semipreemption." *Journal of Health Politics, Policy, and Law* 14, no. 2 (1989): 239–60.

Freeman, Joshua Benjamin. *Working-Class New York: Life and Labor since World War II.* New York: New Press: Distributed by W.W. Norton, 2000.

Gass, Thomas Edward. *Nobody's Home: Candid Reflections of a Nursing Home Aide.* Ithaca: Cornell University Press, 2004.

Geronimo, Jojo. "Reclaiming Education's Role: A Response to Ruth Needleman." *New Labor Forum* 13, no. 3 (2004): 99–105.

Gilroy, Paul. *The Black Atlantic: Modernity and Double Consciousness.* Cambridge, MA: Harvard University Press, 1993.

Goldsmith, Jeff, David Blumenthal, and Wes Rishel. "Federal Health Information Policy: A Case of Arrested Development." *Health Affairs* 22, no. 4 (2003): 44–55.

Gordon, Suzanne. *Nursing against the Odds.* Ithaca: Cornell University Press, 2005.

Gottschalk, Marie. *The Shadow Welfare State: Labor, Business, and the Politics of Health Care in the United States.* Ithaca: Cornell University Press, 2000.

Gray, Bradford H., and Catherine Row. "Safety-net Health Plans: A Status Report." *Health Affairs* 19, no. 1 (2000): 185–93.

Greater New York Hospital Association. *Health Care Statistics 2003.* New York: Greater New York Hospital Association, 2003.

Green, Joshua. "The New War over Wal-Mart." *Atlantic Monthly* June (2006): 38–44.

Grubb, W. Norton. "Evaluating Job Training Programs in the United States: Evidence and Explanations." Berkeley: National Center for Research in Vocational Education, Graduate School of Education, University of California, 1995.

———. "Learning and Earning in the Middle, Part I: National Studies of Pre-Baccalaureate Education." *Economics of Education Review* 21, no. 4 (2002): 299–321.

Grubb, W. Norton. "The Returns to Education in the Sub-Baccalaureate Labor Market, 1984–1990." *Economics of Education Review* 16, no. 3 (1997): 231–45.
——. *Working in the Middle.* San Francisco: Jossey-Bass, 1996.
Gubrium, Jaber. *Living and Dying at Murray Manor.* New York: St. Martin's Press, 1975.
Gusmano, Michael K., Michael S. Sparer, Lawrence D. Brown, Catherine Rowe, and Bradford Gray. "The Evolving Role and Care Management Approaches of Safety-Net Medicaid Managed Care Plans." *Journal of Urban Health* 79, no. 4 (2002): 600–16.
Hacker, Jacob S. "The Historical Logic of National Health Insurance: Structure and Sequence in the Development of British, Canadian, and U.S. Medical Policy." *Studies in American Political Development* 12 (Spring 1998): 57–130.
Hammer, Michael, and James Champy. *Reengineering the Corporation: A Manifesto for Business Revolution.* New York: HarperCollins, 1993.
Handel, Michael J. "Skills Mismatch in the Labor Market." *Annual Review of Sociology* 29 (2003): 135–65.
Haslanger, Kathryn. *Medicaid Managed Care in New York: A Work in Progress.* New York: United Hospital Fund, 2003.
——. "Radical Simplification: Disaster Relief Medicaid in New York City." *Health Affairs* 22, no. 1 (2003): 252–58.
Health Resources and Services Administration (HRSA). *State Health Workforce Profiles 2000: New York.* Washington, DC: U.S. Department of Health and Human Services, HRSA, 2004.
Health/PAC Bulletin. "What Course for Health Workers?" In *Prognosis Negative: Crisis in the Health Care System,* edited by David Kotelchuck, 247–55. New York: Vintage Books, 1976.
Henwood, Doug. "Old Party, New Bottle." *Left Business Observer* (April 1993).
Herman, Bruce. "How High-Road Partnerships Work." *Social Policy* (Spring 2001): 11–19.
Hevesi, Alan G. *Current Trends in the New York City Economy.* Albany: New York State, Office of the State Comptroller, 2004.
Heyes, Anthony. "The Economics of Vocation, or 'Why Is a Badly Paid Nurse a Good Nurse'?" *Journal of Health Economics* 24, no. 3 (2005): 561–69.
Hiles, David R.H. "Health Services: The Real Jobs Machine." *Monthly Labor Review* 115, no. 11 (1992): 3–17.
Himmelstein, David U., James P. Lewontin, and Steffie Woolhandler. "Medical Care Employment in the United States, 1968 to 1993: The Importance of Health Sector Jobs for African Americans and Women." *American Journal of Public Health* 86, no. 4 (1996): 525–28.
Hirsch, Michael. "Titanic." *Village Voice,* January 20, 1998.
Hochschild, Arlie. "The Nanny Chain." *American Prospect* 11, no. 4 (January 3, 2000): 32–36.
——. *The Managed Heart: Commercialization of Human Feeling.* Berkeley: University of California Press, 1983.
Hollinger-Smith, Linda, Anna Ortigara, and David Lindeman. "Developing a Comprehensive Long-Term Care Workforce Initiative." *Alzheimer's Care Quarterly* 2, no. 3 (2001): 33–40.

Ilan, Amos, and Catherine Lanier. *Journal of Health and Human Services Administration.* New York: Greater New York Hospital Association, 1999.

James, Nicky. "Emotional Labour: Skill and Work in the Social Regulation of Feelings." *Sociological Review* 37, no. 1 (1989): 15–42.

Kincheloe, Joe. *How Do We Tell the Workers? The Socioeconomic Foundations of Work and Vocational Education.* Boulder, CO: Westview Press, 1999.

Klein, Jennifer. *For All These Rights: Business, Labor and the Shaping of America's Public-Private Welfare State.* Princeton, NJ: Princeton University Press, 2003.

———. "The Politics of Economic Security: Employee Benefits and the Privatization of New Deal Liberalism." *The Journal of Policy History* 16, no. 1 (2004): 34–65.

Krajcinovic, Ivana. *From Company Doctors to Managed Care: The United Mine Worker's Noble Experiment.* Ithaca: Cornell University Press, 1997.

Lafer, Gordon. "Hospital Speedups and the Fiction of a Nursing Shortage." *Labor Studies Journal* 30, no. 1 (2005): 27–46.

———. *The Job Training Charade.* Ithaca: Cornell University Press, 2002.

———. "What Is 'Skill'? Training for Discipline in the Low-Wage Labour Market." In *The Skills That Matter,* edited by Chris Warhurst and Irena Grugulis, 109–27. New York: Palgrave MacMillan, 2004.

Langer, Elinor. "The Hospital Workers: 'The Best Contract Anywhere'?" In *Prognosis Negative: Crisis in the Health Care System,* edited by David Kotelchuck, 266–85. New York: Vintage Books, 1976. [orig. published in *The New York Review of Books*].

Lathrop, J. Philip. *Restructuring Health Care.* San Francisco: Jossey-Bass, 1993.

Lavin, David E., and David Hyllegard. *Changing the Odds: Open Admissions and the Life Chances of the Disadvantaged.* New Haven, CT: Yale University Press, 1996.

Lazes, Peter, Stephen L. Walston, Maria Figueroa, and Patricia Garcia Sullivan. "The Use and Impact of Re-Engineering and Restructuring in Acute Care Hospitals." Research report by Cornell and Indiana Universities, 2003.

Lichtenstein, Nelson. "From Corporatism to Collective Bargaining: Organized Labor and the Eclipse of Social Democracy in the Postwar Era." In *The Rise and Fall of the New Deal Order, 1930–1980,* edited by Steve Fraser and Gary Gerstle, 122–52. Princeton, NJ: Princeton University Press, 1989.

Livingstone, David W. *The Education-Jobs Gap: Underemployment or Economic Democracy.* Aurora, Ontario: Garamond Press, 2004.

———. "Lifelong Learning and Underemployment in the Knowledge Society: A North American Perspective." *Comparative Education* 35, no. 2 (1999): 163–86.

Lopez, Steven Henry. "Culture Change Management in Long-Term Care: A Shop-Floor View." *Politics and Society* 34, no. 1 (2006): 55–79.

Markowitz, Gerald, and David Rosner. "Seeking Common Ground: A History of Labor and Blue Cross." *Journal of Health Politics, Policy, and Law* 16, no. 4 (1991): 695–717.

McCormick, Lynn. "Reshuffling of Immigrant Nursing Aide Ladders in New York City." Unpublished paper, Hunter College, City University of New York, n.d.

McGee, Micki. *Self-Help, Inc.: Makeover Culture in American Life.* New York: Oxford University Press, 2005.

McNally, David. *Even Eagles Need a Push: Learning to Soar in a Changing World.* New York: Dell, 1994.

Meagher, Gabrielle. "What Can We Expect from Paid Carers?" *Politics and Society* 34, no. 1 (2006): 33–53.

Mishel, Lawrence, Jared Bernstein, and Heather Boushey. *The State of Working America 2002/2003.* Ithaca: Cornell University Press, 2003.

"Mission Possible? New York City's Municipal Hospitals in an Era of Declining Resources." *Hospital Watch* 13, no. 1 (2002): 1–6.

Moss, Philip, and Chris Tilly. *Stories Employers Tell: Race, Skill, and Hiring in America.* New York: Russell Sage Foundation, 2001.

Munts, Raymond. *Bargaining for Health: Labor Unions, Health Insurance and Medical Care.* Madison: University of Wisconsin Press, 1967.

Nash, Al. "Local 1199, Drug and Hospital Union: An Analysis of the Normative and Institutional Orders of a Complex Organization." *Human Relations* 27, no. 6 (1974): 547–66.

Needleman, Jack, Peter Buerhaus, Soeren Mattke, Maureen Stewart, and Katya Zelevinsky. "Nurse-Staffing Levels and the Quality of Care in Hospitals." *New England Journal of Medicine* 346 (2002): 1715–22.

Needleman, Ruth. "Going Back to School: What Should Union Education Be About?" *New Labor Forum* 13, no. 2 (2004): 101–10.

Nelson, Julie A., and Nancy Folbre. "Why a Well-Paid Nurse Is a Better Nurse." *Nursing Economics* 24, no. 3 (2006): 127–30.

Newfield, Jack. "Rivera Rules (Interview with Union Leader Dennis Rivera)." *Tikkun* 12, no. 6 (1997): 19–22.

Nissen, Bruce. "Alternative Strategic Directions for the U.S. Labor Movement: Recent Scholarship." *Labor Studies Journal* 28, no. 1 (2003): 133–55.

Paraprofessional Healthcare Institute. "The Role of Training in Improving the Recruitment and Retention of Direct-Care Workers in Long-Term Care." *Workforce Strategies,* no. 3 (January 2005).

——. *Training Quality Home Care Workers.* New York: PHI Technical Series Publication, August 2003.

Pearce, Diana, with Jennifer Brooks. *The Self-Sufficiency Standard for the City of New York.* New York: Women's Center for Education and Career Advancement, 2000.

Pew Health Professions Commission. *Critical Challenges: Revitalizing the Health Professions for the Twenty-First Century.* Pew Health Professions Commission, December 1995.

Phillips-Fein, Kim. "Does That Elephant Bite? Union Alliances with the GOP." *New Labor Forum* 12, no. 1 (2003): 7–16.

Pincus, Fred. "The False Promises of Community Colleges: Class Conflict and Vocational Education." *Harvard Educational Review* 50, no. 3 (1986): 332–61.

Pindus, Nancy M., Patrice Flynn, and Demetra Smith Nightingale. *Improving the Upward Mobility of Low-Skill Workers: The Case of the Health Industry.* Washington, DC: The Urban Institute, 1995.

Quadagno, Jill S. *One Nation, Uninsured: Why the U.S. Has No National Health Insurance.* New York: Oxford University Press, 2005.

Reich, Robert B. *The Work of Nations: Preparing Ourselves for 21st Century Capitalism.* 1st ed. New York: Alfred A. Knopf, 1991.

Robbins, Tom. "Blue Cross Hijacked." *Village Voice,* February 13, 2002.

——. "Hospital Holiday." *Village Voice,* May 29, 2003.

——. "Labor's Cheap Date with Pataki." *Village Voice,* September 10, 2002.

Robinson, James C. "The Curious Conversion of Empire Blue Cross." *Health Affairs* 22, no. 4 (2003): 100–18.

Rosner, David, and Gerald Markowitz. "The Struggle over Employee Benefits: The Role of Labor in Influencing Modern Health Policy." *Milbank Quarterly* 81, no. 1 (2003): 45–73.

Rothman, David J. "A Century of Failure: Health Care Reform in America." *Journal of Health Politics, Policy, and Law* 18, no. 2 (1993): 271–86.

Ruggie, Mary. "The Paradox of Liberal Intervention: Health Policy and the American Welfare State." *American Journal of Sociology* 97, no. 4 (1992): 919–44.

Ruzek, Jennifer Y., Lindsey E. Bloor, Jennifer L. Anderson, Mai Ngo, and the Center for the Health Professions. *The Hidden Health Care Workforce: Recognizing, Understanding and Improving the Allied and Auxiliary Workforce.* San Francisco: UCSF Center for the Health Professions, July 1999.

Salit, Sharon, Steven Fass, and Mark Nowak. "Out of the Frying Pan: New York City Hospitals in an Age of Deregulation." *Health Affairs* 21, no. 1 (2002): 127–39.

Schweikhart, Sharon Bergman, and Vicki Smith-Daniels. "Reengineering the Work of Caregivers: Role Definition, Team Structures, and Organizational Redesign." *Hospital and Health Services Administration* 41, no. 1 (1996): 19–35.

Scott, Robert A., Linda H. Aiken, David Mechanic, and Julius Moravcsik. "Organizational Aspects of Caring." *Milbank Quarterly* 73, no. 1 (1995): 77–95.

Scott, W. Richard, Martin Ruef, Peter J. Mendel, and Carol A. Caronna. *Institutional Change and Healthcare Organizations: From Professional Dominance to Managed Care.* Chicago: University of Chicago Press, 2000.

Sennett, Richard, and Jonathan Cobb. *The Hidden Injuries of Class.* New York: Vintage Books, 1973.

Sered, Susan Starr, and Rushika J. Fernandopulle. *Uninsured in America: Life and Death in the Land of Opportunity.* Berkeley: University of California Press, 2005.

Smith, David Barton, William Aaronson, and Richard L. Jones Jr. "The Perils of Healthcare Workforce Forecasting: A Case Study of the Philadelphia Metropolitan Area." *Journal of Healthcare Management* 48, no. 2 (2003): 99–111.

Shortell, Stephen M., Robin R. Gillies, and Kelly J. Devers. "Reinventing the American Hospital." *Milbank Quarterly* 73, no. 2 (1995): 131–59.

Sochalski, Julie, Linda H. Aiken, and Claire M. Fagin. "Hospital Restructuring in the United States, Canada, and Western Europe—an Outcomes Research Agenda." *Medical Care* 35, no. 10 (1997): OS13–OS25.

Sparer, Michael S., and Lawrence D. Brown. "Nothing Exceeds Like Success: Managed Care Comes to Medicaid in New York City." *Milbank Quarterly* 77, no. 2 (1999): 205–23.

——. "Uneasy Alliances: Managed Care Plans Formed by Saftey-Net Providers." *Health Affairs* 19, no. 4 (2000): 23–35.

Sparer, Michael S., Lawrence D. Brown, Michael K. Gusmano, Catherine Rowe, and Bradford H. Gray. "Promising Practices: How Leading Safety-Net Plans are Managing the Care of Medicaid Clients." *Health Affairs* 21, no. 5 (2002): 284–91.

Spratley, Ernell, Ayah Johnson, Julie Sochalski, Marshall Fritz, and William Spencer. *The Registered Nurse Population, March 2000: Findings from the National Sample Survey of Registered Surveys.* U.S. Department of Health and Human Services, Health Resources and Services Administration, Bureau of Health Professions, Division of Nursing, 2001.

Starr, Paul. *The Social Transformation of American Medicine.* New York: Basic Books, 1982.

Stashenko, Joel. "Spitzer: Tobacco Payments Will Be Lower Than Projections." *Associated Press Newswire,* December 27, 2000.

Stern, Andrew L. "Labor Rekindles Reform." *American Journal of Public Health* 93, no. 1 (2003): 95–98.

Stevens, Beth. "Labor Unions, Employee Benefits, and the Privatization of the American Welfare State." *Journal of Policy History* 2, no. 3 (1990): 233–60.

Stone, Deborah. "Care and Trembling." *American Prospect* 43 (March–April 1999): 61–67.

Stone, Robyn. *Frontline Workers in Long-Term Care: A Background Paper.* Washington, DC: Institute for the Future of Aging Services, American Association of Homes and Services for the Aging, 2001.

Takahashi, Beverly, and Edwin Meléndez. "Union-Sponsored Workforce Development Initiatives." In *Communities and Workforce Development,* edited by Edwin Meléndez, 119–50. Kalamazoo, MI: W.E. Upjohn Institute for Employment Research, 2004.

Tronto, Joan. *Moral Boundaries: A Political Argument for an Ethic of Care.* New York: Routledge, 1993.

Uchitelle, Louis. *The Disposable American: Layoffs and Their Consequences.* New York: Alfred A. Knopf, 2006.

United Hospital Fund. "Trends through December 1997." *Hospital Watch: A Quarterly Report on Hospitals in New York City* 9, no. 3 (1998).

———. "Operating Margins Drop for Second Consecutive Year." *Hospital Watch: A Quarterly Report on Hospitals in New York City* 10, no. 3 (1999).

Van Maanen, John, and Gideon Kunda. "'Real Feelings': Emotional Expression and Organizational Culture." *Research in Organizational Behavior* 11 (1989): 43–103.

Walston, Stephen Lee, Lawton Robert Burns, and John R. Kimberly. "Does Reengineering Really Work? An Examination of the Context and Outcomes of Hospital Reengineering Initiatives." *Health Services Research* 34, no. 6 (2000): 1363–88.

Walston, Stephen Lee, Linda D. Urden, and Patricia Sullivan. "Hospital Reengineering: An Evolving Management Innovation: History, Current Status and Future Direction." *Journal of Health and Human Services Administration* 23, no. 4 (2001): 388–415.

Weber, David. "At New York City's Mount Sinai, Reengineering Is a Way to Grow, Not a Special Project." *Strategies for Healthcare Excellence* 12, no. 12 (1999): 1–8.

Weeden, Kim A. "Why Do Some Occupations Pay More Than Others? Social Closure and Earnings Inequality in the United States." *American Journal of Sociology* 108, no. 1 (2002): 55–101.

Weinberg, Dana Beth. *Code Green: Money-Driven Hospitals and the Dismantling of Nursing.* Ithaca: Cornell University Press, 2003.

Willis, Ellen. "The Writer's Voice: Intellectual Work in the Culture of Austerity." In *Post-Work: The Wages of Cybernation,* edited by Stanley Aronowitz and Jonathan Cutler, 257–74. New York: Routledge, 1998.

Willis, Paul. "Labor Power, Culture, and the Cultural Commodity." In *Critical Education in the New Information Age,* 139–69. Lanham, MD: Rowman & Littlefield, 1999.

Woolhandler, Steffie, Terry Campbell, and David Himmelstein. "Costs of Health Care Administration in the United States and Canada." *New England Journal of Medicine* 349, no. 8 (2003): 768–75.

Wouters, Cas. "The Sociology of Emotions and Flight Attendants: Hochschild's Managed Heart." *Theory, Culture & Society* 6 (1989): 95–123.

Zelizer, Viviana A. "Intimate Transactions." In *The New Economic Sociology,* edited by Mauro F. Guillen, Randall Collins, Paula England, and Marshall Meyer, 274–300. New York: Russell Sage Foundation, 2002.

Zuboff, Shoshana. *In the Age of the Smart Machine: The Future of Work and Power.* New York: Basic Books, 1988.

INDEX

reform and restructuring of health care,
63–64, 65, 72
soft skills training, 134, 135, 137
Training and Upgrading Fund financing, 183
training for health care workers, 75–79,
82–84
upgrading, 139–40
complex *vs.* simple jobs, myths about, 104–5
computer literacy training, 83–84
Conference Board of Canada, 136, 166, 206, 226
Congress of Industrial Organizations (CIO).
See American Federation of Labor and
Congress of Industrial Organizations
Consortium for Worker Education, 79, 82–83,
85, 92, 148, 160, 225
consultants
for reform and restructuring efforts, 71,
259n43
for training industry, 75–76, 78–79
continuous quality improvement (CQI),
62–63
cost control and cost cutting
allied health care workers blamed for failures
of, 34–36, 37, 43, 45–46
financial problems of hospitals, analysis of,
197–200
health care reform and restructuring, at heart
of, 62, 73–74
moral imperative, austerity as, 242, 278n11
multiskilling as means of, 89, 91–93
training industry and, 87
universal health care and rising health care
costs, 221–22
wages of allied health care workers as reason
for high health care costs, 13, 24
counterculture of 1960s, 278n11
CQI (continuous quality improvement), 62–63
credential inflation, 98–101
cultures of solidarity, 279n15
CUNY (City University of New York), 9–10,
79–81, 148, 152–53, 170, 209, 226–27
Cuomo, Mario, 184, 187
customer service programs. *See* soft skills training

Davis, Leon, 184
Davis, Ossie, 228
DC37 (District Council 37), 4, 27, 38, 78, 92, 152,
223, 269n27
Dee, Ruby, 228
Depression, 230–31
deskilling, multiskilling as, 94–96
devaluation of caring labor
allied health care workers' sense of, 7, 21–24
means of redressing, 234–35
multiskilling contributing to, 101–3, 157
race discrimination, as form of, 156
upgrading and, 140, 155–57
Diamond, Timothy, 43, 52

dietary jobs, 144–47
District Council 37 (DC37), 4, 27, 38, 78, 92, 152,
223, 269n27
double diapering, 34–35
downsizing. *See* layoffs and downsizing

economic viability of training strategy, 161–64,
167–68, 178–79
education and training
alternative approaches to, 233–43
as employment-based benefit. *See under*
employment-based benefits
industry in NYC. *See* health care workforce
training industry in NYC
EKGs (electrocardiograms), 11, 82, 89–90, 92, 98,
101, 102, 106, 152, 161, 205, 235
electrocardiograms (EKGs), 11, 82, 89–90, 92, 98,
101, 102, 106, 152, 161, 205, 235
emotional burdens of allied health care work,
49–53
emotional labor, concept of, 131, 278n8
Empire Blue Cross and Blue Shield, 194
employment-based benefits, 16, 208–32
education
1199 bureaucracy of, 228–29
1199 health care benefits situation compared
to training program, 222–23
fracturing of system, 224
marketing of, 224–27
significance of, 209–10
as threat to public education, 208–10,
240–41
health care
in 1199, 218–21
centrality to union viability as institutions, 217–18
inadequacy of current system, 221–22
lessons to be learned from history of, 208–9
universal. *See* universal health care
history of collective bargaining for, 211–17,
230–32
limitations of, 229–32
Employment Retirement Income Security Act
(ERISA), 275n58
Employment, Training and Job Security
Program (ETJSP), 77, 82, 183, 187,
189, 191–92
enjoyment of training by health care workers,
112, 118, 174–76
ERISA (Employment Retirement Income
Security Act), 275n58
ETJSP (Employment, Training and Job Security
Program), 77, 82, 183, 187, 189, 191–92

Family Health Plus program, 192, 193, 198, 221,
275n54
Fantasia, Rick, 214, 265n15
federal government. *See* government